Sport and Exercise Medicine for Pharmacists

Sport and Exercise Medicine for Pharmacists

Edited by

Steven B Kayne

BSc (Pharm), PhD, MBA, LLM, MSc (Sp Med), DAgVetPharm, FRPharmS, FCPP, FIPharmM, MPS (NZ), FNZCP, FFHom

Independent Consultant Pharmacist

Visiting Lecturer, School of Pharmacy
University of Strathclyde, Glasgow

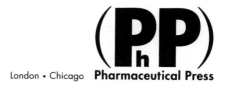

London • Chicago **Pharmaceutical Press**

Published by the Pharmaceutical Press
Publications division of the Royal Pharmaceutical Society of Great Britain

1 Lambeth High Street, London SE1 7JN, UK
100 South Atkinson Road, Suite 206, Grayslake, IL 60030-7820, USA

© Pharmaceutical Press 2006

 is a trade mark of Pharmaceutical Press

Typeset by Type Study, Scarborough, North Yorkshire
Printed in Great Britain by TJ International, Padstow, Cornwall

ISBN 0 85369 600 4

Contents

Foreword

You don't need to be an elite athlete to enjoy participating in sport and exercise. The benefits of regular exercise are well documented and – providing you don't overdo it – can be exhilarating and improve well-being.

Most people see their local community pharmacist more regularly than all other healthcare professionals put together, so this is a good first point of contact for advice. The pharmacist can also help with minor injuries and sports-related illness and should be aware of the over-the-counter medicines that contain substances banned by the World Anti-Doping Agency (WADA).

A quarter of this book is dedicated to doping – a problem that will not go away. Opportunities to impress on youngsters the potential long-term dangers to health of taking performance-enhancing drugs, as well as stressing the futility of cheating in sport, should not be missed. Pharmacists can play an important part in the promotion of clean sport and good health and this book will support them in this important role.

Steve Backley OBE
August 2005

Steve Backley, from Sidcup in Kent, turned to the javelin after initially starting out in athletics as a cross-country and middle-distance runner. Now, 25 years later, he's the four times European javelin champion, three times Commonwealth Games champion and twice World Championships runner-up. He also became the first Briton to mount the podium in an athletics event at three separate Olympic Games (1992, 1996 and 2000), winning a bronze and two silver medals.

Preface

I believe every human has a finite number of heart beats. I don't intend to waste any of mine doing exercises!
Neil Armstrong, US astronaut and the first man to walk on the moon

Far too many members of the public have expressed sentiments similar to those attributed to Neil Armstrong above who, given the high degree of physical fitness necessary to participate in a space programme, must have been speaking tongue-in-cheek! When combined with obesity and smoking, a lack of exercise has been shown to contribute to ill health and premature death. With the greatly expanded responsibilities for healthcare delivery taken on by pharmacy in recent years, promoting a healthy lifestyle has become an important element of the new community pharmacy contract. Supplementary and independent prescribing also present challenges and opportunities to expand our activities into previously unexplored areas of practice.

Research has shown in the UK that the public do not think of pharmacies as a potential port of call for advice on sport- and exercise-related problems, despite the fact that in many cases these closely resemble the very things pharmacists are dealing with on a day-to-day basis as a result of domestic mishaps. For example, soft tissue injuries and abrasions account for the majority of injuries sustained by non-elite athletes, yet only 2% admit to consulting a pharmacist (Kayne and Reeves, 1994). The main reason given for this was "not believing the pharmacist had sufficient knowledge". Personal experience would suggest that the position has not changed materially in the last ten years. It is hoped that this book will provide the knowledge that pharmacists need to take up confidently the many opportunities associated with sport and exercise and encourage them to make their new interest known to potential clients.

For most pharmacists, sports-related activities will form part of a portfolio of services to the community. However, for some colleagues, a new speciality called 'sport and exercise pharmacy' is emerging in the UK. Its practitioners seek to apply their skills to help meet the particular needs of clients involved in competitive sports and exercise at the highest levels. With the successful London Olympic bid for 2012, and the resulting heightened interest in sport at all levels, opportunities for developing such activities by pharmacists should not be missed.

The objectives of this book are to:

- create an awareness of the importance of exercise in the promotion and maintenance of public health;
- provide background information on the disciplines that comprise sport and exercise medicine;
- provide practical advice on how pharmacists can integrate sports care into their daily practice and be more proactive, as well as responding to requests for advice on the prophylaxis and treatment of minor problems;
- encourage pharmacists to become more proactive in preventing drug abuse in sport and provide advice on nutrition, food supplements and herbal remedies.

The book is not designed to be read from cover to cover at one sitting, but to be a resource to dip into as the need arises. There is some repetition of important material, to obviate the need to flick back and forth through different chapters, although references to the other entries for a topic are given.

I consider myself extremely fortunate to have secured contributions from so many well-qualified colleagues and to them and the Pharmaceutical Press, I offer my sincere thanks.

Steven Kayne
August 2005

Reference

Kayne S B, Reeves A (1994). Sports care and the pharmacist – an opportunity not to be missed. *Pharm J* 253: 66–67.

Acknowledgements

My thanks to the following for kindly allowing me to take photographs:

Dr John MacLean, Ceri and Evelyn of the Sports Injuries Clinic, Scottish National Stadium, Hampden Park, Glasgow (Chapter 4).

Dr David Cowan and Dr Paul Levy of King's College London (Chapter 8).

Noel and Jonathan and their staff at Campus Pharmacy, Stirling (Chapter 10).

About the editor

Steven Kayne spent almost 30 years as a Community Pharmacist in Glasgow, with a special interest in health promotion through sport and exercise. He graduated from Glasgow University with a Master's degree in Sports Medicine in 2002. He writes and lectures widely in the UK and overseas on a variety of topics of interest to pharmacists. Dr Kayne is a visiting lecturer at the University of Strathclyde, Glasgow, and holds a number of advisory positions as well as being a member of the Scottish Executive of the Royal Pharmaceutical Society of Great Britain and Chairman of the College of Pharmacy Practice in Scotland. He has written, edited and contributed to, several pharmacy textbooks.

Contributors

J Stuart Anderson MCSP, AACP, ACPSM, SRP
Stuart Anderson has extensive experience working within the elite athletic environment, lecturing internationally and providing expertise in coordinating training cycles with physical rehabilitation and performance conditioning. Stuart worked as Physiotherapist in Athletics at the 2004 Athens Olympic Games and the 2002 Manchester Commonwealth Games, and has advised and toured with several professional athletic teams and dance companies. He studied physiotherapy at the University of Manchester, followed by numerous postgraduate courses addressing various aspects of the clinical management of elite athletes, and has worked within sports medicine teams in Canada, Sweden and the UK. Stuart is currently physiotherapist and lecturer in body conditioning and health maintenance for the Royal Ballet in London.

Pamela Mason BSc, MSc, PhD, MRPharmS
Pamela Mason has been an Independent Pharmaceutical and Nutrition Consultant since 1994. She is a regular contributor to the *Pharmaceutical Journal* and other pharmaceutical publications. She is the author of the *Handbook of Dietary Supplements* (Pharmaceutical Press, 2001), *Nutrition and Dietary Advice in the Pharmacy* (Blackwell Science, 2000) and *Locum Pharmacy* (Pharmaceutical Press, 2004). Between 1989 and 1994, she worked as an editorial assistant on the British National Formulary and as a writer of training material at the National Pharmaceutical Association. She has nearly 20 years' experience as a practising community pharmacist in Manchester, North Wales and London.

Anthony C Moffat BPharm, PhD, DSc, CChem, FRSC, FRPharmS
Anthony Moffat graduated in pharmacy (1965), followed by a PhD (1969) and DSc (1984), degrees all from Chelsea College, University of London, England. During 1969 and 1970 he was Assistant Professor at Baylor College of Medicine, USA. This was followed by 23 years in the Forensic Science Service, England. Since 1994 he has been Chief Scientist at the Royal Pharmaceutical Society (RPSGB), London, and Head of

the Centre for Pharmaceutical Analysis at The School of Pharmacy, University of London. In 2004 he retired from his role at the Royal Pharmaceutical Society. He has had over 200 publications, including the co-authorship of seven books.

His awards include the British Pharmaceutical Conference Science Award, Society of Analytical Chemistry Silver Medal, Philip Allen Award of the Forensic Science Society and the joint award of the BUCHI 2002 Award. He is a member of the British Pharmacopoeia Commission.

David Mottram BPharm, PhD, FRPharmS

David Mottram is a pharmacy graduate from Cardiff University, where he also obtained his PhD in pharmacology. After two years as a Medical Research Council Postdoctoral Fellow he has pursued a career in academic pharmacy and is currently Professor of Pharmacy Practice at Liverpool John Moores University. He became a Fellow of the RPSGB in 1997. His major areas of research have centred on aspects of neuro-pharmacology, postgraduate education in pharmacy, pharmacy practice and drug use in sport. He has published over 120 research papers, contributed a number of book chapters and is the editor of the book *Drugs in Sport*, first published in 1988 and now in its third edition.

Mark C Stuart BPharm, PGDipCDDS, DipBotMed, MRPharmS

Mark was Superintendent Pharmacist for the Manchester 2002 Commonwealth Games, pharmacist for the Sydney 2000 Olympic Games and worked with doping-control for the Athens 2004 Olympics. He studied pharmacy at Sydney University and has postgraduate qualifications in clinical drug dependence and botanical medicine. He has worked in community and hospital pharmacy in both Australia and England.

Mark is currently Senior Medical Editor for the National Institute for Health and Clinical Excellence and was previously a staff editor of the British National Formulary and Senior Resident Pharmacist at the London Clinic in Harley Street. He has also worked closely with UK Sport on resources for athletes, including the online UK Sport Drug Information Database. Mark has had numerous articles published in journals and magazines about drugs in sport and regularly lectures on the topic. He manages a website for pharmacists and other healthcare professionals on sports medicine and anti-doping issues (http://www.sportspharmacy.com).

Trudy Thomas BSc, MSc, MRPharmS
Trudy Thomas is Senior Lecturer in Pharmacy Practice at the Medway School of Pharmacy. Previously she worked at Canterbury and Coastal PCT as a Prescribing Advisor. She has been the Centre for Pharmacy Post-graduate Education (CPPE) Tutor for West Kent since 1991. As a consultant she has written and delivered training for healthcare professionals including nurse and pharmacist prescribers. In the 1990s she was a training officer for the National Pharmaceutical Association. A keen runner, Trudy has always been interested in exercise and sport. Her MSc looked at the role of the community pharmacist in supporting people undertaking physical activity. She was project leader for the three CPPE workshops on sport and fitness.

Part One

Introduction

1

The physiology of exercise

Steven B Kayne

Introduction

To appreciate how sport and exercise can be a benefit it is necessary to understand the physiology of exercise. This chaper describes the fundamentals of sports physiology.

Energy is necessary to enable all functions of the body to be carried out, and is derived from the oxidation of glucose. Glucose is obtained from the metabolism of carbohydrates, fats and proteins and undergoes oxidation in all cells of the body (cellular respiration) to produce carbon dioxide, water and energy. These processes are driven by the efficient utilisation of oxygen through respiratory and cardiovascular processes.

Complete oxidation of glucose proceeds through three stages (Figure 1.1):

- glycolysis to produce pyruvic acid
- the Krebs cycle
- the electron transport chain.

The resultant energy is used to convert adenosine diphosphate (ADP) to adenosine triphosphate (ATP), from which it is liberated during exercise (see below).

Respiration and exercise

The respiratory process

The total lung capacity (TLC) in adult males is approximately 6 litres, but at rest only about 10% of this is used. The tidal volume (TV) is the amount of air that moves into and out of the lungs with each breath, and at rest is 500 mL. Of this, 150 mL (known as the residual volume) occupies the inactive space (i.e. those parts of the airway not involved in gaseous exchange), which means that only 350 mL reaches the alveoli.

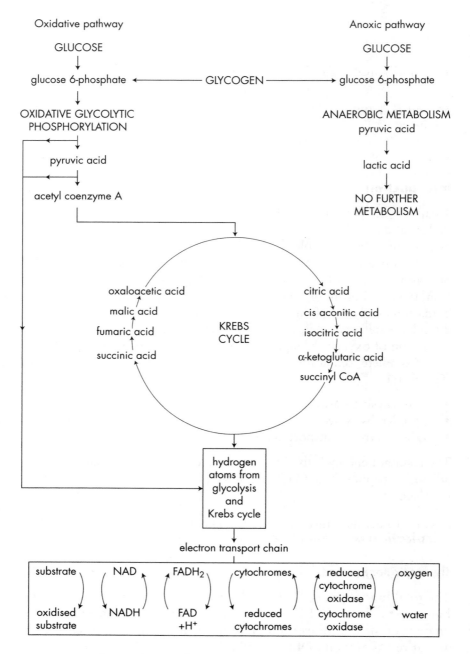

Figure 1.1 Outline pathways of glucose metabolism. Reproduced from Kayne S B, Sport and Exercise. In: Harman R J, ed., *Handbook of Pharmacy Health Education*; published by Pharmaceutical Press, 2001.

During exercise, the TV increases, and at maximal breathing, when the largest proportion of the TLC is used, it is referred to as the vital capacity (VC). This may be between 3 and 5 litres in adult males, which still leaves a residual volume of 1–1.5 litres. The VC of males is 50% greater than that of females. The effort required for respiration is minimal at rest, but increases as activity increases and additional muscles are employed.

The average rate of respiration at rest is 12 respirations/minute. The TV is 500 mL, and so the average volume of air inspired every minute is 6 litres. The maximum breathing capacity (maximum ventilation volume) in adult males in a normal sea-level atmosphere is 125 litres/minute. The volume of air taken in during a deep inspiration may be as much as 3.6 litres. Exercise increases the rate of respiration and the volume of air inspired per minute.

The rate of respiration is controlled primarily by the concentration of carbon dioxide in the blood. If the concentration falls, then respiration rate decreases until the carbon dioxide concentration in the blood rises to normal levels. Oxygen only acts as a stimulus if there is a severe reduction in blood oxygen concentration, because haemoglobin remains at least 85% saturated with oxygen until quite low oxygen concentrations are inhaled. Further reductions in oxygen will affect the inspiratory area in the medulla, causing breathing to stop altogether.

Overbreathing immediately before an event is thought by some athletes to improve performance because a few vital seconds may be gained by temporarily removing the desire to breathe. Carbon dioxide is flushed out of the lungs, reducing its blood concentration to such an extent that respiration temporarily stops. The oxygen remaining in the lungs diffuses slowly into the blood but eventually a very low blood oxygen concentration stimulates breathing. At about the same time, or shortly afterwards, the blood carbon dioxide concentration rises sufficiently to act as a further stimulus. The interaction of both stimuli is required to maintain respiration. It is possible to hold one's breath for up to a minute after a deep inspiration, and this too may be used to gain time, especially in swimming. Eventually, respiration is stimulated by rising blood carbon dioxide concentrations. Athletes may combine breath-holding with overbreathing in an effort to further increase the time of non-breathing. This practice should not be encouraged as it may lead to a fainting, i.e. a temporary loss of consciousness and posture, something that is particularly dangerous for swimmers.

Alveolar diffusion capacity, which is a measure of the gaseous exchange efficiency of the alveoli, varies even among healthy subjects, and training cannot increase this function above an individual's inherent maximum. Thus, the oxygen saturation of blood will be different among highly trained athletes. However, through intensive training, the muscles can adapt to a certain amount of oxygen deprivation (see below).

Respiration during exercise

Aerobic respiration

Exercise involving aerobic respiration requires the oxygen demands of the active muscle to be fully met once the initial period of adjustment is over. Oxygen is taken into the body during respiration at the same time that carbon dioxide is expelled. The heart pumps oxygenated blood received from the pulmonary circulation to the rest of the body and deoxygenated blood to the lungs for oxygenation. Oxygen binds with haemoglobin in the erythrocytes for transportation in the systemic circulation to the tissues. It therefore follows that during exercise, the overall energy demand is increased. The efficiency of all these processes must increase to meet the greater oxygen requirements.

To achieve this, there must be increases in respiration rate and depth, cardiac output, and blood flow to the muscles. Regular aerobic exercise induces adaptive changes so that future exercise becomes comparatively easier. However, this is not a long-term effect, and previous levels of fitness will return if exercise sessions are discontinued.

The capacity to follow these activities reflects an ability to take in and use oxygen and depends on three factors:

- effective breathing
- effective oxygen transport from the lungs to cells
- effective use of oxygen within the cells.

Aerobic capacity is usually referred to as $VO_{2(max)}$ – the maximum rate of utilisation of atmospheric oxygen during continuous activity. It is expressed as mL/min/kg of body weight. The scale for a man in his twenties might range from 33 (very poor) to 60 (outstanding) and for a woman from 24 (poor) to 45 (outstanding). For a man in his sixties the range would be from 20 to 45 and for a woman of the same age 17.5 to 32 (see http://www.brianmac.demon.co.uk/vo2max.htm). A person's $VO_{2(max)}$ may be determined under laboratory conditions using a treadmill and apparatus to collect the expired air. Inactivity decreases $VO_{2(max)}$ whereas aerobic training for a few weeks can improve it substantially. $VO_{2(max)}$ improves as the maximum cardiac output increases (see below). $VO_{2(max)}$ starts to decline after 20 years of age, but the rate of decline can be decreased by regular exercise.

Aerobic exercise is of relatively low intensity but can be of fairly long duration. It involves the movement of groups of large muscles and causes participants to breathe more deeply, adding to the workload of the heart and lungs and raising the heart rate. Such exercise, if performed regularly, will improve the cardiovascular and respiratory systems. Examples include walking, jogging, dancing and swimming.

Anaerobic respiration

This occurs during sustained muscle activity when there is insufficient oxygen to meet the requirements of aerobic respiration. The pyruvic acid produced by the oxidation of glucose cannot be completely oxidised, and is converted to lactic acid (see Figure 1.1). Approximately 80% of the lactic acid is transported to the liver for conversion to glucose or glycogen, and the remainder accumulates in the muscles.

Exercise involving anaerobic respiration does not rely on a supply of oxygen to the muscles from the circulation, but can only be sustained for 1–2 minutes, in contrast to aerobic exercise, which in a fit subject can be sustained for hours. Anaerobic respiration occurs during short bursts of extremely strenuous activity (e.g. a 100-metre sprint), when the supply of oxygen is insufficient to keep up with the exercising muscles. Most forms of exercise utilise both aerobic and anaerobic respiration.

Isotonic and isometric exercise

Exercise may be classified as isotonic or isometric:

- Isotonic (endurance or dynamic) exercise involves muscle work during movement (e.g. cycling, running or swimming) and is of value in improving stamina and endurance. Isotonic exercise is dependent mainly on aerobic respiration.
- Isometric (power or static) exercise (e.g. handgrip or weightlifting) involves a sustained increase in contraction of antagonistic muscles without movement and is primarily used to increase muscle strength. As a result, people who train regularly using isometric exercises are likely to be heavier than endurance athletes. They also tend to have more deposits of body fat. Isometric exercise is dependent mainly on anaerobic respiration.

The cardiovascular system and exercise

The cardiac output (CO) is the volume of blood pumped from the left ventricle of the heart into the aorta every minute. It is equal to the pulse rate (PR) multiplied by the stroke volume (SV), which is the volume of blood ejected by the ventricles at each heartbeat:

$$CO = PR \times SV$$

In a normal adult heart, the resting pulse rate is about 70 beats/minute, and the stroke volume about 70 mL. The cardiac output at rest is therefore about 5.25 litres/minute. To increase oxygen perfusion of the tissues to cope with the increased demand created by exercise or in response to exercise at altitude, the cardiac output must be increased by raising the stroke volume or the pulse rate.

The pulse rate is controlled in part by the autonomic nervous system: the sympathetic component increases the rate and the parasympathetic component lowers it. In people who have not been used to regular vigorous exercise, the cardiac output is mainly raised by an increase in the pulse rate. Physical training, however, increases the parasympathetic tone of the vagus nerve, and there is a much smaller rise in pulse rate for a given workload. Subjects who have undergone training for a period of time previously feel more comfortable than untrained individuals. In order to achieve the desired increase in cardiac output, trained individuals show a greater rise in stroke volume, which is produced by an increased ventricular capacity of up to 30%. This causes the heart to enlarge, but must be distinguished from enlargement caused by cardiac disease, in which the increased size is a result of muscular hypertrophy. The increase in size of the ventricular chamber reduces the pressure developed during systole. The resting pulse rate of highly trained individuals also falls, and may be as low as 40 beats per minute in elite athletes.

The cardiac reserve is the maximum that the cardiac output can be increased above normal during vigorous activity, and is expressed as a percentage. In the average adult, this reserve is around 400%, but trained athletes may achieve a 600% cardiac reserve. The cardiac output in trained athletes may reach 30 litres/minute or more during exercise. These cardiac changes reduce the work that the heart has to perform for a given workload and makes exercising progressively easier. These effects occur as a result of long-term isotonic exercise and may be apparent after a few weeks of training.

The optimum level of aerobic exercise needed by individuals varies with age, general health and fitness and how active the person has been in the past. In order to make appreciable gains in aerobic fitness, the heart rate during exercise must be raised above the resting heart rate by about 60% of the difference between an individual's resting and maximum heart rate. This is called the critical threshold, and above this exercise is said to have a significant effect. In most subjects, movement should be sufficiently robust to raise the pulse to between 140 and 160 beats per minute in order to exceed the critical threshold.

In isometric exercise, the arterial pressure rises, which increases the tension on the wall of the left ventricle. The cardiac output changes little and isometric exercise does not greatly improve stamina. Cardiac output increases linearly with increases in the intensity of aerobic exercise up to exhaustion. This is the result of increases in heart rate and stroke volume. The latter increases because the heart muscle contracts more forcefully, facilitating a more complete emptying of the ventricles with each heartbeat. Harmful effects are unlikely provided that exercise levels increase slowly over a period of weeks. This precaution is particularly important if people have had an inactive lifestyle.

The 'athletes' heart' represents a gradual enlargement of the ventricles, but without a corresponding thickening of the walls. The heart beats slower but with greater force to eject a larger volume of blood in its stroke volume. Healthy asymptomatic athletes are likely to alarm their physicians because of seemingly dangerous disturbances of heart rate and/or conduction. Arrhythmias in highly trained athletes are in fact common.

Cardiovascular monitoring

The occurrence of occasional sudden and premature death in both amateur and professional athletes who appear to exhibit all the attributes of cardiorespiratory health and fitness has raised the consciousness of the underlying causes. Concern has been expressed as to the correct evaluation of conditioned athletes (Ferst and Chaitman, 1984).

In a study looking at the causes of sudden death in 46 competitive athletes under the age of 35, 37 were found to be exercise-related, occurring during or immediately following a sports activity (Kahn, 1996). Eighteen of the sudden deaths were preceded by warning symptoms or electrocardiographic changes. A conservative estimate suggests that 13 out of 2.7 million US high-school athletes die suddenly each year from a non-traumatic cause during sports participation (Fuller et al., 1997).

The implication is clear – some or all of these deaths could (and perhaps should) have been avoided with an appropriate screening programme. However, identifying all athletes at risk of exercise-related sudden death is difficult, particularly if they are asymptomatic.

Of all the cardiovascular measurements carried out on patients in hospital, the electrocardiogram (ECG) is considered to be one of the most important. Interpretation of the ECG trace allows causal identification of an abnormal heart rhythm or an evolving heart attack. Physiological adaptations of the heart to prolonged intense physical exercise produce a range of changes in the ECG trace. In particular, water polo athletes have been shown to have substantial cardiac hypertrophy and often present with bradycardia and abnormalities in their ECG traces (Zakynthinos *et al.*, 2001).

These changes are of interest because of their frequency and close resemblance to pathological changes occurring in certain organic heart diseases. The heart reacts to acute physical stress with a rapid increase in heart rate and a resulting increase in contractility. Regular physical training results in a permanent adaptation process in the heart that is not immediately reversible. The amount of training necessary to obtain adaptations in the ECG trace is unclear. An athlete who has ceased involvement in a moderate level of training within the past few months will still exhibit ECG changes associated with physical exercise.

One way of differentiating between a 'normal' athletic heart and an athletic patient is to instruct the individual to stop training for some months. If the ECG abnormalities persist, they are more likely to be the result of pathological processes than of physical conditioning. Such action is unlikely to gain an athlete's immediate co-operation!

Studies in the literature that interpret ECG data from athletes vary widely, involving anything from 20 subjects up to several thousand, but all demonstrate that the process is not without problems (Holly *et al.*, 1998). Adaptations in the athletic heart that result in vagotonia and increased cardiac mass and volume account for most of the normal variants in the athlete's ECG. Accompanied by normal blood pressure and cardiac examination these findings should be considered normal variants and need be followed up only if a risk is perceived. Family history is particularly important in this respect. However, it is sometimes difficult to differentiate the healthy athlete with athletic heart from the athletic patient with a diseased heart. The ECG cannot be considered a 'gold standard' indicator of the presence or future likely development of coronary artery disease. However, the technique is valuable in determining whether non-athletic individuals planning to take on intense exercise are safe to do so. In these circumstances the ECG will provide useful information regarding the diagnosis of coronary artery disease and allow identification of a high-risk individual.

Effects of exercise on haemoglobin

The principal function of haemoglobin, which is contained in erythrocytes, is to transport oxygen in the blood. The normal blood haemoglobin concentration is 14–18 g per 100 mL of blood for males, and 12–16 g per 100 mL of blood for females. A constant enhanced demand for oxygen by the tissues (e.g. as a result of physical training) increases the number of erythrocytes, and consequently the amount of haemoglobin, present. Plasma volume may also rise, with the result that the haemoglobin concentration remains constant or may even drop, suggesting anaemia ('sports anaemia'). However, the actual oxygen-carrying capacity is higher because the total amount of haemoglobin present is greater.

In highly trained individuals these increases may approach 40% above average values. Carbon monoxide, present in tobacco smoke and exhaust fumes from motor vehicles, binds with haemoglobin much more strongly than oxygen and therefore substantially reduces the oxygen-carrying capacity of the blood. Exercise can aid the removal of carbon monoxide from haemoglobin.

Effects of rise in body temperature

The core temperature, which is the deep body temperature measured by the oral or rectal method, may increase to 41°C during intensive exercise. In order for this heat to be lost by conduction, convection and radiation from the skin, the volume of blood perfusing the skin increases during strenuous activity. Heat is also lost by the evaporation of sweat. If any of these mechanisms are blocked, or the individual is unfit, heat stroke or even sudden death may occur.

Sport and exercise at high altitude

The main effects of sport and exercise at high altitude result from the lower availability of oxygen in the air. Lower oxygen pressure in the inspired air causes a lower oxygen pressure in the alveoli and this in turn leads to less oxygen in the blood. At sea level, blood haemoglobin is 96% saturated, while at an altitude of 2300 metres saturation falls to 90%.

Below about 1500 metres there is little appreciable fall in $VO_{2(max)}$ but thereafter there is a 10% drop per 1000 metre gain in height. Physiological adaptation results in an increased pulmonary ventilation. Simultaneously the heart increases its output by up to a third, raising both pulse rate and stroke volume. With time the body produces new erythrocytes and the blood oxygen-carrying capacity rises. Muscle enzymes also adapt and become more efficient.

Gastrointestinal effects of exercise

The heart, brain and skeletal muscles have increased oxygen demands during exercise, and blood must be redirected to these organs away from other parts of the body (e.g. the gastrointestinal tract). In vigorous activity, the blood supply to the heart tissue is increased by up to four or five times. The need for diversion of the systemic blood flow decreases with training because the oxygen-extracting ability of the muscles improves (see below). The individual feels more comfortable during exercise as a result of fewer gastrointestinal symptoms.

Energy requirement of the muscles

As explained above, the energy that is utilised in muscular activity is produced from the oxidation of glucose achieved following anaerobic and aerobic respiration. Energy is stored in the phosphate bonds of ATP, which is liberated during exercise by hydrolysis of the terminal bond, reforming ADP in the process.

The role of creatine

Creatine (Cr) or methylguanidine-acetic acid, is a physiologically active substance necessary for muscle contraction. The normal daily intake of dietary Cr is less than 1 g, obtained mainly from meat and fish and other animal products. However, the estimated average daily requirement is double that amount. The balance in the body is maintained mainly by the kidneys, together with smaller amounts from the liver and pancreas. The intake of exogenous Cr in the diet appears to play a role in the control of endogenous Cr synthesis by means of a feedback mechanism. Cr is formed from three amino acids, arginine, glycine and methionine, and it reaches the muscle cells by an active membrane transport system.

Almost all the Cr in the body is located in skeletal muscle in either the free (Cr: ~40%) or phosphorylated (PCr: ~60%) form and represents an average Cr pool of about 120–140 g for an average 70 kg person (Bemben and Lamont, 2005). The concentrations of PCr and free Cr in resting human skeletal muscle vary widely. The fast twitch fibres (see page 14) have a higher total Cr content than the slow fibres. For reasons not yet understood, females appear to have slightly higher resting levels of Cr than males. PCr is present in resting muscle in a concentration three to four times that of ATP, the immediate energy source for muscle contraction. If cellular ATP concentration falls too far, fatigue occurs.

The rate of ATP hydrolysis to adenosine diphosphate (ADP) and free phosphorus (P) is set by the power output of the muscles, i.e. the intensity of the exercise. Regeneration of ATP at a rate close to that of its hydrolysis is vital if fatigue is to be delayed. Indeed, a decline in the rate of resynthesis of ATP as a result of depletion of PCr is recognised as a possible cause of reduction in muscle power in maximal intensity exercise. In the regeneration of ATP, transfer of the phosphate group from PCr is catalysed by the enzyme creatine kinase, resulting in the restoration of ATP and the release of free Cr. The mechanisms involved may summarised as follows:

$$ATP \rightarrow ADP + P$$

$$PCr + ADP + H^+ \rightarrow ATP + Cr$$

The creatine kinase reaction is extremely rapid and because the muscle PCr concentration can fall to almost zero it is likely to contribute significantly to the energy supply required for short bursts of high-intensity exercise.

During the recovery stage following exercise, the creatine kinase reaction is reversed using oxygen resulting from a metabolic process in the mitochondria:

$$Cr + ATP \rightarrow PCr + ADP$$

$$ADP + P + metabolism \rightarrow ATP$$

The lactic acid that accumulates as a result of anaerobic metabolism (Figure 1.1) during sustained muscle activity must eventually be catabolised, and the extra oxygen required for this process is termed the 'oxygen debt'. The additional oxygen is 'repaid' at the end of the activity by a continued increase in the depth and rate of respiration.

It is hypothesised that Cr can act through a number of possible mechanisms as a potential ergogenic aid, but it appears to be most effective for activities that involve repeated short bouts of high-intensity physical activity (see Chapter 3). There appears to be no strong scientific evidence to support any adverse effects but it should be noted that there have been no studies to date that address the issue of long-term Cr usage (Bemben and Lamont, 2005) (see also Chapter 8).

Muscle fatigue

The process of fatigue

Muscle fatigue resulting in pain is caused by a combination of factors, including the build-up of lactic acid and carbon dioxide in the tissues, and a reduced supply of oxygen. As fatigue develops, levels of ATP, PCr and high-energy phosphates decrease, and levels of lactate, ADP, inorganic phosphates and hydrogen ions increase. The response of the muscle fibres becomes progressively weaker in the face of sustained contraction, and activity must either cease or switch to the slower aerobic pace.

Types of muscle fibres

There are two types of fibre present in skeletal muscles: fast twitch fibres, which contract quickly and with great strength, and are suitable for anaerobic exercise; and slow fibres, which are more suitable for aerobic exercise. The proportion of each type of fibre present in the muscles of an individual is genetically determined, and someone who naturally has a greater number of slow fibres is unlikely to become an elite marathon runner. However, training does improve performance above baseline in both types.

Anaerobic metabolism

Anaerobic metabolism is a means of allowing short periods of sustained high-intensity muscle contraction. Glycolysis results in the formation of pyruvate at a rate higher than that at which it can be removed by oxidative metabolism. This leads to a build-up of lactate within the muscle. Muscle pH falls as a result of the glycolysis and is thought to be involved in the development of fatigue. The breakdown of PCr acts as a buffer mechanism within the cell, delaying the point at which a critically low pH is reached. An increased availability of PCr for breakdown may increase the buffering capacity in the muscles.

Sprinting is a particular athletic event in which a short distance (e.g. 60 or 100 metres) is run at high speed. However, sprinting may also be employed in everyday life (e.g. in running for a bus or, at its most extreme, to escape from danger). Sprinting requires anaerobic metabolism in the muscles, and for unfit individuals, any increase in activity above their normal level may be comparable to a 'sprint' in terms of muscle metabolism and fatigue. If oxygen were provided at a sufficient rate to keep pace with oxidative processes to produce enough energy for a sprint, the blood supply to the muscles would have to increase to such an extent that there would be no room in the muscles for sufficient myofibrils to sustain the contraction, or enough mitochondria to cope with the oxidative processes.

Aerobic metabolism

Longer periods require aerobic metabolism and the activity must therefore continue at a slower pace (e.g. marathon running). Regular aerobic training will, however, increase the capacity for sprinting by increasing the number of capillaries in the muscles.

References

Bemben M G, Lamont H S (2005). Creatine supplementation and exercise performance: recent findings. *Sports Med* 35: 107–125.

Ferst J A, Chaitman B R (1984). The electrocardiogram and the athlete. *Sports Med* 1: 390–403.

Fuller C M, McNulty C M, Spring D A, *et al.* (1997). Prospective screening of 5615 high school athletes for risk of sudden cardiac death. *Med Sci Sports Exerc* 29: 1131–1138.

Holly R G, Shaffrath J D, Amsterdam E A (1998). Electrocardiographic alterations associated with the hearts of athletes. *Sports Med* 25: 139–148.

Kahn J (1996). Screening can prevent sport-related deaths. *Medical Tribune* 2 May.

Kayne S B (2001). Sport and exercise. In: Harman R J, ed. *Handbook of Pharmacy Health Education*, 2nd edn. London: Pharmaceutical Press, 194.

Zakynthinos E, Vassilakopoulos T, Mavrommati I, *et al.* (2001). Echocardiographic and ambulatory electrocardiographic findings in elite water-polo athletes. *Scand J Med Sci Sports* 11: 149–155.

Further reading

Fentem P H, Turnbull N B, Bassey E J (1990). *Benefits of Exercise: The Evidence.* Manchester: Manchester University Press.

Lamb D R (1984). *Physiology of Exercise. Responses and Adaptations*, 2nd edn. New York: Macmillan.

MacLeod D, Maughan R, Nimmo M, eds (1987). *Exercise: Benefits, Limits and Adaptations*. London: E & FN Spon.

Reilly T, Secher N, Snell P, *et al.*, eds (1990). *Physiology of Sports*. London: E & FN Spon.

2

Physical activity in the community

Trudy Thomas

Introduction

The health benefits of physical activity

There are many benefits associated with participating in physical activity:

- People who engage in regular physical activity – even of a moderate nature – generally have lower mortality rates (Blair *et al.*, 1989).
- People with existing medical conditions, such as type 2 diabetes and coronary heart disease, who exercise have lower levels of mortality than those who do not (Hardman, 1991; Eriksson, 1999).
- Physical activity can promote good mental health and is associated with decreased levels of moderate depression and anxiety (Steptoe, 1992).
- In older people, activity can
  - improve physical functioning and help maintain independence (Young and Dinan, 2000)
  - strengthen bones, thus helping to prevent osteoporosis (Fordham, 2000).
- In recent years, there has been a focus in the UK on obesity as a risk factor for health problems in both adults and children. While the aetiology of obesity is multi-factorial, the increasingly sedentary nature of the UK population is thought to play an important part (National Audit Office, 2002). A combination of diet and an increase in physical activity appears to bring about a greater weight loss than dietary control alone can achieve (National Prescribing Centre, 1998).

Health benefits from exercise are achievable regardless of the age, gender or health status of the individual. For all these reasons, the successful promotion of exercise by health care professionals is seen as an area that could substantially benefit the health of the population (Department of Health, 1993).

Defining physical activity

The key definitions associated with physical activity are given in Box 2.1. It is important to differentiate between physical activity and exercise:

- Physical activity is a general term referring to any bodily movement produced by the skeletal muscles resulting in energy expenditure (Health Education Authority, 1995a). This includes activities undertaken as part of day-to-day living and work. An individual's level of physical fitness relates to their ability to perform physical activity. It may be partly determined by heredity and partly acquired through physical activity and other lifestyle factors.

Box 2.1 Definitions. Source: Caspersen *et al.* (1985)

Physical activity
This refers to all musculoskeletal movement that results in energy expenditure and therefore includes activities undertaken as part of day-to-day living and during the course of work, as well as leisure time activities such as exercise and sport.

Exercise
Defined as 'planned, structured and repetitive movement done to improve or maintain one of the components of physical fitness'. Exercise may also be thought of as physical activity undertaken in leisure time for the purpose of improving or maintaining fitness.

Sport
Defines physical activity involving structured, competitive situations governed by rules. Football and hockey, for example, are considered as sports whereas aerobics is classified as exercise.

Physical fitness
A set of attributes that people have or achieve that relates to their ability to perform physical activity. It may be partly determined by heredity and partly acquired through physical activity and other lifestyle factors. For health-related benefit, frequency, duration and intensity of activity need to be defined.

- Exercise refers to planned, structured activities involving repetitive bodily movements.

The frequency, duration and intensity of activity are factors used to determine the health benefit of exercise and are defined in Box 2.2. For health-related benefits, the frequency, duration and intensity of activity need to be defined. Examples of the kinds of activity designated as light, moderate and vigorous intensity are shown in Box 2.2.

What amount and type of exercise is recommended for health benefit?

UK and international guidance

The exercise guidelines recommended by the American College of Sports Medicine (ACSM), issued in 1978 and revised in 1990, were adopted as the international standards (American College of Sports Medicine, 1990). However, in 1993, new guidelines issued jointly by the ACSM and the US Center for Disease Control and Prevention recognised the mounting evidence that more frequent but moderate exercise was beneficial (Pate *et al.*, 1995). This report recommended that people should

---

Box 2.2 Categorisation of physical activity intensity, with examples. Source: Health Education Authority (1995b)

Light – requiring little exertion and not causing a noticeable change in breathing. Long walks (2 miles+) at a slow pace, lighter DIY or gardening, e.g. decorating, weeding, fishing, darts, snooker, exercises, table tennis, golf.

Moderate – requiring sustained rhythmic muscular movement, at least the equivalent of brisk walking that leaves the person feeling warm and slightly out of breath.

Long walks (2 miles+) at a fast brisk pace, football, swimming, tennis, aerobics, cycling, golf, social dancing, exercises, heavy DIY or gardening (e.g. mixing cement, digging).

Vigorous – involves sustained rhythmic large muscle movements of at least 60–70% of maximum heart rate – makes a person sweaty and out of breath.

Playing squash, running, football, tennis, cycling, aerobics.

accumulate 30 minutes of moderate-intensity physical activity over the course of most days.

In April 1994, the Health Education Authority (HEA) recommended that to achieve health benefits relating to minimising mortality, individuals in the UK should undertake five moderate-intensity sessions per week, each lasting 30 minutes. An alternative was three vigorous-intensity sessions each lasting 20 minutes, in order to maximise aerobic fitness and minimise mortality. It was recognised that some people would combine elements of both recommended sessions (Biddle *et al.*, 1994).

The concept of 'active living'

Taking the international and national guidance literally would imply that when undertaking physical activity a person must carry it out in one continuous daily bout of 20 minutes (vigorous intensity) or 30 minutes (moderate intensity) and that the activity must be at of least moderate intensity to confer any health benefits. There is, however, growing speculation as to whether undertaking several short bouts of activity throughout the day will confer similar health benefits. The premise for this is that it is the total daily energy expenditure that is the determinant for health gains. The limited data available has focused on weight reduction when continuous activity is compared to short bouts of activity. The results suggest that similar weight reductions are possible with long and short bouts of exercise (Hardman, 1999).

There is no firm consensus on the precise health benefits to be gained from light-intensity activities. While the cardiovascular benefits from such activities may be minimal, other aspects of physical fitness such as improved muscular strength, co-ordination, joint mobility and flexibility and mental health gains may be achievable. These health gains may be particularly important for people who are currently sedentary, obese, elderly or disabled. Light- to moderate-intensity activities may make realistic first-stage goals for those who do not regularly exercise but who plan to start.

There has been little research to map the benefits of different types of physical activity. Studies have tended to focus on one age group, such as children or adults. It is thought that different components of activity may be important at different stages of life (Boreham and Riddoch, 2003). Although evidence is lacking, it is proposed that vigorous, varied, intermittent exercise may be most beneficial to children and young adults. In middle age, moderate exercise that works the cardiovascular system may prove the most appropriate. In older age, gentler exercise that focuses on flexibility and improved everyday functioning may help the person stay more 'healthy'. For example, indoor bowling has benefits for the elderly in providing both exercise and social contact (Figure 2.1). More research is needed this area.

Overall, evidence is emerging to support the concept of 'active living', whereby people are encouraged to incorporate physical activity of any kind into daily living at all stages of the lifespan. This change in focus is now reflected in the World Health Organization (WHO) recommendations for the amount of physical activity that is considered beneficial for health, which are shown in Box 2.3 (World Health Organization, 2002).

Many governments, including those of Australia, Canada, New Zealand, the UK and the Republic of Ireland, are promoting the concept of 'active living'. All have health promotion strategies that include

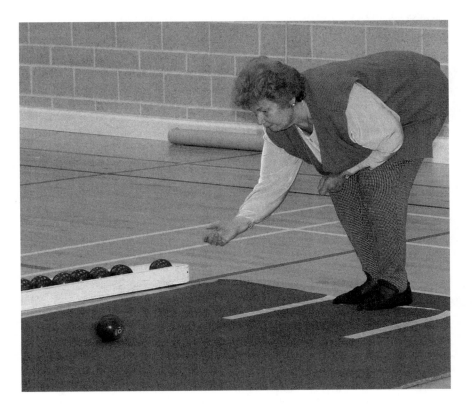

Figure 2.1 Elderly bowlers enjoy exercise and social contact.

Box 2.3 Concepts of health gain. Source: World Health Organization (2002)

Much of the health gain is obtained through of at least 30 minutes of cumulative moderate physical activity every day. This level of activity can be reached through a broad range of appropriate and enjoyable physical activities and body movements in people's daily lives, such as walking to work, climbing stairs, gardening, dancing, as well as a variety of leisure and recreational sports

Additional health gains can be obtained by relevant daily moderate to vigorous physical activities of longer duration, e.g. **children and young people** need an additional 20 minutes' vigorous physical activity three times a week. **Weight control** would require at least 60 minutes every day of moderate/vigorous physical activity.

---

targets to increase participation in physical activity in the general population (see end of chapter for details).

How much exercise is being taken in the UK?

Results from national surveys

The Allied Dunbar National Fitness Survey (ADNFS) is the most comprehensive survey available of the patterns of adult physical activity and levels of fitness in England (Sports Council and Health Education Authority, 1992). It consisted of a questionnaire sent to the homes of over 4300 participants, aged from 16 to 74. This was combined with the HEA National Survey of Activity and Health, which used the same questionnaire as the ADNFS in another 2200 people. The results of the combined survey showed that the majority (70%) of the English population were undertaking levels of physical activity that are below those required for optimum health.

This level required for optimum health was assessed by assigning a target level of activity for three specific age groups for the 4 weeks before the study. The target levels are shown in Table 2.1.

The survey assumed that anyone not achieving the target level of activity would be acquiring no health benefit, which – as already shown – is unlikely to be true. However, more recent studies by the Office for National Statistics (ONS), which looked purely at participation in sport or physical activity, showed that over half of those surveyed had not

Table 2.1 Target levels for the three age ranges studied in the Allied Dunbar National Fitness Survey. Source: Health Education Authority (1995a)

Age range (years)	Number of weekly sessions (of 20 minutes or more) and intensity
16–34	12 sessions of vigorous activity
35–54	12 sessions of moderate to vigorous activity
55–74	12 sessions of moderate activity

taken part in any form of activity in the 4 weeks before the survey (Figure 2.2) (Office for National Statistics, 2000).

Figures from the rest of the UK show a similar trend. The Scottish Health Survey, conducted in 1998, showed that 72% of women and 59% of men are not active enough for health (Scottish Executive, 2000). Only 28% of adults in Wales achieve 30 minutes of moderate-intensity activity on at least 5 days of the week (Chief Medical Officer Wales, 2005).

A sedentary lifestyle is a problem throughout the western world. It has been estimated that up to 60% of adult Americans do not exercise regularly and that some 25% are completely sedentary (US Surgeon General, 1997). A number of comparative studies show that

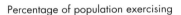

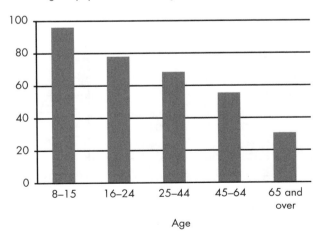

Figure 2.2 Participation in a sport or physical activity by age in the UK 2000–01. Source: Social Trends 34; published by Office for National Statistics (http://www.statistics.gov.uk). Crown copyright material is reproduced with the permission of the Controller of HMSO.

participation in physical activity in the UK is higher than that of other European countries. Direct comparisons are difficult because there is a lack of standardisation of methods, definitions, etc. However, countries most similar to the UK in terms of culture and weather generally achieve greater levels of participation (Department for Culture, Media and Sport, 2002). Compared to Scandinavian countries, participation in sports and physical activity in the UK is low (Figure 2.3).

Not only are the levels of participation in the UK lower than those in Scandinavia, but both the regularity and intensity of participation in the UK is significantly lower (Figure 2.4).

The UK still has a way to go if it is going to match the 70% of the Finnish population reported as undertaking at least 3 hours per week of exercise or physical activity during their leisure time, or the 57% of Australians who report undertaking at least 2.5 hours a week of moderate and vigorous physical activity (includes non-leisure time activity) (Department for Culture, Media and Sport, 2002). National surveys of 12 500 adult New Zealanders found that 68% enjoyed at least 2.5 hours of physical activity a week (Sport and Recreation New Zealand, 2003).

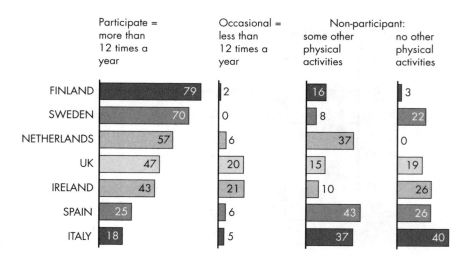

Figure 2.3 Participation in physical activity in the UK compared to other EU countries (percentage of population). Source: Game Plan: A Strategy for Delivering Government's Sport and Physical Activity Objectives; published by the British Government Strategy Unit, 2002. Crown copyright material is reproduced with the permission of the Controller of HMSO.

All adults 16+

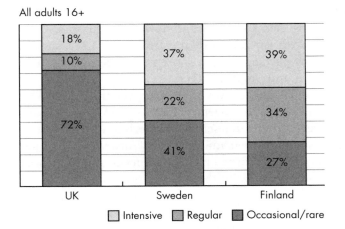

Figure 2.4 Comparison of intensity of activity carried out by UK participants compared to Sweden and Finland. Source: Game Plan: A Strategy for Delivering Government's Sport and Physical Activity Objectives; published by the British Government Strategy Unit, 2002. Crown copyright material is reproduced with the permission of the Controller of HMSO.

Participation in specific population groups

Effect of gender

Overall, UK men were shown to be more active than women in the ADNFS, the 2000 Time Use Survey from the ONS and the Scottish Health Survey, particularly in relation to more vigorous activity (Biddle *et al.*, 1994; Scottish Executive, 2000). The 1998 Social Focus on Men survey from the ONS showed that one-third of all men compared to one-fifth of all women had participated in some form of vigorous activity in the 4 weeks before being interviewed (Office for National Statistics, 1998).

The effect of age

The ADNFS in the UK and the Australian Sports Commission Survey also showed that participation rates fell with increasing age, which might be expected (Sports Council and Health Education Authority, 1992; Australian Institute of Health and Welfare, 2000). However in Finland and Sweden, participation in organised and competitive sport actually increases amongst older people, because of the focus placed on this group in these countries. There is some hope that the figures for the UK may be moving closer to its Scandinavian neighbours. Comparing the 1999 results with similar work undertaken in 1977 shows that more people are now participating in sport as they get older (Department for Culture, Media and Sport, 2002).

The ADNFS only surveyed people over the age of 16. Figure 2.5 from the ONS shows that over 95% of 8- to 15-year-olds are physically active. However, there is a significant decline in these activities by the time the person is in their mid-20s. The Australian Institute of Health and Welfare (2000) recorded participation rates of 88.8% in the 15–24 age group and only 60% in the 65+ age group.

It would appear that any benefits from an active youth are negated by reverting to a sedentary lifestyle as an adult (Paffenbarger *et al.*, 1986). One exception to this is bone density. Bone mass, which peaks in the late 20s, can be influenced by physical activity taken throughout childhood and adolescence. Maximising peak bone mass may provide some protection against osteoporosis in older life, although many other factors will also have an influence (Boreham and Riddoch, 2003).

It might be supposed that individuals who are active as children take this behaviour into adult life and so will enjoy health benefits as a result. However, physical activity is a relatively unstable behaviour and subject to so many influences that this is by no means clear. As such there is a scarcity of long-term studies into this behaviour 'tracking', as it is called.

It is clear that inactive children are more likely to be overweight. A large study in 1992 showed that overweight in adolescence is associated with a wide range of adverse health events in adulthood that are independent of adult weight (Must *et al.*, 1992).

Socioeconomic influences

Physical activity participation varies across social groups, as Figure 2.5 shows. There is an interesting link between gender and social class that warrants further investigation and may assist in targeting physical activity interventions.

The picture in Scotland is similar, with the proportion of sedentary adults (doing 30 minutes or less of physical activity on one day a week or not at all) in the lowest socioeconomic groups being double that among those from the highest socioeconomic groups (Scottish Executive, 2000).

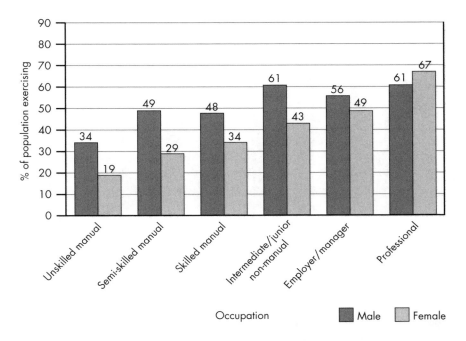

Figure 2.5 Participation rates in physical activity in the previous 4 weeks by socio-economic group. Source: Game Plan: A Strategy for Delivering Government's Sport and Physical Activity Objectives; published by the British Government Strategy Unit, 2002. Crown copyright material is reproduced with the permission of the Controller of HMSO.

Effect of ethnicity

For ethnic minority groups overall, the participation rate in physical activity is 40% compared with a national average of 46% (Sport England, 2000). This varies across both genders and there is significant variation between different ethnic groups (Figure 2.6).

Indian (31%), Pakistani (21%) and Bangladeshi (19%) women in particular have a lower involvement in sport than the UK national female average of 39%. These figures relate to sports participation and do not necessarily mean that physical activity levels per se are lower in these ethnic groups. In a survey in 1998 by the ONS, men from different ethnic minority groups were asked to record their activities. In the general population, 38% of men had participated in sports and exercise (excluding walking), at a moderate intensity level or above. The highest participation rate was for Black Caribbean men (47%), while the

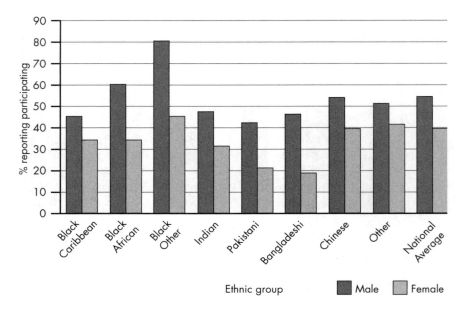

Figure 2.6 Participation in physical activity in ethnic minority groups compared to UK average. Source: Sport England (2000). Crown copyright material is reproduced with the permission of the Controller of HMSO.

lowest was for Bangladeshi men (24%) (Office for National Statistics, 1998).

This pattern is reflected in other countries where minority communities have been found to be less physically active. In a survey of 12 500 New Zealanders in 2002/3, self-reported levels of physical activity had increased by an overall 5%. However, there was a decrease in physical activity levels among Māori and Pacific communities (Sport and Recreation New Zealand, 2003).

Participation in people-specific clinical conditions

A national survey in 2000 by Sport England revealed lower levels of participation in sport among the young disabled compared with the rest of the population (Sport England, 2001). The most popular sports for the young disabled are horse riding and swimming, where participation levels are higher than in the overall population of younger people. However, these are sports that tend to organise events specifically for people with disabilities. Participation in other sports alongside the non-disabled is low.

Type 2 diabetics tend to be overweight and older, and in addition may have coronary heart disease, all risk factors for inactivity. It is also known that people with mental health problems exercise less than those without (Mutrie, 1999).

Obesity

People who are overweight are less likely to participate in physical activity. Dishman and others have established that the most consistent discriminator between adherers and drop-outs in exercise programmes is the percentage of body weight that is fat (Dishman, 1982). This may be because excess weight can cause discomfort and/or fatigue during exertion. Psychological factors also play a part, with overweight people being self-conscious and lacking confidence (Wilfley and Brownell, 1994).

Obesity occurs with a high prevalence in minority populations and in people with lower socioeconomic background. In addition there is an increase in obesity in older people, especially women (Wilfley and Brownell, 1994). Increasing physical activity participation in obese people is a particular challenge.

What motivates people to take up physical activity?

The ADNFS found four main motivating factors for both men and women to take exercise. These were:

- to feel in good shape physically
- to improve or maintain health
- to feel a sense of achievement
- to get outdoors.

An overwhelming majority of people surveyed believed that exercise is important to health. Generally, the benefits of exercise on mental health were less well recognised than the physical benefits of exercise. However in the HEA National Survey of Activity and Health, 'to feel mentally alert' was included as a potential motivating factor and actually scored highly (Health Education Authority, 1995a). If people recognise the benefits of physical activity in terms of health and their own personal beliefs, why is participation so low?

A clue comes from the ADNFS, which showed that the majority of people thought that most other people did not get enough exercise to keep them fit, while less than half thought this was applicable to themselves (Sports Council and Health Education Authority, 1992). Most people believed that they were keeping 'fairly' fit by being 'fairly' active. Generally people overestimated their activity levels, with 4 out of 5 men and women rating themselves as very or fairly fit.

Barriers to participation (the adoption problem)

The ADNFS showed that for people aged 16–69, the most commonly quoted barriers to participation in exercise were marriage, child care, domestic tasks, work pressure and lack of time. Motivational factors were also important: people said they felt they did not have the energy and needed to relax in their spare time. For women especially, emotional barriers were prominent. Reasons quoted included 'I'm not the sporty type', 'I'm too shy or embarrassed', or 'I might get injured'. In addition 18% of men and 15% of women quoted 'I have an injury or disability that stops me'. These barriers suggest that the sedentary population views physical activity, and in particular structured exercise, as requiring time and motivation. They also view participation in physical activity as a situation they will find uncomfortable and possibly dangerous (Sports Council and Health Education Authority, 1992).

Research into different types of exercise has shown specific barriers quoted for individual activities. For example concerns about road safety and air pollution were issues for those contemplating cycling (Bird *et al.*, 1998).

Some population groups may also describe specific barriers. For example, Sidney and Shepherd noticed the importance the elderly attached to programmes especially designed for seniors and accompanying safety instructions (Sidney and Shepherd, 1976). Their observation may be linked to people's age-related fear of injury while exercising (10% of men and women aged 25–44, but 15% of men and 21% of women over 65) (Shepherd, 1994).

The issue of time as the main barrier in most studies could be an area for further investigation. Perhaps people who exercise have more leisure time than those who are less active? Investigating barriers to exercise adoption may be a red herring, as people may simple assign a 'barrier' when they had no intention of taking up physical activity in the first place. However in some cases it could offer genuine insight for those working with sedentary populations. A better understanding may assist in overcoming barriers and make a particular activity more accessible.

Examples include traffic-free cycling areas, and exercise classes for people with a particular health problem, e.g. obesity.

Exercise adherence

Maintenance of exercise as a health behaviour

Exercise as a health behaviour needs to be adopted for as long as possible to achieve any benefits but it seems this is difficult to maintain. Research has shown that approximately 50% of individuals who join an exercise programme will drop out during the first 6 months (Dishman, 1982). In order to try to better understand the reasons for this, exercise psychology has borrowed theories of behaviour change from sociocognitive, behavioural and health psychology. These models have been adapted for exercise adoption, to try to give a better insight into what happens when a person is taking up physical activity. They may also help to target interventions to facilitate the process of adoption and ultimately a perpetuation of the health behaviour. However no one model explains, in full, physical activity or exercise behaviour.

Pharmacists are most likely to be familiar with the trans-theoretical model, which incorporates the cycle of change and is illustrated in Figure 2.7. The trans-theoretical model was developed to describe and understand the processes going on when a person gives up an addictive behaviour. It has been applied widely to smoking cessation. This model of change has also been studied as a method for better understanding the processes individuals go through when introducing physical activity to their lives (Reed, 1999). Similarities have been found between the cessation of risky behaviours such as addiction and acquisition of regular physical activity as a healthy behaviour, including rates of relapse. Interventions to increase adoption of physical activity based on the current predicted stages of change have shown the model to be applicable in some aspects (Marcus *et al.*, 1992). However differences do exist. People taking up exercise may be more unstable at each stage of change than those giving up addictive behaviours.

Most people who try to introduce a lifestyle change will need to experience relapse several times before moving to a more stable state where the healthy behaviour is more habitual. Prochaska and Marcus (1994) speculate that termination of risk behaviour may never be reached with many people taking up physical activity. Relapse is a potential for all but a few, because it is easier to move in and out of the adopted behaviour than it is when quitting a risk behaviour such as smoking. The

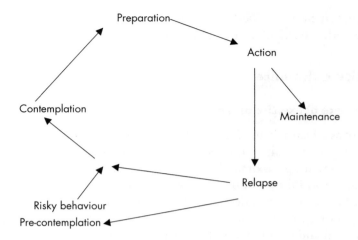

Figure 2.7 The cycle of change. Modified from Prochaska and DiClemente (1983).

role of injury might also play a part, where the most committed habitual exerciser has inactivity imposed because of injury. Likewise those who have an existing clinical condition may have enforced inactivity due to an exacerbation of, or treatment for, the original medical problem.

Risks associated with physical activity

Physical activity-related injury

Physical activity, even of a moderate nature, is not without risk of injury (see also Chapters 4 and 10). It is estimated that 10% of all accident and emergency admissions are sports-related (Kannus, 2000). This figure includes the most severe injuries only, usually as a result of vigorous exercise, and often involving contact sports such as rugby. A 1995 study estimated exercise-related morbidity in England and Wales to be in the order of 29 million incidents a year, resulting in new or recurrent injuries (Nicholl *et al.*, 1995). However this study only included people in the 16–45 age group. A survey conducted in England in 1991 found that a large proportion of injury incidents occurred in young men playing vigorous sports, and that most of these cases were new (as opposed to recurrent) injuries. Most injury incidents (70%) involve men, with almost half of these (48%) occurring in the 16–25 age group. Football was responsible for over a quarter (29%) of the incidents, and no other activity was involved in more than 10% of the incidents, although rugby accounts for by far the highest injury rate (participants sustain almost 100 injuries per 1000 occasions of participation) (Department for Culture, Media and Sport, 2002). In the Netherlands a survey in 1992/3 looked at absolute numbers of injuries (Van Sluijs et al., 2003). There were 2.9 million registered injuries in that time, of which 1.1 million required medical attention. The survey also looked at the number of injuries per 1000 hours, i.e. the injury incidence. Indoor football had the highest injury incidence, with karate, tae kwon do and outdoor football equal in second place. Accurate information regarding the extent of sports-related injury and ailment in the population as a whole is almost impossible to estimate because of the number of people who self-treat or seek alternative treatments.

Sudden cardiac arrest

Physical activity, particularly if vigorous in nature, brings with it an increased risk of sudden death or myocardial infarction (see Chapter 1). The absolute risk of death is low among otherwise healthy middle-aged and older adults. The risk has been estimated to be in the region of one cardiac arrest per 20 000–45 000 exercisers a year (Siscovick et al., 1984). Risk of sudden death during vigorous exercise is higher for those less accustomed to activity than those who exercise regularly (Van Sluijs et al., 2003).

Deaths have occurred in young athletes, and have understandably received much publicity. It is thought that in most of these cases the cause is a congenital heart problem that is allegedly asymptomatic. In people over 35, the most common cause of sudden death during exercise is thought to be coronary artery disease.

It appears that just as the health benefits from regular physical activity increase with an increased amount and intensity of activity, so do the health risks, whether these risks be trauma injury or cardiovascular in nature.

Minimising risks

Consideration of the intensity of exercise undertaken is an important factor in injury prevention. A 1998 study showed the rate of injury from walking, gardening, weightlifting, outdoor bicycling and aerobics to be small (Powell et al., 1998).

The relationship between age and injury rate in relation to physical activity is unresolved. Young to middle-aged persons have a reported injury rate of 10–50% in both novice and veteran exercisers (Pollock *et al.*, 1977; Macera *et al.*, 1989). However, comparison between two studies involving older exercisers showed an increased injury rate with increasing age. In addition there was a greatly increased injury rate (57%) in those older people taking part in a high-intensity, high-impact activity, compared with a much lower injury rate (14%) in a matched age group, taking part in a similar intensity activity but with a lower impact, i.e. jogging compared to walking (Pollock *et al.*, 1991; Carroll *et al.*, 1992).

A question remains as to whether all cases of sudden death from cardiovascular disease could be prevented if every athlete who competed was screened for cardiovascular disease. Certainly the majority of the cardiac conditions that predispose to sudden death during exercise would be detectable using endocardiography. However, this would not be economically viable, as a vast number of athletes would need to be screened in order to detect a small proportion of people at risk from sudden cardiac death. Screening for cardiovascular disease is warranted in athletes with a familial history of early (under 40 years) cardiac death. Likewise any athlete experiencing symptoms such as palpitations, chest pain, inappropriate breathlessness, dizziness or fainting should be examined by a cardiac specialist, although it should be noted that these predisposing cardiac conditions can be asymptomatic.

Recommendations for those involved in planning physical activity interventions to improve health are that the intensity of the exercise must be suitable for the target audience and that ideally this will be tailored to the particular circumstances of each individual.

What is being done to encourage sustained participation in physical activity?

Levels of intervention

King (1994) proposed that there are four levels of intervention that impact on physical activity uptake. These must all be addressed if a coherent and effective approach to increasing physical activity in populations is adopted:

Level 1   **Legislative/policy**
Example: An increase in the amount and type of compulsory exercise in schools, insurance incentives for those who exercise regularly.

Level 2   **Organisational/environmental**
Example: Safe cycling routes, buses to and from schools.

Level 3   **Inter-personal**
Example: Group classes, local walking schemes.

Level 4   **Individual**
Example: Advice and leaflets to patients/clients in primary care settings.

National policy

Making a positive change to the amount of physical activity taken by the population will have a dramatic influence on levels of disease and death. Getting the nation more active is not the job of one person, or even all healthcare professionals. Physical activity promotion and implementation must be led by a coordinated policy that starts with government strategy.

It is recognised that those working in primary care will only be able to make a difference to the physical activity levels of their local populations by working in partnership. Councils, schools, community youth and elders groups will all need to be explored as potential sites for physical activity provision and promotion.

Examples of UK national policies are given below:

England

Many government documents in recent years have highlighted the importance of physical activity in the management of the nation's health. The 2001 National Audit Office report on tackling obesity (National Audit Office, 2002) and *Game Plan: A Strategy for Delivering Government's Sport and Physical Activity Objectives* (Department for Culture, Media and Sport, 2002) both recommended the formation of a cross-government organisation to promote physical activity. The Department for Culture, Media and Sport (DCMS) and the Department of Health are jointly leading this team to develop a national delivery plan for physical activity and sport. The team is called the Activity Co-ordination Team (ACT). ACT's core target, set by *Game Plan*, is to increase participation in sport and physical activity to 70% of the population by 2020, particularly among:

- economically disadvantaged groups
- school leavers
- women
- older people.

The delivery plan intends to provide an evidence-based foundation for a long-term national physical activity and sport strategy for England. ACT aims to develop a joined-up approach to increase levels of participation in physical activity at regional and local level. This will involve incorporating strands from sport and leisure, education, the workplace, travel and the environment, as well as health care.

Local Exercise Action Pilots (LEAPs) have been set up in England to inform the work of ACT. There will be one pilot in each of the nine English regions to test different community approaches to increasing physical activity. These pilots will involve health services working with other organisations such as Sport England and the Countryside Agency, as well as local government departments.

For English health organisations the National Service Frameworks for coronary heart disease, mental health, older people and for diabetes all include recommendations about the important role played by physical activity, not just in the management of medical conditions but in their prevention (Department of Health 2000a, b; 2001a, b).

Scotland

The Scottish Executive Heath Department, through its Physical Activity Task Force, has set targets for 50% of the population aged 16 and over to take part in sport at least once a week by 2022 (Scottish Executive, 2003). Another target is that 80% of all people under 16 years of age will be meeting the minimum recommended levels of physical activity by 2022. The 'Let's Make Scotland more Active' campaign is targeting groups of the population identified as having low participation rates, in particular:

- parents of children under 5
- teenage girls
- men in their mid-years.

Wales

The National Assembly has emphasised the importance of physical activity in policy documents (Chief Medical Officer Wales, 2005). Physical activity is a key area in the framework document for coronary heart disease prevention and treatment.

A Healthy and Active Lifestyles Task Force was set up in November 1999, its role being to investigate ways of encouraging people in Wales to be more active and to prepare a strategy for action. The Task Force report was submitted to Ministers in 2001 and development of an implementation plan is under way.

Northern Ireland

March 1996 saw publication of 'Be active – be Healthy', the Northern Ireland physical activity strategy 1996–2002 (Health Promotion Agency for Northern Ireland, 2000). The strategy aims to increase the level of health-related activity particularly among those who exercise least. A Northern Ireland physical activity action plan was drawn up based on the strategy and proposed the development of a programme of public information to persuade the public of the benefits of physical activity. In 2001, the Health Promotion Agency for Northern Ireland, which was leading this work, joined forces with the Department of Health and Children in the Republic of Ireland to launch an all-island campaign to encourage the public to be more physically active. In the Republic of Ireland in 2003 a new Physical Activity Campaign 'Let it Go, Just for 30 Minutes' was launched. This campaign has been organised by the Health Promotion Unit and is aimed at the 50% of the population that does not engage in any form of regular physical activity.

Health promotion activity

Because of the multi-pronged approach needed to promote physical activity as a benefit to health, one, more or all of the following interventions may be used in a locality.

Interventions by healthcare professionals

General practitioners   There have been a few studies that have looked at the effect of doctors giving advice about exercise adoption (Eaton and Menard, 1999). The overall opinion is that doctors who have been specially trained in giving advice on physical activity give advice more often. However, this has not been directly shown to have any significant long-term effect on physical activity adoption in the patients given advice (Harland *et al.*, 1999). These studies do contribute the knowledge that the provision of written materials and/or following up patients after the initial advice can further increase activity levels (Taylor, 2003). Because long-term benefits are notoriously difficult to achieve in exercise adherence, some authorities view short-term adoption as a success (McMurdo, 1999; Riddoch, 1999).

A study that looked at barriers to physical activity promotion by GPs and nurses showed the main influence on a practitioner's promotion activities is their own participation in physical activity (McKenna *et al.*, 1998). GPs were three times more likely and nurses four times more likely to promote physical activity if they were in the action or maintenance stage of their own physical activity status.

Pharmacists   A joint project between Avon Health Authority and the Avon Health Promotion Unit in 1997 used community pharmacists to promote physical activity through everyday contact with patients (Oxford and Simmons, 1997). This resulted in greater awareness of recommendations surrounding physical activity amongst the pharmacists and an increased number of interactions with patients. There was no attempt to link these results with the amount of physical activity that the recipients of the information undertook.

Nurses   It has been suggested that nurses can make informed recommendations to patients about the ways in which appropriate exercise can bring health-related benefits (Rollo, 2004).

Exercise referral schemes

These schemes involve GPs or other healthcare professionals referring selected patients to a structured exercise programme. The patient is assessed by an exercise specialist who will decide on a planned programme for that individual. This may be a series of sessions at the leisure centre or may involve a local walking scheme. The benefit of exercise referral is that the GP can identify people who would normally not be participating in physical activity and so who are likely to obtain the most health benefit from exercise intervention. These schemes have been shown to result in sustainable improvements in physical activity levels and in health indicators and they are certainly popular with healthcare professionals and providers of leisure facilities (Biddle *et al.*, 1994; Riddoch *et al.*, 1998).

A National Quality Assurance Framework for exercise referral was published in the UK in 2001 (Department of Health, 2001c). A National Framework for Developing GP Exercise Referral in Ireland was developed during 2001/2 (Health Promotion Unit for the Republic of Ireland, 2002). Such structured frameworks may further increase the popularity of exercise referral, and also start to build a greater evidence base about its effectiveness. The current evidence base is scant because in the earlier schemes many GPs were not required to keep a record of their referrals. In addition, schemes were not standardised in any way.

Walking schemes

Walking is widely promoted, because it is considered to be an ideal activity – it is acceptable to the majority of people, it is accessible and low impact/low risk. Many health promotion agencies have incorporated walking schemes within their policy documents on physical activity (see end of chapter for details, and Chapter 10). In Scotland the former captain of the British Lions rugby team, Gavin Hastings, took part in a successful television advertising campaign to promote walking exercise. In some areas the walking schemes are linked to the exercise referrals programme.

It may be that a healthy transport policy for children would do much to encourage physical activity (Roberts, 1996). The journey to school accounts for 35% of all journeys made by children and has the potential to make an important contribution to levels of physical activity. However, since 1975, the average distance walked by schoolchildren has fallen by 27%, largely because of the increasing proportion of journeys to school made by car.

To date there is little evidence on the acceptability and effectiveness of walking schemes. The question has been raised as to whether these programmes will only work for people who are already active and/or gregarious. Proper evaluation of these schemes is needed.

Cardiac rehabilitation

The emphasis after myocardial infarction (MI) or other cardiac illness is for an early resumption of activity. Cardiac rehabilitation addresses the impact of major life-threatening illness and takes a holistic approach. In Britain, cardiac rehabilitation is routine following uncomplicated MI or coronary artery bypass graft surgery. Exercise can address issues of a physiological, psychological and social nature. It has been shown that physical activity as part of a rehabilitation programme will reduce the risk of death after heart attack (O'Connor *et al.*, 1989).

Exercise in pregnancy

A structured training programme for the pelvic floor muscles has been shown to be associated with fewer cases of active pushing in the second stage of labour lasting longer than 60 minutes (Salvesen and Mørkved, 2004). Training of the pelvic floor muscles has also been shown to be effective in the treatment of stress incontinence (Bø *et al.*, 1999).

Other health promotion initiatives

Other initiatives around the world include the Canadian SummerActive events, which provide opportunities for Canadians to walk, roll, run, swim, cycle, dance, jump and skate their way to better health. This campaign also includes initiatives on smoking cessation and healthy eating. The campaign mobilises schools, workplaces, sport or recreation clubs, health centres and other settings to create fun and stimulating environments for healthy living. More than 79 280 Albertans simultaneously walked one kilometre on 26 May 2005 to successfully set a new Guinness Book of World Records for walking. Over 300 walks were organised by Alberta schools, communities and workplaces. Together, they beat the previous world record of 77 500 walkers set by Japan in 2001. The Alberta Active Living Challenge Day is organised annually as part of its mission to encourage Albertans to be physically active and lead healthy lifestyles (Public Health Agency of Canada, 2005).

The WHO urges its members to celebrate a 'Move for Health' day each year to promote physical activity as an essential for health and well-being, and proposes that Member States celebrate the day on 10 May, although they do have the flexibility to choose the time and duration that best suits them for the event. The theme for 2005 was 'supportive environments' – physical-friendly environments that have been shown to encourage physical activity (World Health Organization, 2005).

The British government's policy statement on sport, 'Raising the Game', aimed to help schools to re-establish sport as "one of the great pillars of education", to achieve "the wider social and health benefits of sport", and to assist children to make "informed decisions about adopting healthy and active lifestyles" (Department of National Heritage, 1995). The policy statement proposed a minimum of 2 hours of sport and physical education a week for all children aged up to 16. In 2000, the School Sport Partnerships Programme was initiated to help promote the attainment of this target for 75% of children in England by 2006. Most schools are now committed to securing an entitlement of at least 2 hours per week of high-class physical education and sport within and beyond the curriculum for 5 to 16-year-olds and satisfactory progress is being made towards the target (Office for Standards in Education, 2004).

Conclusion

Currently in the UK the population is not active enough to maximise the health benefits on offer from regular physical activity. Developing initiatives to promote physical activity at all stages of life will be an investment for the future. Many other countries are starting to reap rewards from initiatives that have been running for a number of years. In these countries, much effort has focused on raising awareness of the benefits of physical activity and this is an important first stage before real improvements in participation can be expected. To be successful, any local initiatives must fit with national strategy and involve healthcare professionals working with other community partners. Although the importance of healthcare professionals in these partnerships is recognised, pharmacists are as yet under-used. However the recent focus on the treatment and prevention of obesity has already highlighted the significant role pharmacists have to play in delivering the public health agenda (Anon, 2004).

References

American College of Sports Medicine (1990). American College of Sports Medicine position stand: the recommended quantity and quality of exercise for developing and maintaining cardiorespiratory and muscular fitness in healthy adults. *Med Sci Sports Exerc* 22: 265–274.

Anon (2004) Obesity report prompts calls for greater pharmacy involvement. *Pharm J* 272: 695.

Australian Institute of Health and Welfare (2000). *Physical Activity Patterns of Australian Adults*. Results of the 1999 National Physical Activity Survey (available from: http://www.aihw.gov.au/publications/health/papaa/index.html). Canberra: AIHW.

Biddle S J H, Fox K R, Edmunds L (1994). *Physical Activity Promotion through Primary Health Care in England*. London: Health Education Authority.

Bird S R, Smith A, James K (1998). Adherence and compliance to exercise and rehabilitation programmes. In: Bird S R, Smith A, James K, eds. *Exercise Benefits and Prescription*. Cheltenham: Stanley Thornes, 63–87.

Blair S N, Kohl III H W, Paffenbarger R S, *et al.* (1989). Physical fitness and all-cause mortality. A prospective study of healthy men and women. *JAMA* 262: 2395–2401.

Bø K, Talseth T, Holme I (1999). Single blind, randomised controlled trial of pelvic floor muscle exercises, electrical stimulation, vaginal cones and no treatment in management of stress incontinence in women. *BMJ* 318: 487–493.

Boreham C, Riddoch C (2003). Physical activity and health through the lifespan. In: McKenna J, Riddoch C, eds. *Perspectives on Health and Exercise*. Basingstoke: Palgrave Macmillan, 11–30.

Carroll J F, Pollock M L, Graves J E, *et al.* (1992). Incidence of injury during moderate- and high-intensity walking training in the elderly. *J Gerontol A Biol Sci Med Sci* 47: M61–M66.

Caspersen C J, Powell K E, Christenson G M (1985). Physical activity, exercise and physical fitness: definitions and distinctions for health-related research. *Public Health Rep* 100: 126–131.

Chief Medical Officer Wales (2005). Health Promotion Division. http://www.cmo.wales.gov.uk/content/about-us/hpd-e.htm (accessed 12 August 2005).

Department for Culture, Media and Sport (2002). *Game Plan: A Strategy for Delivering Government's Sport and Physical Activity Objectives*. London: DCMS/Strategy Unit, Cabinet Office.

Department of Health (1993). *Better Living, Better Life*. London: Knowledge House.

Department of Health (2000a). National Service Framework for Coronary Heart Disease: Modern Standards and Service Models. London: DoH.

Department of Health (2000b). National Service Framework for Mental Health: Modern Standards and Service Models. London: DoH.

Department of Health (2001a). National Service Framework for Older People: Modern Standards and Service Models. London: DoH.

Department of Health (2001b). National Service Framework for Diabetes: Standards. London: DoH.

Department of Health (2001c). *Exercise Referral Systems: A National Quality Assurance Framework*. London: DoH.

Department of National Heritage (1995). *Sport: Raising the Game*. London: DNH.

Dishman R K (1982). Compliance/adherence in health-related exercise. *Health Psychol* 1: 237–267.

Eaton C B, Menard L M (1999). A systematic review of promotion of physical activity in primary care. In: MacAuley D, ed. (1999). *Benefits and Hazards of Exercise*. London: BMJ Books, 46–64.

Eriksson J G (1999). Exercise and the treatment of type 2 diabetes mellitus. An update. *Sports Med* 27: 381–391.

Fordham J (2000). Treatment of established osteoporosis. *Pharm J* 264: 593–596.

Hardman A (1991). *Exercise and the Heart. Report of a British Heart Foundation Working Group*. London: British Heart Foundation.

Hardman A E (1999). Intermittent exercise patterns. In: MacAuley D, ed. (1999). *Benefits and Hazards of Exercise*. London: BMJ Books, 322–337.

Harland J, White M, Drinkwater C, *et al.* (1999). The Newcastle exercise project: a randomised controlled trial of methods to promote physical activity in primary care. *BMJ* 319: 828–832.

Health Education Authority (1995a). *Physical Activity Matters*. London: HEA.

Health Education Authority (1995b). *Health Update: Physical Activity*. London: HEA.

Health Promotion Agency for Northern Ireland (2000). Get a life, get active. http://www.healthpromotionagency.org.uk/Work/Physicalactivity/campaigns1.htm (accessed 12 August 2005).

Health Promotion Unit for the Republic of Ireland (2002). National Frameworh for Developing GP Exercise Referral in Ireland.

Kannus P (2000). Nature, prevention and management of injury. In: Harries M, McLatchie G, Williams C, *et al.* (2000). *ABC of Sports Medicine*, 2nd edn. London: BMJ Books, 1–6.

King A C (1994). Clinical and community interventions to promote and support physical activity participation. In: Dishman R K, ed. *Advances in Exercise Adherence*. Champaign, IL: Human Kinetics, 183–212.

Macera C A, Pate R R, Powell K E, *et al.* (1989). Predicting lower extremity injuries among habitual runners. *Arch Intern Med* 149: 2565–2568.

McKenna J, Naylor P J, McDowell N (1998). Barriers to physical activity promotion by general practitioners and practice nurses. *Br J Sports Med* 32: 242–247.

McMurdo M (1999). Newcastle exercise project [electronic response]. 12 October. http://bmj.bmjjournals.com/cgi/eletters/319/7213/828

Marcus B H, Banspach S W, Lefebvre R C, *et al.* (1992). Using the stages of change model to increase the adoption of physical activity among community participants. *Am J Health Promot* 6: 424–429.

Must A, Jacques P F, Dallal G E, *et al.* (1992). Long term morbidity and mortality of overweight adolescents. *N Engl J Med* 327: 1350–1355.

Mutrie N (1999). Exercise adherence and clinical populations. In: Bull S, ed. *Adherence Issues in Sport and Exercise*. Chichester: John Wiley and Sons, Chapter 4.

National Audit Office (2002). *Tackling Obesity in England*. Report by the Comptroller and General Auditor. HC220. Session 20001–2001: 15 February 2001. Executive Summary. London: Stationery Office.

National Prescribing Centre (1998). *Management of Obesity*. Manchester: National Prescribing Centre and UK Drug Information Pharmacists Group.

Nicholl J P, Coleman P, Williams B T (1995). The epidemiology of sports and exercise related injury in the United Kingdom. *Br J Sports Med* 29: 232–238.

O'Connor G T, Buring J E, Yusef S, *et al.* (1989). An overview of randomised controlled trials of rehabilitation with exercise after myocardial infarction. *Circulation* 80: 234–244.

Office for National Statistics (1998). *Social Focus on Men* [Maximum intensity level attained in physical activity by men: by age, available from http://www.statistics.gov.uk/STATBASE/Product.asp?vlnk=7590&More=Y]. London: ONS.

Office for National Statistics (2000). *The UK 2000 Time Use Survey*. Participation in sport or physical activity: by age 2000–01. London: ONS.

Office for Standards in Education (2004). *The School Sport Partnerships Programme. Evaluation of Phases 3 and 4 (2003–4)*. London: OFSTED.

Oxford L, Simmonds G (1997). *Promoting Physical Activity from Community Pharmacies*. Bristol: Avon Health Authority and Health Promotion Service Avon.

Paffenbarger R S, Hyde R T, Wing A L, *et al.* (1986). Physical activity, all-cause mortality, and longevity of college alumni. *N Engl J Med* 314: 605–613.

Pate R R, Pratt M, Blair S N, *et al.* (1995). Physical activity and public health. A recommendation from the Centers for Disease Control and Prevention and the American College of Sports Medicine. *JAMA* 273: 402–407.

Pollock M L, Gettman L R, Milesis C A, *et al.* (1977). Effects of frequency and duration of training on attrition and incidence of injury. *Med Sci Sports Exerc* 9: 31–36.

Pollock M L, Carroll J F, Graves J E, *et al.* (1991). Injuries and adherence to walk/jog and resistance training programs in the elderly. *Med Sci Sports Exerc* 23: 1194–1200.

Powell K E, Heath G W, Kresnow M-J, *et al.* (1998). Injury rates from walking, gardening, weightlifting, outdoor bicycling and aerobics. *Med Sci Sports Exerc* 30: 1246–1249.

Prochaska J O, DiClemente C C (1983). The stages and processes of self-change in smoking: towards an integrative model of change. *J Consult Clin Psychol* 51: 390–395.

Prochaska J O, Marcus B (1994). The trans-theoretical model: application to exercise. In: Dishman R K, ed. *Advances in Exercise Adherence*. Champaign, IL: Human Kinetics, 161–181.

Public Health Agency of Canada (2005). SummerActive 2005 Success Stories. http://www.summeractive.canoe.ca/SummerActiveStories/letters.html (accessed 30 September 2005).

Reed G R (1999). Adherence to exercise and the trans-theoretical model of behaviour change. In: Bull S, ed. *Adherence Issues in Sport and Exercise*. Chichester: John Wiley and Sons, 19–45.

Riddoch C (1999). Conclusions drawn from the Newcastle project findings are misleading (electronic response]. 14 October. http://bmj.bmjjournals.com/cgi/eletters/319/7213/828

Riddoch C, Puig-Ribera A, Cooper A (1998). *Effectiveness of Physical Activity Promotion Schemes in Primary Care: A Review*. London: Heath Education Authority.

Roberts I (1996). Walking to school has future benefits [letter]. *BMJ* 312: 1229.

Rollo I (2004). Understanding the role of exercise in health promotion. *Nurs Times* 100: 36–38.

Salvesen K A, Mørkved S (2004). Randomised controlled trial of pelvic floor muscle training during pregnancy. *BMJ* 329: 378–380.

Scottish Executive (2000). The Scottish Health Survey 1998. Edinburgh Scottish Executive Department of Health. http://www.show.scot.nhs.uk/scottishhealth survey (accessed 20 June 2005).

Scottish Executive (2003). *Let's Make Scotland More Active: A Strategy for Physical Activity*. Edinburgh: SEHD Physical Activity Task Force. http://www.scotland.gov.uk/library5/culture/lmsa.pdf (accessed 20 June 2005).

Shephard R J (1994). Determinants of exercise in people aged 65 years and older. In: Dishman R K, ed. *Advances in Exercise Adherence*. Champaign, IL: Human Kinetics, 343–361.

Sidney K H, Shepherd R J (1976). Attitudes towards health and physical activity in the elderly: Effects of a physical training program. *Med Sci Sports* 8: 246–252.

Siscovick D S, Weiss N S, Fletcher R H, *et al.* (1984). The incidence of primary cardiac arrest during vigorous exercise. *N Engl J Med* 311: 874–877.

Sport and Recreation New Zealand (2003). SPARC Facts '97–'01. http://www.sparc.org.nz/research-policy/research-/sparc-facts-97-01 (accessed 12 August 2005).

Sport England (2000). *Sports Participation and Ethnicity in England. National Survey 1999/2000. Headline Findings.* London: Sport England.

Sport England (2001). *Disability Survey 2000 – Young People with a Disability and Sport: Headline Findings.* London: Sport England.

Sports Council and Health Education Authority (1992). *Allied Dunbar National Fitness Survey: Main Findings.* London: Sports Council/HEA.

Steptoe A (1992). Physical activity and psychological well-being. In: Norgan N G, ed. *Physical Activity and Health.* Cambridge: Cambridge University Press, 207–229.

Taylor A (2003). The role of primary care in promoting physical activity. In: McKenna J, Riddoch C, eds (2003). *Perspectives on Health and Exercise.* Basingstoke: Palgrave Macmillan, 153–180.

US Surgeon General (1997). *Physical Activity and Health.* Washington, DC: US Government.

Van Sluijs E M F, Verhagen E A L M, Van der Beek A J, *et al.* (2003). Risks of physical activity. In: McKenna J, Riddoch C, eds. *Perspectives on Health and Exercise.* Basingstoke: Palgrave Macmillan, 109–130.

Wilfley D E, Brownell K D (1994). Physical activity and diet in weight loss. In: Dishman R K, ed. *Advances in Exercise Adherence.* Champaign, IL: Human Kinetics, 361–393.

World Health Organization (2002). *Pan American Sanitary Bureau/Regional Office of the World Health Organization Physical Activity Sheet.* Geneva: WHO.

World Health Organization (2005). Move for Health Day. http://www.who.int/moveforhealth/about/en (accessed 12 August 2005).

Young A, Dinan S (2000). Active in later life. In: Harries M, McLatchie G, Williams C, *et al.*, eds. *ABC of Sports Medicine*, 2nd edn. London: BMJ Books, 51–56.

Further reading

Harries M, McLatchie G, Williams C, *et al.* (2000). *ABC of Sports Medicine*, 2nd edn. London: BMJ Books.

Blenkinsopp A, Panton R (1999). Physical activity. In: Anderson C, ed. *Health Promotion for Pharmacists*, 2nd edn. Oxford: Oxford University Press.

British Heart Foundation. Physical Activity and Your Heart. Health Information Series Number 1.

Blenkinsopp A, Anderson C (2000). Current thinking on: Exercise and physical activity. *Pharm Mag* CE1, July.

McKenna J, Riddoch C, eds (2003). *Perspectives on Health and Exercise.* Basingstoke: Palgrave Macmillan.

MacAuley D, ed. (1999). *Benefits and Hazards of Exercise.* London: BMJ Books.

Useful addresses

Sport England
3rd Floor Victoria House
Bloomsbury Square
London WC1B 4SE
Tel: +44 (0)8458 508 508
http://www.sportengland.org

sportscotland
Caledonia House
South Gyle
Edinburgh EH12 9DQ
Tel: +44 (0)131 317 7200
http://www.sportscotland.org.uk

Sports Council for Wales
Sophia Gardens
Cardiff CF11 9SW
Tel: +44 (0)29 2030 0500
http://www.sports-council-wales.co.uk

Irish Sports Council
Top Floor, Block A
Westend Office Park
Blanchardstown
Dublin 15
Ireland
Tel: +353 1 8608800
http://www.irishsportscouncil.ie

Sports Council for Northern Ireland
House of Sport
Upper Malone Road
Belfast BT9 5LA
Tel: +44 (0)28 9038 1222
http://www.sportni.org

British Heart Foundation (BHF)
14 Fitzhardinge Street
London W1H 6DH

Tel: +44 (0)20 7935 0185
http://www.bhf.org.uk

BHF National Centre for Physical Activity and Health
Loughborough University
Loughborough
Leicestershire LE11 3TU
Tel: +44 (0)1509 223259
http://www.bhfactive.org.uk

British Association of Sport and Exercise Science (BASES)
Chelsea Close
Off Amberley Road
Armley
Leeds LS12 4HP
Tel: +44 (0)113 289 1020
http://www.bases.org.uk

Countryside Agency Head Office
John Dower House
Crescent Place
Cheltenham
Gloucestershire GL50 3RA
Tel: +44 (0)1242 521381
E-mail: info@countryside.gov.uk

3

Sports nutrition

Pamela Mason

Introduction

The role of nutrition in sports is well accepted, and is now one of the most heavily researched areas of nutrition. In recent years, athletes and sports enthusiasts have benefited enormously from the advances made in sports nutrition and trainers increasingly recognise the role played by nutrition in sports performance. However, because interest among athletes in improving performance is understandably huge, research in this area may be misinterpreted, generating recommendations that are often incorrect, unsubstantiated or detrimental to health or sports performance.

In athletes, nutrition affects both health maintenance and sports performance, influencing the ability to train and recover from training, to compete and maximise performance. The main dietary principles in sport are based on the principles of healthy eating, but some aspects require particular emphasis:

- Energy intake – with an appropriate balance of carbohydrate, protein and fat.
- Fluid intake – with consideration given to both the quantity and type of fluid.
- Timing of food and fluid consumption – with appropriate gaps (neither too long nor too short) between food and fluid consumption and sporting activity.

Sources of energy

The main sources of energy are carbohydrate 16.8 kJ/g (4 kcal/g), fat 37.8 kJ/g (9 kcal/g) and protein 16.8 kJ/g (4 kcal/g). Alcohol also supplies energy 29.4 kJ/g (7 kcal/g). The two main fuels for physical activity are carbohydrate and fat, although protein can also be used if necessary.

Energy is stored in the body as:

- Glycogen – this is derived from dietary carbohydrate and stored in the muscle (up to a maximum of approximately 600 g) and in the liver (approximately 100 g).
- Fat – this is stored mainly in the form of triglyceride in the adipose tissue.
- Creatine phosphate – in the muscle.

The biochemical pathways associated with energy storage and utilisation are summarised in Chapter 1.

Energy requirements

Energy requirements are primarily determined by energy expenditure, which comprises:

- Basal metabolic rate (BMR) – the amount of energy expended by the body to maintain basic physiological functions over a period of 24 hours and constitutes 60–75% of energy expenditure. BMR, which can be calculated from the equations in Table 3.1, is principally determined by:
  — Body weight. Larger people have a higher BMR than smaller ones. Adipose tissue has a lower BMR than lean tissue, but the energy cost of moving an overweight or obese person tends to counteract the lower BMR of body fat.
  — Gender. Men tend to have a greater body mass than women, so have a higher BMR.
  — Age. Children have a higher BMR per unit surface area than adults.
  — Miscellaneous factors, such as pregnancy, anxiety and disease (e.g. fever, sepsis, tissue injury, hyperthyroidism, diarrhoea, impaired absorption) may increase BMR, while hypothyroidism or undernutrition results in a fall in BMR.

Table 3.1 Calculation for basal metabolic rate (BMR)

Age (years)	Men BMR (kcal/day)	Women BMR (kcal/day)
10–18	17.5 × weight (kg) + 651	12.2 × weight (kg) + 746
18–30	15.3 × weight (kg) + 679	14.7 × weight (kg) + 496
30–60	11.6 × weight (kg) + 879	8.7 × weight (kg) + 829
> 60	13.5 × weight (kg) + 487	10.5 × weight (kg) + 596

- Physical activity. This can account for 20–40% of daily energy expenditure and up to 75% during intense training of long duration. Energy requirements can therefore vary from 7.56 MJ (1800 kcal)/day for young female gymnasts to 25.2 MJ (6000 kcal)/day for marathon runners.
- Dietary-induced thermogenesis. This is the rise in metabolic rate (and hence heat production) that occurs following food consumption and accounts for about 5–10% of energy expenditure over a period of 24 hours.

Energy metabolism during physical activity

Sporting activity depends on the availability of both glycogen and fat and the proportions used depend on the intensity and duration of the activity (see Chapter 1).

During intense physical activity, when the body needs energy quickly, glycogen is the main energy source. However, stores of glycogen are not large compared with needs, being sufficient to run for about 32 km (20 miles). When glycogen stores become depleted, glucose can be obtained from glycerol and amino acids.

During prolonged sporting activity, the body has to use fat in addition to glycogen. Stores of fat are far greater than those of glycogen, even in lean athletes, and the potential energy yield from fatty acid oxidation is enormous. Training enhances the ability of the muscles to produce a greater proportion of energy from free fatty acids, while sparing the limited glycogen stores. However, the rate of ATP production from fat is relatively slow compared with that from glycogen, making fat a less readily available source of energy.

Carbohydrate requirements during exercise

During any physical activity, the aim is to conserve glycogen, and the intake of dietary carbohydrate must be sufficient to maximise glycogen levels during training and competition (see also Chapter 1). Every time an athlete trains, the amount of glycogen within the working muscles falls. Muscle glycogen becomes depleted after 2–3 hours of continuous endurance exercise, such as marathon running or cycling, but can also be severely depleted after periods of 15–30 minutes of higher intensity exercise.

Glycogen reserves must be completely restocked before the next training session. After physical activity, glycogen is restored to the muscle at a rate of about 5–7% per hour and after prolonged exercise, it can take up to 20 hours to fully replenish glycogen stores. If complete refuelling is not achieved between training sessions, and this is repeated over successive days of training, glycogen will become progressively depleted, leading to difficulty in participating in physical activity, with continual lethargy and tired, heavy muscles.

Carbohydrate is therefore the most important fuel for sporting activity and performance. This applies not only to athletics and endurance sports but also to those taking part in team sports, such as football, hockey and tennis. Current healthy eating guidelines recommend that carbohydrate should provide approximately 50–55% of dietary energy, with an emphasis on starchy, complex carbohydrates rather than sugary foods. The optimum diet for most sports is likely to provide higher quantities of carbohydrate (i.e. 70% of total energy requirements).

In quantitative terms this approximates to an intake of 500–600 g of carbohydrate each day. However, carbohydrate requirements can also be estimated according to the weight of the individual. Athletes training regularly usually require a daily intake of 6–10 g/kg body weight, depending on the type, length and intensity of training. Such levels should be sufficient to replenish and maintain glycogen stores of athletes.

Both starchy and sugary carbohydrates seem to be equally effective for glycogen refuelling. A diet providing 70% of total energy as starchy carbohydrates will prove to be too physically bulky for many athletes, so the use of more sugary carbohydrates may therefore be necessary, especially for those with high energy requirements. As this advice is contrary to current healthy eating guidelines, pharmacists may need to explain the reasons for it, emphasising the importance of all carbohydrate in the diet.

An athlete's lifestyle may make it difficult to consume the required amount of carbohydrate. For example, training straight after work may leave little time for buying, cooking and eating food. Ease and speed of food preparation are important but the athlete should be discouraged from eating excessive quantities of fast food and takeaways. Bread, baked potatoes, pasta, rice and breakfast cereals are healthier choices.

The timing of carbohydrate intake can be crucial, and it is vital that the athlete begins a training session, game or competition with adequate glycogen stores. The recommended method of achieving this, particularly before a competition, is to increase carbohydrate intake over the 3–5 days before the event and to taper training. This method has reduced the traditional 'carbohydrate loading' method popular during the 1970s.

Increasing glycogen stores by increasing carbohydrate in the days before the event benefits all sports people, including athletes, distance cyclists, marathon runners, football players and those taking part in tournaments lasting several days (e.g. tennis tournaments). However, glycogen is stored in association with water, thereby increasing body weight. This may be a disadvantage where an athlete competes in a weight-category sport such as boxing or judo.

Carbohydrate may be consumed before, during and after the competition as follows.

Before competition

For optimum performance it has been suggested that approximately 200–300 g of carbohydrate should be consumed during the 4 hours before a competition. Consumption of carbohydrate immediately before the event (i.e. during the last hour) can be considered. There seems to be little support now for the traditional idea that sugary foods and drinks consumed immediately before exercise can induce hypoglycaemia and impair performance.

In addition to being high in carbohydrate, pre-competition foods and drinks should be low in fat, without large quantities of fibre; they should contain some (but not excessive) protein and be readily digestible.

During competition

Consumption of carbohydrate during competitions of long duration or between bouts of intermittent competition enhances performance. Although ingestion of carbohydrate can be difficult during a competition, athletes should make every effort to do so where the type of activity allows. Drinks containing carbohydrate can fulfil the twin objectives of maintaining hydration and topping up glycogen levels and are quick and easy to consume. Solid food can also be consumed if desired – like pre-competition food, this should be high in carbohydrate and low in fat.

After competition

Refuelling of the carbohydrate stores should begin as soon as possible after the competition. Around 50 g of carbohydrate (or 0.7–1.0 g/kg body weight) may be consumed within the first 2-hour period and repeated every 2 hours (Table 3.2 lists foods that contain 50 g of

Table 3.2 Foods containing 50 g carbohydrate

3–4 slices of bread	8 tablespoons cooked pasta
1 bagel	4 tablespoons cooked rice
2–3 slices malt loaf	1 medium jacket potato
1 large bowl breakfast cereal	5 small boiled potatoes
2–3 cereal bars	7 heaped tablespoons mashed potato
2 currant buns	400 g tin baked beans or spaghetti
6 Jaffa cakes	1 litre milk
2 bananas	425 g tin rice pudding
3–4 medium apples, oranges or pears	800 mL isotonic sports drink
15 dried apricots	50 g sugar or glucose
2 tablespoons dried fruit (e.g. raisins)	330 mL bottle fruit smoothie
500 mL fruit juice	

carbohydrate). However, many athletes find it difficult to consume solid food immediately after exercise, and drinks containing carbohydrate (e.g. glucose, sucrose, fructose or maltodextrin) in concentrations of 6 g/100 mL or higher are usually more acceptable (see p. 55). Repeating the 50 g amount every 2 hours can also be difficult as such frequent consumption of meals is not always practical. Meals and snacks should therefore provide sufficient carbohydrate to cover the time to the next meal. Thus, if a further meal is planned in 4 hours' time, 100 g of carbohydrate may be consumed for optimum performance.

Glycaemic index

Athletes must include carbohydrates to provide prolonged energy for sports performance and optimal recovery, and during recent years the type of carbohydrate has become an area of increasing focus in sports nutrition. According to traditional thinking, simple carbohydrates, such as those found in high-sugar foods and fruit, trigger a rapid and large rise in blood glucose levels, followed by a rapid and often greater fall. In contrast, complex carbohydrates, such as bread, pasta and starchy vegetables, were thought to induce a more sustained blood glucose response.

However, this classification does not reflect the diversity in glucose response to carbohydrate. For example, many fruits provide a more sustained glucose response than some types of pasta. Over the last 20 years, the glycaemic index (GI) has emerged as a tool to rank carbohydrate-containing foods based on their glucose response following consumption. Table 3.3 lists the GI of some common carbohydrate-containing foods, and the number assigned to each food represents the

Table 3.3 Glycaemic index of some common foods

Food	GI
White bread, wholemeal bread	100
Mashed potatoes	100
Shredded Wheat	99
Muesli	90
Sucrose	87
Porridge oats	87
Chocolate	84
Banana	83
White rice	81
Boiled potatoes	80
Orange juice	80
Brown rice	79
Crisps	77
Peas	71
Baked beans	69
All Bran	65
Spaghetti	59
Orange	55
Apple	52
Lentils, chick peas, kidney beans	50
Milk	50
Peanuts	21

speed at which the food is digested and subsequently absorbed, with higher numbers reflecting faster introduction of glucose into the bloodstream.

Debate remains as to the appropriate use of the GI before, during and after sport, but foods with a high GI are generally thought to be beneficial during the post-exercise period. The issue is complicated by the fact that foods are usually eaten in combinations and the GI of a meal is usually lower than that of the food with the highest GI. The presence of protein in a meal slows the absorption rate of carbohydrates, so blunting the glucose response. Although GI is emerging as a tool to guide selection of carbohydrates, particularly in diabetes and weight loss, its value in sports nutrition is not yet proven.

Fluid

During exercise, the rate of heat production and sweating increases. Sweat contains fluid and electrolytes, so when sweating is prolonged, the body loses both. When losses exceed replacement, the circulatory system is unable to cope, and skin blood flow falls, with the result that sweating and the ability to lose heat are reduced. Body temperature can rise, with possibly fatal consequences.

Athletes should therefore take care to ensure adequate hydration before, during and after exercise. This applies to periods of training and competition and to those exercising indoors. The fluid consumed should contain sodium, as this helps the absorption of water and thus the process of rehydration. In addition, sodium prevents the drop in plasma sodium and osmolality that would occur with the consumption of plain water.

Athletes should be encouraged to use a sports bottle and to use training sessions to grow used to drinking sufficient fluid. At one time, cold drinks were believed to more efficient at rehydration on the basis that they left the stomach more rapidly than warm drinks. However, recent research has cast doubt on this idea and the athlete's preference is the best guide. Above all, the drink must be palatable, otherwise the athlete will not consume it.

Before exercise

Athletes should be fully hydrated before taking any exercise. This can be achieved by:

- Drinking about 500 mL of fluid during the last 10–30 minutes before competition. Consuming fluid earlier than this will cause inconvenience because of the need to pass urine.
- Ensuring that fluid intake is high during the days leading up to the competition as well as on the day of the competition.
  Avoiding large amounts of alcohol the night before a competition.
- Monitoring fluid status by checking the colour of the urine (it should be the colour of pale straw).

During exercise

During exercise, hydration can be maintained by:

- Drinking at an early stage, before thirst is experienced.
- Drinking small amounts of fluid frequently (e.g. 150 mL every 15 minutes, stomach capacity permitting).

After exercise

After exercise, rehydration should be started immediately. Fluid intake should exceed loss by about 50% because fluid loss continues during recovery.

Sports drinks

There are several commercial sports drinks available to athletes (see Chapter 10 for information on the formulation and choice of sport and energy drinks). These can be divided into two main categories:

*   Fluid replacement drinks. These contain 10–25 mmol/L of sodium and sugars (e.g. glucose, sucrose, fructose and maltodextrins). The main function of these drinks is to replace fluid (which they achieve more rapidly than plain water), although the added sugars help to maintain blood glucose levels and spare glycogen.
*   Carbohydrate (energy) drinks. These provide more carbohydrate per 100 mL than fluid replacement drinks (and they provide fluid as well). Carbohydrate is in the form of maltodextrins, which are able to provide larger amounts of carbohydrate at an equal or lower osmolality than the same concentration of glucose.

There are three main types of sports drinks:

*   Isotonic. These usually contain carbohydrate at a level of 4–8 g/100 mL. This is sufficient to provide a small amount of carbohydrate as energy during sport, but not an excessive amount, which would impair absorption of fluid.
*   Hypotonic. These typically contain < 4 g carbohydrate/100 mL. They help fluid replacement, especially if sodium is present, but will not make any major contribution to carbohydrate intake.
*   Hypertonic. These contain > 10 g carbohydrate/100 g. They impair fluid absorption and are not generally to be recommended during sport because they can exacerbate dehydration.

Protein

Many athletes believe that consumption of large amounts of protein is required to build muscle, increase strength and enhance performance. Intensive training results in deposition of protein in the muscle, which leads to an increased requirement for protein. There is no consensus on recommendations for protein requirements for athletes, but current evidence suggests that endurance athletes require 1.2–1.4 g protein/kg body weight per day, while strength or speed athletes may require 1.7 g protein/kg body weight per day. However, unless energy intake is insufficient to meet requirements, such quantities of protein can usually be obtained from the diet (see Chapter 10 for product information).

Athletes at the higher end of the energy spectrum will find it easy to meet these requirements, while those at the lower end of the energy intake range may require guidance. For example, a strength athlete weighing 80 kg may need around 140 g of protein a day. This may be difficult to obtain from food alone if energy intake is low or the athlete is a vegetarian. (Typical daily intakes of protein in UK adults are around 85 g in men and 62 g in women.) In such cases, a protein supplement may be useful to make up a shortfall in the diet, although it is not a substitute for a poorly planned diet.

Vitamins and minerals

Athletes consuming high-energy healthy diets should be obtaining all the vitamins and minerals they require. However, some athletes have poor eating habits, including foods of low nutrient density in order to achieve their carbohydrate and energy requirements without making too much effort to choose and prepare healthier food. Such individuals may benefit from a multivitamin and mineral preparation containing around 100% of the recommended daily allowance (RDA) of a wide variety of vitamins and minerals.

Iron and calcium deserve particular mention. Some athletes, particularly women, are at risk of poor iron status because of low intakes, heavy menstrual periods or because dietary iron is predominantly in the form of non-haem iron. Iron supplementation may be recommended. Female athletes with amenorrhoea or dysmenorrhoea have an increased risk of developing osteoporosis because of reduced levels of oestrogen. Calcium is particularly important in athletes with low bone density, low calcium intakes and menstrual irregularities because stress fractures are common in this group of individuals.

Weight control

Weight management is important for many athletes, especially for some sports where a specific body image is required (e.g. female gymnastics, bodybuilding, dancing) or where a sport requires the athlete to compete in a weight category (e.g. judo, boxing, lightweight rowing, wrestling). Athletes sometimes resort to rapid weight loss methods such as fasting, dehydration, exercising in sweat suits, saunas, self-induced vomiting, diuretics, laxatives or 'slimming pills', and weight losses of 4.5 kg in 3 days are not uncommon.

However, such practices will lead to diminished glycogen reserves, which will more than offset any advantages of competing in a lower weight category. Athletes, particularly women, competing in weight category sports or sports where body image is important may develop eating disorders. Menstrual dysfunction, decreased bone density and iron-deficiency anaemia are also risks.

Weight loss should be carefully planned and the diet should provide sufficient carbohydrate to restock and maintain the glycogen stores. Body fat should be lost without lean tissue being affected. The diet should therefore be low in fat, but high in carbohydrate, and should provide all the essential nutrients in an energy intake that will achieve weight loss.

Athletes who need to gain weight will want to increase muscle rather than body fat. This can best be achieved by regular training. Training is best supported by consuming a diet with a high enough pro-portion of carbohydrate to maximise glycogen stores.

Sports supplements

There is a huge variety of sports supplements on the market (see Chapter 10). Examples of the supplements offered for sale in an American store (some of which are available in the UK) are shown in Figures 3.1 and 3.2. Products are available through the Internet as well as from mail order companies, health food stores and sports shops. Many of the supplements are known as ergogenic aids, i.e. substances that supposedly raise athletic performance above what would normally be expected.

Many athletes believe that these products are essential for sports success and providing a competitive edge. However, the most effective way to achieve fitness and performance goals is through efficient training and optimal nutrition, and there is a lack of scientific evidence to support the performance-enhancing claims for many sports supple-ments.

There is no guarantee that supplements, including vitamins and minerals, ergogenic aids and herbal remedies, are free from banned substances (see also Chapter 6). Athletes should therefore be advised to

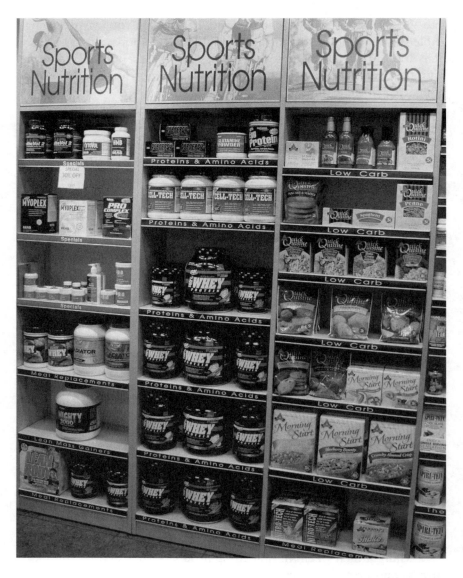

Figure 3.1 Examples of sports nutrition products on sale in a New Orleans health store (2004).

be extremely cautious about the use of any supplements and should consult a qualified accredited sports dietitian or sports doctor before taking them. Supplements are taken at the athlete's own risk and are their personal responsibility. Further guidance on the use of nutritional

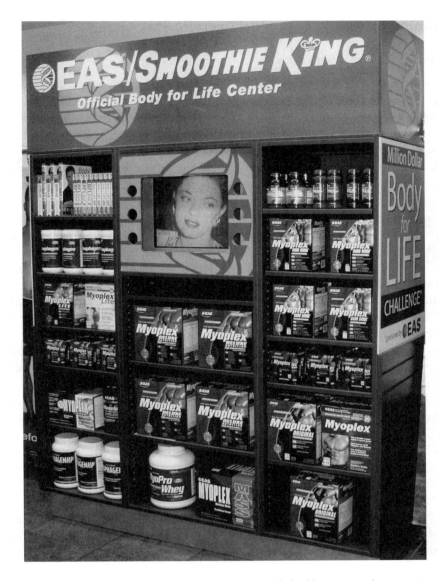

Figure 3.2 Examples of supplements used in body-building, on sale in a New Orleans health store (2004).

supplements may be found on the UK Sport website (http://www. uksport.gov.uk).

Some of the most popular supplements are discussed in the following sections.

Amino acids and amino acid derivatives

Branched-chain amino acids

Branched-chain amino acids (BCAAs) are a group of essential amino acids (isoleucine, leucine, valine) that have been studied for their potential role in delaying central nervous system (CNS) fatigue, particularly in athletes. When ingested, BCAAs are not readily degraded by the liver but instead circulate and compete for uptake into the brain with the amino acid, tryptophan. Tryptophan is a precursor to serotonin (5-hydroxytryptamine), which may depress the CNS and produce symptoms of fatigue. Research has shown that exercise increases the ratio of free tryptophan to BCAA, thus raising serotonin levels in the brain. There is also evidence that plasma BCAA levels decrease during exercise.

It has been suggested that supplementing BCAAs will lower this ratio and result in improved mental and physical performance, although the evidence to date is inconclusive. Many field studies that have shown that BCAA administration enhances performance have been criticised on methodological grounds, including failure to control variables such as dietary intake and exercise intensity, lack of matched controls and subject bias (Davis, 1995). Moreover, controlled laboratory studies have not demonstrated any positive performance effect with BCAA supplementation (Van Hall *et al.*, 1995; Madsen *et al.*, 1996) although some have shown improved mental performance (Bloomstrand *et al.*, 1991). Research investigating the effect of BCAA supplementation on body composition and the muscle breakdown that occurs with exercise suggest that BCAAs may be beneficial (Mourier *et al.*, 1997), although studies to date have generally involved only small numbers of subjects.

BCAA supplements are available in tablet and powder forms, ranging from 7 to 20 g per serving. Some sports beverages also contain amounts ranging from 1 to 7 g/L.

No long-term studies have assessed the safety of BCAA supplementation. However, large doses of BCAAs (> 20 g) may impair water absorption across the gastrointestinal tract and cause abdominal discomfort and at these doses may also increase plasma ammonia to toxic levels. Acute ammonia toxicity is reversible, but during the time it exists, it may be serious enough to impair performance or induce central fatigue.

Carnitine (L-carnitine)

Carnitine (L-carnitine) is a short-chain carboxylic acid, synthesised in the body from the amino acids lysine and methionine. It is also obtained from the diet and is found in protein-containing foods such as meat, poultry, fish and dairy produce. It plays a central role in fatty acid metabolism by transporting long-chain fatty acids into the mitochondria for beta-oxidation. Approximately 95% of the body's carnitine is located in skeletal and cardiac muscle.

Supplemental carnitine can increase muscle carnitine content, which gave rise to the idea that it could enhance sports performance. There is some scientific basis for this in that increased carnitine intake may increase fatty acid oxidation, thus sparing glycogen and glucose. Carnitine may also enhance conversion of pyruvate to acetyl CoA, which would decrease lactic acid production and improve exercise performance. However, the few controlled trials conducted so far have provided no scientific evidence that carnitine supplements enhance physical performance in athletes (Heinonen, 1996).

Carnitine is available in the form of tablets and capsules and at doses ranging from 0.5 to 6 g/day, no serious adverse effects have been noted. However, doses exceeding 6 g daily have been associated with nausea and diarrhoea. Athletes should be warned not to use the D or D,L forms of carnitine as they are associated with impaired exercise performance.

Creatine

Creatine supplements increase the storage of creatine phosphate, potentially making more ATP available to the working muscles and enabling them to work harder before becoming fatigued (see Chapter 1). However, evidence for benefit of creatine supplementation in sports performance is slight and appears to be limited to highly specific forms of exercise.

Several small double-blind studies have found that creatine can enhance performance in sports that involve repeated short bursts of high-intensity activity (e.g. swimming, cycling, football) and resistance training (Volek *et al.*, 1997; Williams and Branch, 1998; Leenders *et al.*, 1999; Mujika *et al.*, 2000; Finn *et al.*, 2001). However, studies of endurance (e.g. marathon running) (Balsom *et al.*, 1993) or non-repetitive aerobic exercise (e.g. single sprints) (Mujika *et al.*, 1996) have not found benefits with creatine supplementation.

Creatine is available mainly in the form of powder (see Chapter 10). The usual dose regimen employed in studies is 5 g creatine monohydrate four times daily as a loading dose, then 2–5 g daily as maintenance for no longer than 30 days. These doses should not be exceeded because of the risk of adverse effects. Reported side-effects of excessive doses have included diarrhoea, vomiting, seizure, myopathy, atrial fibrillation, cardiac arrhythmias, shortness of breath, deterioration in renal function and deep-vein thromboses.

Creatine supplementation often causes weight gain, but whether this is due to increased muscle mass is debatable. Increased intracellular creatine may cause an osmotic influx of water into the cell because creatine is an osmotically active substance. It is therefore possible that the weight gained is a result of water retention, and not of increased muscle.

Beta-hydroxymethylbutyric acid

Beta-hydroxymethylbutryic acid (HMB) is a metabolite of the branched-chain amino acid leucine. Leucine is found in particularly high concentrations in muscles and during physical activity, and muscle damage can lead to breakdown of leucine and high HMB levels. There is some evidence to suggest that taking HMB reduces the destruction of muscle tissue (Slater and Jenkins, 2000).

HMB has therefore been investigated as a supplement for enhancing strength and muscle in athletes and, in doses of 3 g daily, it has been shown to increase muscle growth response to weight training and also strength (Nissen *et al.*, 1996; Panton *et al.*, 2000; Slater and Jenkins 2000). There is also preliminary evidence to suggest that HMB may protect muscles from exercise-induced damage. However, all the studies conducted so far have been small, and larger well controlled studies will be required to confirm whether HMB can enhance muscle mass and strength in adults.

Glutamine

Glutamine is a non-essential amino acid and is the most abundant free amino acid in skeletal muscle and plasma. It is found in protein-rich foods and is also synthesised in the body from glutamic acid. Its main function is as a fuel source for the gut mucosal cells, renal tubular cells, lymphocytes, macrophages and endothelial cells. Strenuous exercise is associated with reduced plasma glutamine levels and impaired immune function. In these circumstances, requirements appear to exceed supply, and glutamine is therefore considered by some researchers to be conditionally essential.

Studies investigating the role of glutamine supplements on immunity after intense activity have yielded inconsistent results, but as they have used only small numbers of subjects they are difficult to interpret. Data summarised from eight double-blind, placebo-controlled studies of 151 athletes indicate that glutamine supplementation after endurance exercise may reduce the incidence of self-reported infection (Castell and Newsholme, 1997), but laboratory studies have not shown improvements in immune parameters with glutamine ingestion. There is some evidence that adequate carbohydrate consumption (which is vital for replenishing glycogen stores) helps to reduce the decrease in plasma glutamine.

Other amino acids

A number of other amino acids and amino acid derivatives are used by athletes, sometimes individually and sometimes in combination. These include alanine, arginine, aspartic acid, N-acetylcysteine, and also ornithine alpha ketoglutarate (OKG), which is ornithine and glutamine combined.

Alanine is a glucogenic amino acid and it has been suggested that it could spare muscle. Plasma levels of alanine increase during exercise, but there is currently no evidence that supplemental alanine spares muscle during exercise or enhances exercise performance.

Aspartic acid is also a glucogenic amino acid, which is involved in urea synthesis. The hypothesis that aspartic acid could enhance athletic performance was developed because this amino acid spares glycogen by increasing the availability of free fatty acids for fuel and potentially reduces exercise fatigue by clearing excess ammonia from the blood through urea synthesis. However, the ergogenic effects of aspartate salts are debatable. Trials to date have involved small numbers of subjects and suffered from methodological problems such as failure to evaluate serum aspartate levels. Until larger controlled trials are conducted, supplementation is not warranted.

N-acetylcysteine (NAC) is a derivative of the sulphur-containing amino acid cysteine. First introduced as a mucolytic drug in the 1960s, NAC has been shown more recently to have antioxidant activity *in vitro*. It has therefore been investigated for its potential to reduce oxidative stress and muscle fatigue and to enhance immunity in athletes. However, the few trials conducted so far have been small in size and have provided conflicting data.

Evidence for benefit of arginine and OKG is similarly sparse and the few clinical trials performed have not shown positive results.

Protein supplements

Although adequate protein can be obtained from a well-planned diet, protein supplements may be beneficial in athletes with particularly high protein requirements (e.g. strength and power athletes) or those with low energy intakes. Protein supplements (which should be distinguished from amino acid supplements) contain whey, casein, soya, egg or a mixture of these proteins.

Whey protein has a high biological value – higher than any protein-containing food. This means that a high percentage of the amino acids are utilised for tissue growth. In addition, it is easily digested, resulting in a rapid increase in blood levels of amino acids. Casein also has a high biological value, although not as high as whey, and it is absorbed more slowly, thereby helping to maintain high levels of plasma amino acids over a prolonged period. For athletes trying to maximise protein accretion, it may be best to take a whey-based protein immediately after training to achieve a rapid uptake of protein and a casein-based protein at night or at times when there may be a gap of several hours before the next meal (see Chapter 10).

Antioxidants

Physical activity increases free radical production, and maintaining or enhancing the body's antioxidant status may help to prevent tissue damage from free radical attack. Whether athletes benefit from antioxidant supplements is unclear. Studies using antioxidant supplements have produced conflicting results. Mixtures of antioxidants (e.g. vitamin C, vitamin E, flavonoids and carotenoids) may provide better protection than single nutrients, but antioxidants are best obtained from food, of which fruit and vegetables are the most concentrated sources.

Boron

Boron has been proposed as a sports supplement because it is thought to increase testosterone levels. However, research to date has provided

no significant evidence that boron supplementation influences testosterone levels, lean body mass or strength in bodybuilders.

Chromium

Athletes may require additional chromium in their diets because of
increased losses from exercise, but there is currently no evidence that
supplements are anabolic or have other benefits for healthy athletes. Two
well-controlled studies found no benefits of chromium supplementation
(around 200 micrograms daily) on strength or body composition in
sports performers (Clancy *et al.*, 1994; Hallmark *et al.*, 1996). However,
one double-blind, placebo-controlled study in weight trainers showed
that supplementation resulted in a statistically significant increase in
body weight in female weightlifters, but resulted in no change in male
weightlifters (Hasten *et al.*, 1992).

Chromium is an essential nutrient, but the long-term effects of
increased intakes are not known. There is particular concern in relation
to chromium picolinate, which may have the potential to cause cancer,
and is commonly found in sports supplements. In 2003, the UK Food
Standards Agency's Expert Vitamin and Mineral (EVM) report advised
that chromium should not be taken in this form, but that having 10 mg
a day or less in total of chromium in other forms is unlikely to cause
harm.

Colostrum

Colostrum is the first milk produced by all mammals, and has long been
regarded as the most beneficial, immune-boosting nutrition for
newborns. Dairy colostrum has attracted the attention of international
sports scientists for its powerful effect on fitness levels and was one of
the favoured food supplements taken by the Australian Olympic
swimming team at the Athens 2004 games.

It has been suggested that a daily supplement of colostrum can
increase strength and stamina by up to 20%, as well as improving
endurance, exercise performance and increasing lean body mass.

Coenzyme Q10

Coenzyme Q10 (ubiquinone 10; ubidecarenone) supports the synthesis of
ATP in the lipid phase of the mitochondrial membrane by transporting

electrons and protons. In addition, it is thought to be a free radical scavenger, an antioxidant and to have membrane stabilising properties.

This substance is synthesised endogenously, particularly in the heart, liver, kidney and pancreas. Tissue levels peak around the age of 20 and decline after that. Coenzyme Q10 is also found in food, especially fatty fish, such as sardines and mackerel, wholegrain cereals, meat and poultry, soya beans, nuts and vegetables such as spinach and broccoli. The relative significance of biosynthesis and dietary intake to coenzyme Q10 status has not been clarified.

Because of its involvement in ATP production and potential antioxidant role, coenzyme Q10 has been investigated for possible benefit in exercise performance. However, controlled studies in athletes have been disappointing in that coenzyme Q10 does not appear to enhance exercise performance or reduce oxidative stress induced by exercise.

Coenzyme Q10 is available in capsules and tablets in dose ranging from 15 to 60 mg per dose. No adverse effects have been reported except for mild nausea.

Dehydroepiandrosterone

Dehydroepiandrosterone (DHEA; Prasterone) is the most abundant hormone secreted by the adrenal glands, which in the peripheral tissues can be converted into androgens (e.g. testosterone, dihydrotestosterone, androstenedione) and oestrogens. Athletes use DHEA in the belief that it might increase lean body mass, including muscle tissue. However, studies in human beings have not demonstrated a beneficial effect of DHEA on body composition or exercise performance.

Ginseng

There are three different herbs commonly called ginseng. These are Asian or Korean ginseng (*Panax ginseng*), American ginseng (*Panax quinquefolius*) and Siberian ginseng (*Eleutherococcus senticosus*). *Panax ginseng* has shown some promise as an ergogenic supplement, but studies to date have been criticised on methodological grounds and evidence remains incomplete and contradictory. According to a review, there is a lack of sound evidence demonstrating the ability of ginseng to consistently enhance physical performance in humans (Bahrke and Morgan, 1994) (see also Chapter 6).

Phosphatidylserine

Phosphatidylserine is a naturally occurring phospholipid, which is a component of cell membranes. It influences neurotransmitters including acetylcholine, norepinephrine, serotonin and dopamine and plays a role in the functioning of brain cells. In addition, it may retard the production of cortisol and corticotrophin associated with physical stress.

Because raised cortisol levels have a catabolic effect on skeletal muscle and have been associated with overtraining, phosphatidylserine supplementation has been proposed for bodybuilders. However, in addition to breaking down skeletal muscle, cortisol suppresses the inflammatory process and blunting its production may lead to delay in the repair of damaged tissues and/or the recovery from exercise. Moreover, there is no direct evidence to show that phosphatidylserine actually helps athletes to build muscles.

Pyruvate

Pyruvate is produced in the end stages of glycolysis and some researchers have suggested that pyruvate supplementation may spare oxidation of glucose, thus sparing glycogen and enhancing sports endurance. Pyruvate supplements have become popular with athletes and bodybuilders. However, evidence in relation to pyruvate as an ergogenic aid or that it can improve body composition is weak and contradictory. In addition, athletes should be cautioned that pyruvate supplementation has been associated with wind and diarrhoea, which could interfere with sports performance.

Stimulants

A number of plant-derived stimulants are used by athletes to improve performance. These include caffeine (from coffee, tea or cola) and guarana (which contains caffeine-like substances). Caffeine is a CNS stimulant, which appears to improve performance during endurance exercise. There is some evidence that it preserves muscle glycogen, encouraging the metabolism of fats first. Until January 2004 caffeine was among the substances banned by the World Anti-Doping Agency (WADA) and the International Olympic Committee (IOC). The former WADA caffeine limit was 12 mg/mL urine (roughly equivalent to 6–8 cups of coffee). The agency continues to test for caffeine, but a positive result does not result in a penalty. WADA is currently studying whether to introduce new caffeine thresholds.

Tribulis terrestris

Tribulus terrestris is a tropical plant with a long history of medicinal use. One of its components, protodioscine, is converted to DHEA (see above), a finding that has led bodybuilders and strength athletes to try the herb for increasing muscular development. However, evidence is lacking, which is not surprising given that DHEA has not been shown to be an effective sports supplement. One placebo-controlled study in 15 men found that *Tribulus terrestris* did not improve body composition and endurance in resistance training (Antonio *et al.*, 2000).

Vanadium

The trace mineral vanadium has been marketed for use by bodybuilders, based on its apparent ability to improve insulin sensitivity in patients with type 2 diabetes. However, preliminary research in 40 weight-trained athletes found no benefit of supplementation on muscle strength and mass (Fawcett *et al.*, 1996). The dose used was 0.5 mg vanadyl sulphate/kg/day (more than 1000 times the nutritional dose), and there are serious safety concerns about taking vanadium at such high doses.

Animal studies indicate that vanadium can induce haematological and biochemical changes, reproductive and developmental toxicity and pro-oxidant effects. However, vanadium had no effects on haematology or biochemistry in athletes taking vanadium for 12 weeks, but it was associated with side-effects including cramping, diarrhoea and abdominal pain (Fawcett *et al.*, 1997).

Regulation of food supplements

Sports supplements are generally regarded as food supplements and are regulated and labelled according to food law. This means that they cannot make medicinal claims. They are often marketed without adequate evidence of efficacy and safety. To begin to address this issue, the EU Scientific Committee on Food has produced a report on the composition and specification of foods intended to meet the expenditure of intense muscular effort (Scientific Committee on Food, 2001). An EU Directive to regulate sports nutrition products is now being planned and is expected to propose legislation covering:

- carbohydrate-rich energy food products
- carbohydrate-electrolyte solutions
- food supplements (e.g. vitamins, minerals, trace elements, essential fatty acids, caffeine, creatine, carnitine, BCAAs.

References

Antonio J, Uelmen J, Rodriguez R, *et al.* (2000). The effects of Tribulus terrestris on body composition and exercise performance in resistance-trained males. *Int J Sport Nutr Exerc Metab* 10: 208–215.

Bahrke M S, Morgan W P (1994). Evaluation of the ergogenic properties of ginseng. *Sports Med* 18: 229–248.

Balsom P D, Harridge S D R, Soderlund K, *et al.* (1993). Creatine supplementation per se does not enhance endurance exercise performance. *Acta Physiol Scand* 149: 521–523.

Bloomstrand E, Hassmen P, Ekblom B, *et al.* (1991). Administration of branched-chain amino acids during sustained exercise – effects on performance and plasma concentration of some amino acids. *Eur J Appl Physiol* 63: 83–8.

Castell L M, Newsholme E A (1997). The effects of oral glutamine supplementation on athletes after prolonged exhaustive exercise. *Nutrition* 13: 738–742.

Clancy S P, Clarkson P M, DeCheke M E, *et al.* (1994). Effects of chromium picolinate supplementation on body composition, strength, and urinary chromium loss in football players. *Int J Sport Nutr* 4: 142–153.

Davis J M (1995). Carbohydrates, branched-chain amino acids and endurance: the central fatigue hypothesis. *Int J Sport Nutr* 5: S29–S38.

Fawcett J P, Farquhar S J, Walker R J, *et al.* (1996). The effect of oral vanadyl sulphate on body composition and performance in weight-training athletes. *Int J Sport Nutr* 6: 382–390.

Fawcett J P, Farquhar S J, Thou T, *et al.* (1997). Oral vanadyl sulphate does not affect blood cells, viscosity or biochemistry in humans. *Pharmacol Toxicol* 80: 202–206.

Finn J P, Ebert T R, Withers R T, *et al.* (2001). Effect of creatine supplementation on metabolism and performance in humans during intermittent sprint cycling. *Eur J Appl Physiol* 84: 238–243.

Hallmark M A, Reynolds T H, DeSouza C A, *et al.* (1996). Effects of chromium and resistive training on muscle strength and body composition. *Med Sci Sports Exerc* 28: 139–144.

Hasten D L, Rome E P, Franks B D, *et al.* (1992). Effects of chromium picolinate on beginning weight training students. *Int J Sport Nutr* 2: 343–350.

Heinonen O J (1996). Carnitine and physical exercise. *Sports Med* 22: 109–132.

Leenders N, Sherman W M, Lamb D R, *et al.* (1999). Creatine supplementation and swimming performance. *Int J Sport Nutr* 9: 251–262.

Madsen K, MacLean D A, Kiens B, *et al.* (1996). Effects of glucose, glucose plus branched-chain amino acids or placebo on bike performance over 100 km. *J Appl Physiol* 81: 2644–2650.

Mourier A, Bigard A X, de Kerviler E, *et al.* (1997). Combined effects of caloric restriction and branched chain amino acid supplementation on body composition and exercise performance in elite wrestlers. *Int J Sports Med* 18: 47–55.

Mujika I, Chatard J K, Lacoste L, *et al.* (1996). Creatine supplementation does not improve sprint performance in elite swimmers. *Med Sci Sports Exerc* 28: 1435–1441.

Mujika I, Padilla A, Ibanez J, *et al.* (2000). Creatine supplementation and sprint performance in soccer players. *Med Sci Sports Exerc* 32: 518–525.

Nissen S, Sharp R, Ray M, *et al.* (1996). Effect of leucine metabolite beta-hydroxy-beta-methylbutyrate on muscle metabolism during resistance-exercise training. *J Appl Physiol* 81: 2095–2104.

Panton L B, Rathmacher J A, Baier S, *et al.* (2000). Nutritional supplementation of the leucine metabolite beta-hydroxy-beta methylbutyrate (HMB) during resistance training. *Nutrition* 16: 734–739.

Scientific Committee on Food (2001). *Report of the Scientific Committee on Food on Composition and Specification of Food Intended to Meet the Expenditure of Intense Muscular Effort, Especially for Sportsmen.* SCF/CS/NUT/SPORT/5 Final (corrected). Brussels: SCF.

Slater G, Jenkins D (2000). Beta-hydroxy beta-methylbutyric acid (HMB) supplementation and the promotion of muscle growth and strength. *Sports Med* 30: 105–116.

Van Hall G, Raaymakers J, Saris W, *et al.* (1995). Ingestion of branched-chain amino acids and tryptophan during sustained exercise in man: failure to affect performance. *J Physiol* 486: 789–794.

Volek J S, Kraemer W J, Bush J A, *et al.* (1997). Creatine supplementation enhances muscular performance during high-intensity resistance exercise. *J Am Diet Assoc* 97: 765–770.

Williams M H, Branch J D (1998). Creatine supplementation and exercise performance: an update. *J Am Coll Nutr* 17: 216–234.

Further reading

Bean A (2003). *The Complete Guide to Sports Nutrition*, 4th edn. London: A & C Black.

Coleman E (2003). *Eating for Endurance*, 4th edn. Palo Alto, CA: Bull Publishing Co, 2003.

Stear S (2004). *Fuelling Fitness for Sports Performance: Sports Nutrition Guide.* London: Sugar Bureau.

Williams M (1997). *The Ergogenic Edge*. Champaign, IL: Human Kinetics.

Williams M H (2004). *Nutrition for Health, Fitness and Sport*, 7th edn. Boston, MA: WCB/McGraw-Hill.

Useful addresses

Sports Nutrition Interest Group of the British Dietetic Association
5th floor, Charles House
148–9 Great Charles Street

Queensway
Birmingham B3 3HT
Tel: +44 (0)121 200 8080
http://www.bda.uk.com (this site has a factsheet entitled *Fuel for Sports*)

Dietitians in Sport and Exercise Nutrition (DISEN)
PO Box 22360
London W13 9FL
http://www.disen.org.uk (this site contains information about nutrition
for sports and athletics)

Eating Disorders Association
1st floor, Wensum House
103 Prince of Wales Road
Norwich NR1 1DW
http://www.edauk.com

Food Standards Agency
Room 621, Hannibal House
PO Box 30080
London SE1 6YA
http://www.foodstandards.gov.uk

British Nutrition Foundation
High Holborn House
52–54 High Holborn
London WC1 6RQ
http://www.nutrition.org.uk (this website has a factsheet on *Nutrition
and Sport*)

SPRIG
http://www.sprig.org.uk/htfo/htfonutrution.html (this website provides
information on leisure and sports and includes a section on nutrition that
has details of relevant organisations, books and journals)

Part Two

Treatment and prevention of sports-related problems

4

Soft tissue injury

Stuart J Anderson

Introduction

Pharmacists have an important role in emphasising the need for immediate treatment to prevent further damage to soft tissue injuries. This chapter covers the identification of a range of soft tissue injuries but in many cases the management of these injuries should be referred to fully trained colleagues in other disciplines. The importance of adequate rehabilitation should always be impressed upon the client.

Injuries are generally caused by trauma or 'overuse' and are loosely categorised as acute, subacute and chronic, but it is not unusual to have an acute flare-up of a chronic injury. Acute soft tissue trauma is often found in contact sports and can sometimes be attributed to the 'playing conditions', such as a muddy pitch leading to knee ligament injury, or the hazards of a particular sport such as downhill skiing. Overuse injuries are common in activities that involve repeated movements such as tennis and long-distance running, and often involve tendons and related bursae, nerves or periosteum. Different tissues heal at different rates and some less completely than others, often dependent on the pathological nature of the injury, the adequacy of the patient's nutrition, or the blood supply to the tissue involved. With some injuries, pain often improves when the tissues warm up and the individual continues training – this only increases the likelihood of a chronic 'overuse' injury and can be very debilitating.

Muscles, tendons and ligaments tear when they are subjected to forces greater than their inherent strength, and may be injured if they are too weak or too tight for the exercise demands being placed on them. Different tissues have varying elastic limits, and cannot return to their original length after being stretched beyond this limit. This deformative change in length correlates to minor tissue damage (Alter, 1996). This is how joint laxity and instability can be caused by minor strains and sprains.

Muscle injuries such as lacerations, contusions and strains constitute the most common injuries in sports (Jarvinen *et al.*, 2000). If muscle is injured it is vital to differentiate between a strain, tear, rupture (complete tear) or avulsion (tendon torn from bone). Tears can have serious long-term implications if they are not treated thoroughly, as calcified deposits can form within the muscle itself and may later have to be excised. Bleeding and swelling within muscles can put pressure on the associated nerves and can cause an uncomfortable, numbing sensation.

Muscular injuries

Tears and strains

Partial tears imply that only some of the fibres are damaged and may occur in either the central portion ('belly') or the peripheral edge of the muscle, which often can only be differentiated in the post-acute phase of the injury. With peripheral tears, a haematoma is drained by gravity along tissue planes, often resulting in diffuse bruising away from the site of injury. Relative to central tears, the injured site is less tender and responds to movement quickly. Although central tears are often more painful and bring more loss of function, bruising is usually minimal unless there is superficial contact injury. Bruising is often indicative of an intermuscular haematoma, while intramuscular haematomas present with much more movement impairment. Complete tears often present as a 'bunching' of the muscle with attempted contraction and obvious loss of strength.

Contusions

This is a common injury caused by collision in sports, often from a direct blow, which causes localised damage and bleeding. Treatment focuses initially on minimising the bleeding and swelling. Care must be taken to assess the severity as early massage and heat can worsen the bleeding. Complications include myositis ossificans, a disease process characterised by bony deposits or ossification of muscle tissue. Most of these injuries are not significant enough to limit participation in sport, however athletes should consider the use of protective padding to minimise the risk of further injury.

Treatment

Muscle injuries should be treated regularly and often. Treatment will generally involve massage techniques, ice/heat therapy (see p. 114), stretching regularly throughout the day, strengthening as appropriate, and addressing causative factors such as kinetic dysfunction related to muscle imbalance and athletic technique. The extent and sequence of these treatment parameters can depend on the extent of the injury.

Complications

Myositis ossificans may occur when there is a direct blow to the muscle and periosteum, and can result in the formation of bone plaques within the deep muscle. This commonly occurs with impact to the thigh or forearm. This is a very painful condition and the patient often has a feeling of density in the tissues, swelling, and movement limitation. The suspected injury should be X-rayed promptly. If the diagnosis is confirmed, absolute rest is required, often for weeks, and the swelling is minimised. Once the bone is stable or surgically removed, physiotherapy can commence and usually results in good recovery. Resisted work is the last exercise to be started and protective padding should be worn for the athlete's return to sport.

Joint and connective tissue injuries

Sprains refer to injuries of connective tissue such as ligament or capsular tissue, and are graded according to the extent of the damage (see Table 4.1).

Furthermore, moderate or severe sprains can have complications, including:

- Capsular sprains often feature with marked oedema, and internal injury to the joint must be ruled out as quickly as possible.
- Synovial effusion causes pain and swelling, and haemarthrosis must receive medical attention immediately; aspiration is helpful in determining the nature of the swelling.

Table 4.1 Classifications of ligament damage

Grade 1 sprain	Minor tissue damage without related joint laxity
Grade 2 sprain	Presents with some joint laxity but has connective fibres intact
Grade 3 sprain	Presents as a rupture and the ligament(s) in question are torn apart completely. Surgical repair is case-dependent

- Joint subluxation refers to an incomplete dislocation as some degree of contact between articular surfaces is present.
- Neural damage (i.e. common peroneal nerve) related to the sprain may give ongoing symptoms of pain and neuralgia and is sometimes relieved by a local anaesthetic.
- Reflex sympathetic dystrophy or RSD (Sudeck's atrophy) can occur after a severe sprain and causes severe pain between the ankle and foot and swelling. The patient must be encouraged to continue to walk. Physiotherapy, analgesics, nerve block and corticosteroids may help.
- Sinus tarsi presents as chronic pain between the talus and the calcaneus. Corticosteroid and local anaesthetic often help.
  - Synovitis can persist, particularly in chronically unstable joints.
  - Deposits may form in the ligament after healing and cause constant friction and chronic inflammation.

These pathological variations and grades of injury can have very different implications for rehabilitative management. Splinting or bracing may be required for unstable joints or related soft tissue damage. X-ray, MRI and arthroscopy can be helpful in diagnosis of internal derangement or joint fractures.

Peripheral neuropathies

Nerve lesions may be a result of acute trauma injury or chronic injury secondary to repetitive microtrauma, such as entrapment. Common mechanisms of injury also include compression, traction, laceration and ischaemia. Injuries are graded according to the severity of neurophysiological change, ranging from neuropraxia (Grade 1) to axonal degeneration (Grade 2) and nerve transaction (Grade 3). Entrapment injuries are more common in the upper extremities and proximal nerve injuries have a poorer prognosis for neurological recovery (Feinberg *et al.*, 1997). Many entrapment injuries have a sport-specific biomechanical element and remain unrecognised until permanent neurological change has occurred. The timing of diagnosis via manual testing and nerve conduction studies (EMG) is crucial for diagnosis and rehabilitative success. Management also depends on the severity of the symptoms.

Bursitis

The role of bursae is to reduce excessive friction between muscles and tendons over bone. Bursitis can be caused by trauma or by overuse. A bursae may fill with fluid when inflamed and the sites most commonly affected are the shoulder, hips, pelvis, knees, elbows, heels and toes. Bursitis presents as pain through movement, however the specific symptoms are dependent on the specific anatomical site. Acute bursitis often presents with local inflammation and is tender on palpation. Chronic bursitis tends to thicken and calcify as a result of successive acute episodes. Investigative procedures include taking a fluid sample to rule out other possible causes (i.e. gout, infection) or imaging to detect calcium deposits. Non-infectious acute or chronic bursitis can be treated with electrotherapy, soft tissue massage to release associated muscle, NSAIDs or corticosteroids (see Chapter 5), rest, mobilisation, and strengthening as indicated.

Tendinopathies

Tendonitis and tenosynovitis

Tendonitis is defined as inflammation of a tendon; tenosynovitis is inflammation of both the tendon and the protective sheath that surrounds some tendons. Tendonitis is often present with pain on movement and palpation, and the tendon sheaths may be visibly swollen or create a grating sound when actively used. There are a number of causative factors including overuse, tissue degeneration, and biomechanical considerations. Specific joint positions are more likely to place tensile stress on certain areas of the tendon (Almekinders *et al.*, 2003). Treatment generally consists of immobilisation or relative rest, biomechanical correction, electrotherapy, ice/heat therapy (see p. 114), NSAIDs (see Chapter 5), appropriate mobilising and eccentric strengthening exercises, and occasionally corticosteroid injection.

Overuse tendinosis vs tendonitis

Overuse tendonopathies are common and often stubborn to resolve. Research has shown that the underlying pathology associated with these conditions is not commonly inflammatory but is evident of collagen degeneration and tendinosis, which therefore has significant implications for its treatment and management (Khan *et al.*, 2002). There is a strong likelihood of full recovery to sport from tendonopathy but the recovery time often varies considerably, from a few days for acute tendonitis to months in the case of chronic tendinosis.

Paratenonitis

Differential diagnosis of tendonopathy can often reveal an inflammation of the outer layer of tissues, called the paratenon. This condition can obstruct free movement of the tendon and is often found with cases involving major tendons such as the Achilles and patellar tendons.

Partial tendon rupture

This is a much more common injury than total rupture, as the tendon integrity is compromised but is still intact. Adequate rehabilitation can help avoid surgical intervention but this is case-dependent.

Total tendon rupture

Rupture is a relatively uncommon injury. The major tendons are more commonly affected, such as the Achilles tendon, which can rupture spontaneously at any age. There is generally complete loss of associated movement. Avulsion may occur, such as the extensor tendon of a finger when forced into flexion from impact. Surgical repair is often necessary for athletes, followed by extensive rehabilitation.

Compartment syndromes

Although most myofascial compartments are able to cope with exercise-related compartmental pressure, swelling and congestion may block off blood supply and lead to the need for immediate surgical decompression. Compartment syndromes vary in location and according to the cause, rate of onset, and severity of symptoms. Pain can be elicited by passive stretching of the involved muscles and the condition is possibly quite advanced if paraesthesia can be objectively confirmed. Posterior compartment syndrome of the calf can be difficult to differentiate from a deep vein thrombosis without a venogram, and they can be mutually implicated.

The stages of traumatic compartment syndrome are as follows:

- Traumatic compartment syndrome – associated with a crush injury to soft tissue or fracture and becomes symptomatic within the acute period (24–48 hours).
- Sub-acute traumatic compartment syndrome – can become evident after the acute period, such as when a cast is applied too tightly.

- Chronic trauma-induced compartment syndrome (Volkmann's ischaemic contracture).

Exercise-induced compartment syndrome can usually be managed with RICE (see p. 114) methodology, massage, modification of activities, and biomechanical correction if needed. Persistent symptoms can be relieved by surgical fasciotomy of the compartment.

Common soft tissue injuries and considerations

It is beyond the scope of this chapter to outline all soft tissue injuries, complications or treatments. The following is a brief summary of injuries that are frequently seen amongst the athletic population. Adequate management of injuries is dependent on an accurate diagnosis.

The shoulder region

The structure of the shoulder region is shown in Figure 4.1.

Acromioclavicular (AC) joint

There are several grades of injury to the AC joint and immediate orthopaedic referral is wise for an accurate diagnosis. Some sprains can disrupt the joint and give the characteristic step deformity. The unstable joint should have bracing, strapping or a shoulder harness applied as

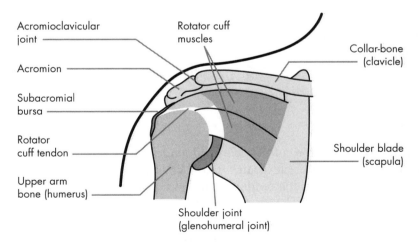

Figure 4.1 Diagram of shoulder region.

soon as possible. Surgical fixation may be indicated if function remains impaired after several weeks.

Shoulder (glenohumeral) joint

Shoulder dislocation is a result of a number of biomechanical considerations. Recurrent dislocation is a sign of instability, which may need surgical correction. Secondary implications of violent shoulder dislocation include fractured head or neck of humerus, nerve damage (circumflex, axillary), or capsular damage. Reduction, support as needed, stability exercises and pain control are all part of early management.

Axillary nerve injury

Shoulder dislocations commonly involve axillary nerve injury, often resulting in secondary deltoid paralysis. The axillary nerve is also susceptible to injury from direct compression. Athletes who sustain this injury typically have a good prognosis for recovery provided contracture is avoided. Surgical intervention is indicated if nerve recovery is not observed 3–4 months post-injury (Perlmutter and Apruzzese, 1998).

Stinger

A stinger is a sports related injury to the nerves about the neck or shoulder. It occurs most commonly in contact and collision sports and is sometimes called a burner or nerve pinch injury, but the term stinger is most descriptive of the symptoms that the athlete experiences including painful electrical sensations radiating through one of the arms. Treatment for acute pain may include activity restriction, ice or heat, anti-inflammatory and analgesic medications, a cervical collar and cervical traction.

Rotator cuff lesions

Injuries to the rotator cuff muscles and tendons vary in their pathology. Acute injuries are muscle strains and partial or complete tendon tears. Overuse injuries include tendinopathy and often involve impingement due to correlated weakness and instability. Treatment for mild acute problems include a broad sling and NSAIDs for 2–3 days. It should be noted that the cervical and upper thoracic spine commonly refer pain to the shoulder, and patients with chronic symptoms often have a number of biomechanical factors involved. A lesion of the suprascapular nerve can mimic a rotator cuff tear (Lorei and Hershman, 1993).

Capsulitis ('frozen shoulder')

This painful condition can be caused by trauma but may also occur spontaneously and presents with disturbed scapular-humeral 'rhythm', because the scapula does not move independently from the humerus as it should. Adhesive capsulitis describes the clinical finding of capsular contraction, thickening and adhesions. It is very important to mobilise shoulder injuries to avoid this complication, as it is very debilitating and can last for a year or more. Treatment could also include anti-inflammatories and steroid injection. This condition may be associated with a variety of systemic diseases such as diabetes and thyroid dysfunction.

Painful arc

Pain is present through the mid-range of abduction and can be caused by a number of conditions including supraspinatus tendinopathy, subacromial bursitis, and fracture of the humeral head.

Biceps tendonitis

Inflammation of the long head of the biceps tendon is the most common cause of pain at the front of the shoulder. Pain is commonly felt with external rotation of the arm in a fully abducted position. Tendon dislocation may occur with a violent overhead action and the athlete feeling subsequent weakness.

Triceps avulsion

The triceps tendon is capable of withstanding forces that make an avulsion a more likely injury in weightlifters and athletes performing similar high-resistance exercise.

The elbow region

Triceps strain

Pain is usually located at the back of the elbow at the point of insertion and is seen in javelin throwers and weightlifters. Posterior impingement of the olecranon may be present with martial arts and weightlifting athletes, and radiograph may reveal a cortical thickening or osteophyte. Medial collateral ligament strain may also be implicated with repetitive throwing or poor technique.

Brachialis strain

This presents as anterior pain, often radiating towards the wrist, and may require differential diagnosis from biceps injury. Treatment should be cautious as there is the potential for development of myositis ossificans.

Epicondylitis (tennis elbow)

There is a wide variety of causative pathologies associated with elbow pain, but it commonly involves the common extensor origin involving the tenoperisteal or musculotendinous junction. It can present as medial or lateral epicondylitis with pain radiating from the elbow to the relevant aspect of the wrist. Treatment includes physiotherapy, ice therapy (see p. 114), strapping/brace for the forearm muscles (see Table 4.6), and NSAIDs (see Chapter 5). Contributing factors include equipment (i.e. racquet strings are too tight), faulty technique, or weak shoulder, wrist or elbow muscles. Medial epicondylitis (forehand tennis elbow) may also be caused by a racquet handle that is too small or forceful throwing movements.

Medial collateral ligament

This is a common injury with throwing athletes and may be treated conservatively or with surgical correction for inherent instability.

Olecranon bursitis

The usual cause is a direct blow or sustained resting pressure.
    Elbow and wrist related neuropathies are summarised in Table 4.2.

Wrist and hand

Wrist strain often presents with a 'crunching sensation' as the tendons move, and is caused by repetitive or unaccustomed use of the wrist. Splinting and avoidance of movements that cause symptoms may help. Scaphoid fracture must be ruled out if the injury is the result of a fall.

Table 4.2 Elbow- and wrist-related neuropathies

- Musculocutaneous nerve palsy is seen in weightlifters with weakness of the elbow flexors and dysesthesias of the lateral forearm.
- Posterior interosseous nerve entrapment is common among tennis players and results in weakness of the wrist and metacarpophalangeal extensors.
- Ulnar neuritis at the elbow is common amongst throwing athletes, tennis players, weightlifters.
- Paralysis of the ulnar nerve at the wrist is seen among cyclists resulting in weakness of grip and numbness of the 4th and 5th fingers.
- Carpal tunnel syndrome may have to be differentiated from pronator teres syndrome, which is entrapment of the median nerve in the forearm.
- Radial nerve injury may be present with tennis elbow often due to poor technique.
- Hypothenar hammer syndrome is a vascular compromise injury to the ulnar nerve seen in martial arts and racquet sports.

Sprained fingers and thumbs are very common in sport and firm strapping can often prevent the undesired movement for return to play, depending on the demands. A severe sprain may rupture ligaments (i.e. ulnar collateral ligament of the thumb) and leave the lax joint susceptible to further problems. Surgical repair is then indicated. Dislocations, avulsions (i.e. mallet finger) and ligament rupture (i.e. Boutonniere deformity) require orthopaedic referral and splinting. Mobilisation of the hand is important to avoid secondary complications and can involve intensive physiotherapy. Hand rehabilitation is often neglected by athletes, particularly by those who do not require the full use of their hands for their sport.

Tenosynovitis (DeQuervain's disease)

This condition is an inflammation of the synovium of the abductor pollicis longus and extensor pollicis brevis tendons as they pass through the dorsal compartment of the wrist near the radial styloid. It is particularly prominent in athletes engaging in racquet sports, rowers, golfers and bowlers. It may present concurrently with intersection syndrome, which is a related bursitis. There is often localised swelling and tenderness, which may extend along the course of the tendons. Treatment includes splinting, physiotherapy and NSAIDs (see Chapter 5). Corticosteroids may be helpful for symptom relief. Surgical release is not often necessary.

Wrist tendinopathies

Any of the flexor or extensor tendons may become injured because of overuse, with associated tenderness, swelling, and possibly crepitus. Physiotherapy and functional rehabilitation should bring resolution.

Gymnast's wrist

This is an impingement syndrome caused by repetitive forced wrist dorsiflexion occurring in the radiocarpal joint. It is very important not to overlook other causes of dorsal wrist pain, such as aseptic necrosis of carpal bones, carpal fractures, lunate subluxation, or radial epiphysis injury.

Carpal tunnel syndrome

Carpal tunnel syndrome (CTS) is a common neuropathy associated with sport and a number of diseases and conditions (Sternbach, 1999). In sport the causative factor is often repeated or sustained wrist flexor activity such as is associated with gymnasts, weightlifters and cyclists. CTS involves compression of the median nerve under the carpal ligament, and presents as aching on the palmer aspect of the wrist with grip weakness and paraesthesia of the middle three fingertips. Symptoms often include nocturnal paraesthesias or burning pain. Treatment includes splinting, mobilisation of the carpals and tissues, and steroid injection. Thenar muscular weakness and atrophy are also common features, which increase the disability and prolong rehabilitation. Surgical intervention is often needed for persistent symptoms.

Ulnar collateral ligament sprain and rupture

This injury occurs as a result of the thumb being forced excessively into abduction, and is common amongst skiing populations. Grade 1 injury follows RICE methodology (see p. 114) with subsequent mobilisation. Grade 2 injuries require splinting or strapping and a cast may be required in severe cases. Complete ruptures generally require surgery followed by immobilisation and rehabilitation.

Spinal injuries

Spinal overuse injury

Despite the common occurrence of back pain in many sports, it must always be taken seriously and not treated complacently. Pain and problems can be caused by a multitude of pathologies, including stress fractures, disc injury, sciatica, spondylosis, spondylolisthesis, muscle imbalance and overuse, nerve root compression, instability, Scheuermann's disease (see p. 112), and spinal structural changes caused by the demands of the sport. Injury to trunk muscles such as the abdominals and erector spinae must not be overlooked.

Acute cervical or head injury/concussion

This is a potentially very serious injury that should be assessed medically as promptly as possible. The athlete should be very closely monitored for loss of consciousness or shortness of breath.

Acute thoracic injury

Injury to the thoracic spine often involves trauma to the ribs, intercostal muscles, or the rib joints attaching to the sternum or spine. Trunk flexion will often induce pain from intercostal tears and extension will open the rib cage and cause related pain. Rib fractures are painful largely because of the tearing of intercostal muscles. In the acute phase elastic wrapping can relieve pain by restricting rib cage expansion. Sprains to sternocostal and costochondral joints causes localised tenderness and swelling, and can occur with weight training and gymnastic movements that force the arms into extension and abduction.

Acute lumbar injury

Lower back injuries are often a result of pushing or pulling against resistance and/or twisting. Often the pain is not severe and activity is continued. However, after the injury has bled for 2–3 hours and muscle spasm begins, it can cause severe pain independent of movement direction. Predisposing factors to lumbar injury include increased lumbar lordosis and associated anterior pelvic tilt, poor postural control and spinal stability often due to weak muscles, hypo or hyper-mobility of spinal joints, arthritic changes and poor alignment. A neoprene spinal support, NSAIDs (see Chapter 5) and relative rest may provide some immediate relief.

Buttock pain

Differential diagnosis can be challenging as pain may be referred from the lumbar spine or sacroiliac joint. The concurrence of groin pain may suggest sacroiliac pathology. Buttock pain is most frequently associated with kicking and running activities and symptom behaviour is often helpful with diagnosis: well-localised pain is often evidence that the source is in the buttock, such as hamstring tendinopathy, ishiogluteal bursitis, gluteal or piriformis muscle pathology. Adolescents may have an apophysitis or avulsion fracture of the ischial tuberosity caused by overuse of the associated hamstring. Buttock pain can also be evidence of systemic disorders and spondyloarthropathies.

Piriformis muscle syndrome

This condition must be differentiated from piriformis strain. Piriformis syndrome involves an impingement of the sciatic nerve, usually as it passes through the muscle. This can give rise to local and referred pain as well as related neurological symptoms. Treatment consists of physiotherapy and surgery if required. Piriformis strain usually presents with pain in the sacral or gluteal region and worsens with prolonged sitting or standing. Treatment is conservative.

Sacroiliac joint dysfunction

This refers to a hyper- or hypomobility of the joint which places stress in and around the structure. It may contribute to pain in the region of the lumbar spine, hamstrings and groin. Pain is thought to arise from the stretching of surrounding soft tissue, which may bring on a secondary inflammatory component (Brukner, 1993).

Groin pain

Groin pain is very common in sporting injuries and may cause chronic problems for the athlete. Accurate diagnosis can be difficult as a variety of pathologies can give similar groin pain and are often elicited by resisted hip flexion. Most groin injuries in athletes are a result of overstretching, twisting, kicking or lunging and can involve partial or complete rupture of tendons. Overuse groin strain can also be correlated with repetitive hip flexion such as in sit-ups.

Groin strain implies muscular injury to any of the following: abdominals, adductors, sartorius, iliopsoas, or the long head of rectus femoris. The standard principles of RICE (see p. 114) should be applied in acute cases and the use of crutches should be considered. Although conservative treatment is often effective for strains, surgical repair is indicated for the reattachment of significant ruptures or avulsions. Differential diagnosis of chronic injuries is often more complex and may involve more than one pathological process. Plain films may not reveal pathology and are often aided by ultrasound scan, bone scanning, MRI and herniography. Systemic disease can also be a cause of pain in this region and should be considered.

Adductor muscle tears and strains

This is a common injury in sport and any of the adductor muscles could be involved. If this injury is not treated adequately it could become chronic and career-threatening. A tear of the adductor muscles usually occurs near the musculotendinous junction about 5 cm from the pubis, or at the tendo-osseous junction producing pain around the pubic tubercle or superior ramus. The injury is often the result of external rotation and abduction injuries. It must be emphasised that successful rehabilitation, particularly of chronic injury, is often dependent on a strengthening programme for the adductor group. Surgical intervention is available if non-operative treatment fails for 6 months or longer. Adductor release and tenotomy has been reported to have limited success in athletes (Nicholas and Tyler, 2002).

Osteitis pubis

Chronic overuse strain of the adductors can lead to osteitis pubis. This condition is related to instability and inflammation of the pubic symphysis and is seen in athletic young adults and adolescents. Pain and tenderness is experienced over the pubic symphysis or along the pubic ramus. Radiography shows widening and fragmentaion or sclerotic changes of the pubic symphysis. MRI can be used to confirm the diagnosis. Osteitis pubis is often best managed by rest, often for several months, and physiotherapy. With presentation of significant pelvic instability on weight-bearing, grafting or plating surgical fixation may be considered.

Obturator neuropathy

This entrapment condition is related to adductor tendinopathy as it is trapped in the adductor fascia. It presents as groin pain, which extends further down the inner thigh with increased exercise and with possible associated weakness. Conservative treatment is generally unsuccessful and surgical fascial release is then indicated.

Bursitis

Of the eight bursae at the hip joint, the trochanteric bursae and the bursae around the insertion of iliopsoas are the most commonly affected. Athough this pathology can be difficult to diagnose without imaging, it is usually associated with muscular damage related to the corresponding deep tendons.

Inguinal ligament

Pathology presents as diffuse pain and inflammation at the insertion to the pubic bone, which can lead to chronic pain.

Hernia

The three most likely types of hernia associated with groin pain are the inguinal, femoral and obturator hernias. High abdominal pressure can force the tissues in the groin to open, such as in weightlifting, and those with inguinal hernia have localised swelling, a palpable lump with cough impulse, and often have discomfort with walking. Symptomatic patients require corrective surgery.

Sports hernia (Gilmore's groin)

This is a complex injury thought to be linked to overuse and muscle imbalance. It is a combination of pathologies, thought not to be necessarily concurrent, which can involve the inguinal ligament and external obliques aponeurosis among other structures. Conservative management is often unsuccessful and surgical intervention is then indicated, followed by strict adherence to rehabilitation.

Nerve entrapment

The ilioinguinal, iliohypogastric, genitofemoral, obturator and the lateral cutaneous nerves of the thigh can become involved in entrapment syndromes. Often there is a history of previous surgery, which may be associated with nerve injury, subsequent entrapment and neuroma. Local anaesthetic may be used as a diagnostic test. Treatment is initially conservative, with an altered training programme for several weeks. Entrapment may be relieved by surgical release.

Degenerative changes in hip or spine

Osteoarthritis of the lumbosacral spine or hip joint and intervertebral disc prolapse are common causes of groin pain.

Fracture of the pelvis or neck of the femur

Stress fractures are frequently seen in long-distance runners, and stress fracture of the femoral neck is also commonly seen in hurdlers, skiers and footballers. Pain is felt to the anterior thigh and possibly to knee. X-ray may not confirm the diagnosis in initial weeks. Pelvic fractures are usually at the inferior pubic ramus close to the symphysis and pain is felt in the groin, buttock or thigh. Compression fractures are not uncommon and are usually seen in younger athletes. A slipped upper femoral epiphysis should also be considered for the adolescent.

Hip pain

Avulsions

Violent blows can cause bony avulsion, especially during adolescence before epiphyses have fully fused. For example, a violent lunging or sprinting-type force can avulse the ASIS and the sartorius and TFL origins. A jumping or sprinting movement can cause an avulsion of the lesser trochanter of the femur by the iliopsoas tendon. Avulsion at the ischium can happen via the hamstrings origin, and similarly, the adductor muscles at the pubic ramus. These conditions require very careful clinical consideration but not necessarily surgical intervention, and have a good prognosis for recovery.

Trochanteric bursitis

The patient presents with localised pain near the greater trochanter, which may radiate down the lateral aspect of the thigh. It often coexists with gluteus medius tendinopathy and is commonly seen in long-distance runners. It can be aggravated by relatively simple activities such as climbing stairs or stretching the related muscle. Treatment includes physiotherapy to address related tightness, ultrasound, NSAIDs (see Chapter 5), and corticosteroid injection if persistent.

Less common causes of hip pain

Hip joint injuries   Pain is usually a dull ache and is felt in the groin, buttock region, and the anterior aspect of the knee. Rheumatological and arthritic disease must be considered. Labral tears can be difficult to diagnose without the benefit of MRI and arthroscopy. Dysplasia, femoral stress fractures of the pubic ramus, and avascular necrosis of the femoral head are possible causes of hip pain.

Snapping hip   This refers to the sound and feeling in the hip region commonly associated with ballet dancers. There are two forms of this condition. Firstly, the TFL or gluteus maximus may slide over the greater trochanter and produce a normally painless noise. Secondly, the patient may complain of painful hip flexion as the psoas tendon passes over the hip joint. Physiotherapy treatment is appropriate.

Quadriceps injury   Contusions are common in contact sports. Treatment includes NSAIDs (see Chapter 5), RICE (see p. 114) and physiotherapy. If there is a lot of swelling and pain within 24 hours patients should attend an emergency department. Complications include myositis ossificans. It is not advisable to massage before medical advice is sought.

The knee

An anterior view of a knee joint is illustrated in Figure 4.2.

Differential diagnosis and management of acute or chronic knee injuries is often complex. It is imperative that an accurate history is taken, as the mechanism of injury is often a strong indicator of pathology. The speed at which effusion develops is also indicative of the nature of the damage. Rapid effusion is often indicative of cruciate ligament tear, whereas swelling developed over a day or so can be due to a

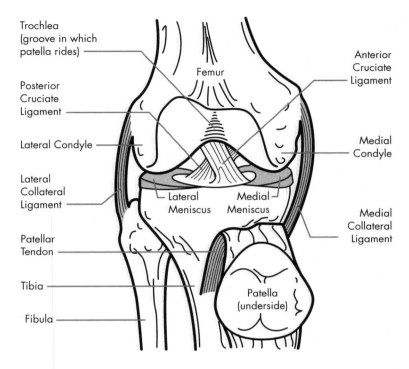

Figure 4.2 Front view of knee joint.

capsular sprain. Internal derangement is often indicated by gross swelling, 'locking' or 'giving way'. Pain at the patello-femoral joint, tibial-femoral joint or patellar tendon is often due to improper biomechanics and overuse, and may be aided by appropriate strapping or bracing. Knee pain can be an indicator of hip disease, particularly during adolescence.

Signs of internal knee derangement

'Locking' and 'giving way' It is important to distinguish between a 'true' locking or giving way and movement inhibited by pain or induced by pain avoidance. True locking is a sign of mechanical blockage, due either to torn cartilage, meniscus, or a loose body, whereby the knee cannot be voluntarily bent or straightened. Often the joint can be manipulated to free it, but the injury should be assessed as quickly as possible as this can often help with differential diagnosis. Giving way is often caused by a sudden relief of mechanical obstruction.

Loose bodies The two most common causes of knee locking or giving way in athletic individuals are torn cartilage and loose bodies from osteochondritis dissecans. Surgical removal or reattachment of the loose body may be successful.

Meniscal tears The menisci help to stabilise and distribute load within the knee joint (tibia and femur) and also act as lubricators and shock absorbers. Meniscal tears are common injuries and can be the result of degenerative change or trauma. Traumatic tears often occur during twisting forces on the knee, and are associated with ligamentous injury. Degenerative tears are usually related to worn articular cartilage and osteoarthritis.

A tear is classified according to whether it is complete or incomplete, stable or unstable, and by its shape. Some types of tear may create a meniscal cyst, which is treated in the same way. Arthroscopic partial menisectomy is indicated for the majority of symptomatic tears and patients can resume activities within a few weeks. Repaired meniscal tears require an adequate blood supply and a stable joint – repair may be performed dependent on the nature and location of the tear and the expected outcome and activity level of the patient. Post-operative protocols do vary, but rehabilitation is generally a lengthier procedure than menisectomy and contact sports should be avoided for 6 months.

Cartilage tears Cartilage is susceptible to partial or complete tears when the knee is subjected to forced rotation with the foot fixed in a weight-bearing position. Symptoms vary from aching and feelings of instability to effusion, locking and 'giving way'. Orthopaedic manual tests and MRI help confirm diagnosis. Arthroscopic investigative surgery to remove damaged tissue such as partial meniscectomy and cartilage removal is often indicated. Adequate rehabilitation is imperative to prevent reinjury.

Cruciate ligament tears Violent injuries may tear either of the cruciates, and may not accompany other soft tissue damage. Specific stability tests are used for injury assessment, however normal knee joint laxity varies considerably and can lead to diagnostic difficulty, particularly with the extrasynovial posterior cruciate ligament.

Anterior cruciate ligament tear Anterior cruciate ligament (ACL) tears are not an uncommon injury in sport yet their management is controversial. Injury history is important in a differentiating this injury from other forms of knee trauma. The mechanism of injury is usually pivoting, sudden deceleration, landing from a jump, or impact trauma, and the patient often hears a cracking sound at the time of injury. A prominent haemarthrosis usually develops within the first few hours. Athletes will sometimes continue activity after the initial pain settles, however most complete tears are very painful. An avulsion of the ligament from the tibia may be evident on X-ray, and periosteal injury often accompanies an ACL tear, which may have implications for rehabilitation. An MRI scan can be useful in establishing a clear diagnosis. Arthroscopy is often performed to assess potential damage to articular cartilage or meniscal tears. Several aspects of the management of ACL tears are debated, ranging from surgical intervention and conservative management, to the use of braces and different rehabilitative protocols (Francis et al., 2001; Beynonn et al., 2002; Birmingham et al., 2002; Karmani and Ember, 2004). The young athlete is often treated conservatively regardless of the grade of injury, provided a ligamentous avulsion is not present. For cases of rupture, reconstructive surgery is usually recommended for those patients who participate in high-speed sports involving pivoting and directional changes, and the average time for return to sport after reconstructive surgery is 6–9 months. It is important to note that re-habilitation should commence from the time of injury and secondary issues may arise during the rehabilitative process, such as low back pain, patellofemoral problems, and lower limb stiffness.

It is well established that people with ACL injuries or reconstruc-tion have decreased proprioceptive skill and a decreased ability to detect passive knee movement (Ageberg, 2002; Beynnon et al., 2002; Bonfim et al., 2003). Braces are commonly used to help provide stability, prevent rotation and excessive movement, and to protect injured or post-operative ligaments. Athletes should be rehabilitated beyond the need for a brace, and there is some evidence that usage may inhibit the re-habilitative process (Birmingham et al., 2002; Ramsey et al., 2003). For the ACL-deficient knee, it has been found that functional braces do not stabilise but perhaps offer proprioceptive feedback to the user (Ramsey et al., 2003). Supportive neoprene sleeves or elasticated bandages may be helpful in providing some proprioceptive sense without limiting movement (Beynnon et al., 2002). Beynnon et al. (2002) advocate the use of a neoprene sleeve support for the first year post-reconstruction and maintain that after 2 years there is no longer a need for artificial support.

Posterior cruciate ligament tear   Damage to this structure usually requires significant force such as a direct anterior blow to the tibia with a flexed knee or a hyperextension injury. It presents as vague posterior pain, but with minimal swelling as the PCL is extrasynovial. Tears are often linked with tears of the posterior joint capsule. MRI may be required to confirm the diagnosis. PCL ruptures can generally be managed conservatively, however X-ray may reveal an avulsion from the tibial insertion and indicates the need for surgical repair.

Cysts   There are three common cysts in the knee, including Baker's cyst (posterior synovial pouch), cartilage cyst (may pop in and out of joint as knee is moved), or on the inner aspect of the knee, which may be the semi-membranosus bursa. Baker's cyst presents as a chronic effusion and is commonly secondary to degenerative or meniscal abnormality.

Medial knee pain

Medial collateral ligament   A medial collateral ligament (MCL) strain is the most common of all knee injuries and can occur simultaneously with a meniscal tear, cartilage damage or ACL injury. Violent injuries of this nature can include ruptured ligaments, forming what is known as a 'triad'.

Medial meniscus   This is often implicated in other knee injuries such as MCL strain.

Pes anserinus tendinopathy/bursitis   This refers to medial knee pain at the site of combined insertion of sartorius, gracilis and semi-membranosus tendons. This is an overuse injury associated with runners, cyclists and swimmers.

Consideration should be given to the source of pain being hip pathology such as Perthes' disease or a slipped femoral epiphyses in adolescents.

Lateral knee pain

Iliotibial band friction syndrome   This is an overuse injury that occurs as a result of the friction between the ITB and the underlying lateral femoral condyle. It often presents as a clicking pain at approximately 30° knee flexion over the lateral side of the knee.

It particularly affects those running long distances or downhill. It has been thought that this syndrome is a tendinopathy, however it has been shown to be related to a secondary bursae (Muhle *et al.*, 1999).

Lateral collateral ligament   Pain and clicking on the lateral aspect of the knee may be due to a lateral ligament sprain caused by twisting or a direct blow.

Hamstring injury   Various overuse injuries are related to musculature on the lateral aspect of the thigh, such as biceps femoris tendinopathy due to excessive acceleration/deceleration activities. Hamstring tendon insertion strains often occur as a result of kicking, sprinting or dancing. Injury to the hamstring muscles can be significantly prolonged by inappropriate management.

Popliteus tendonitis   This condition often presents as pain and soreness on the posterolateral aspect of the knee and may be linked to excessive foot pronation, excessive acceleration/deceleration activities, running downhill, or as a secondary compensatory injury. It is often helped by rest (especially from downhill running), stretching and strengthening relevant musculature (i.e. hamstrings), and corrective orthotics as necessary.

Lateral meniscus   Patients complain about lateral knee pain aggravated by running, especially up hills.

Anterior knee pain

Patellofemoral syndrome (chondromalacia patella)   This is a generalised term to describe pain in and around the patella. There are two principal theories that help to explain the related pathology. Firstly, it has long been thought that the cause of chondromalacia patella was malalignment between the patella and the underlying femur. However, as there is often poor correlation between malalignment and painful symptoms, patellofemoral problems have more recently been thought to be caused by excessive loading and chemical irritation, leading to inflammation and peripatellar synovitis (Dye, 1996).

Numerous biomechanical factors involving other lower limb weight-bearing joints, and related muscle imbalance, may have a significant bearing on clinical presentation and causation. An increase in training parameters (intensity, frequency) may also be predisposing factors. Treatment must address the acute process (relevant rest, ice therapy, NSAIDs, ultrasound, etc.) and biomechanical considerations with relevant treatment and taping. Strengthening, braces and orthotics can help alleviate recurring symptoms. The use of surgical interventions such as lateral retinacular release and chondroplasty is decreasing, and are only used when conservative intervention has failed.

Patellofemoral instability (recurrent patellar subluxation) This condition presents with subluxation of the patella and an acute episode may present with effusion and haemarthrosis. Patients may complain of a painful slipping of the patella with movement. A patella that is located higher in the femoral groove predisposes the patient to this condition. Treatment mirrors that of patellofemoral syndrome, although crutches may be useful to avoid full weight bearing on the acute and unstable injury. Dislocation requires immediate reduction. Radiograph may reveal osteochondral damage and arthroscopy may be required to remove loose fragments.

Patellar tendinopathy Although this degenerative condition has historically been known as 'jumper's knee', it also occurs in sports people who do not jump repetitively. Treatment consists of physiotherapy, ice therapy, relative rest, modified activity, biomechanical correction, strapping or bracing, and progressive eccentric strengthening exercises. Surgery may be indicated if conservative management fails and acute partial tears may be sufficiently large to warrant surgical repair. MRI and ultrasound imaging are useful for investigating this condition.

Fat pad impingement or irritation The infrapatellar fat pad can be impinged between the patella and the femoral condyle as a result of a direct blow, and is often a very painful injury. Chronic irritation of the fat pad is a common secondary pathology associated with patellar tendinopathy.

Bursa The prepatellar bursa may swell due to pressure and friction (housemaid's knee) and must be differentiated from effusion of the knee joint.

Other causes of knee pain Less common causes of knee pain include:

- Synovial plica – often requires differential diagnosis from patellofemoral syndrome.
- Quadriceps tendinopathy – presents as pain above the patella originating from the patellofemoral joint.
- Infrapatellar bursitis – can cause anterior knee pain that mimics patellar tendinopathy.

Shin pain

Causes of shin soreness

Shin soreness is commonly caused by increased shock-absorptive stresses on tissues due to hard training surfaces, hard-soled shoes, running spikes, running on slopes, poor lower limb alignment, unaccustomed footwear or changes in training habits. Novices can be particularly susceptible. Helpful advice for the athlete may include rotating two or three different types of training and training surfaces over a 3–4 day rota, so that repetitive movements are minimised. Treatment includes biomechanical correction, physiotherapy, possibly local steroid injection for tenosynovitis, or surgical decompression in cases of compartment syndrome.

Exercise-induced compartment syndrome

Although blockage of the blood supply associated with compartment syndrome can cause ischaemia, most soft-tissue compartments are large enough to accommodate extra tissue fluid after exercise and essential treatment includes RICE methodology (see p. 114). Differential diagnosis of exercise-induced compartment syndrome is crucial as pain may also be evidence of a stress fracture, periostitis, tendinopathy, or inflammation of the muscular attachment to bone.

Table 4.3 details common overuse injuries below the knee.

Tibialis anterior tendinopathy

This condition is often caused by downhill running, excessive tightness of shoelaces over the tendon itself, or dorsiflexor overuse related to joint restriction.

Table 4.3 Common over-use injuries below the knee

- Medial pain may be due to tibial stressing or stress fracture, long flexor muscle tear or strain, or tenosynovitis of the long flexors.
- Lateral pain in the lower third of the fibula is often evident of fibular stressing or fracture (common in runners).
- Tibial compartment syndrome often presents as swelling with severe pain and sometimes numbness between the first and second toes.
- Posterior compartment syndrome presents as pain on the medial and posterior aspects of the tibia and can be difficult to differentiate from a deep vein thrombosis without a venogram.

Calf and Achilles complex

Figure 4.3 shows the anatomy of the leg and foot and the position of the Achilles tendon.

Calf strains/tears

The calf and Achilles mechanism is often strained by a sudden change of movement direction, and the tendon is particularly stressed because of its dual function of shock absorption and foot leverage. There can be some anatomical variation in calf musculature, such as the position of the plantaris muscle, which can create diagnostic confusion when ruptured. Calf muscle tears are common in middle-aged people returning to sport and it is important to differentiate serious tears from milder strains.

Overuse Achilles tendinopathy

Achilles tendinopathies in competitive athletes often involve the paratenon and, less commonly, bursitis, calcaneal tendinopathy, and

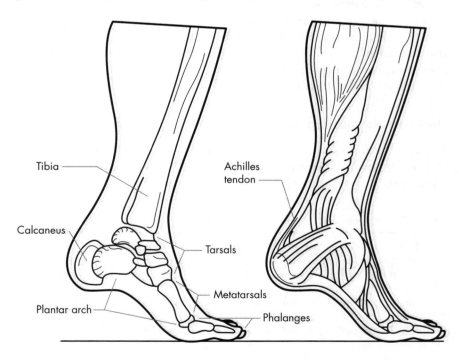

Figure 4.3 Anatomy of the foot and position of Achilles tendon.

the musculotendinous junction. With Achilles tendinopathies there is often no swelling present but it is tender on palpation and pain is felt during or after exercise. This condition often progresses to more debilitating injury if it is left untreated. Achilles paratenonitis is often associated with tendinosis and is an inflammation of the tissue surrounding the tendon, often with swelling and palpable creaking. Stiffness after rest is particularly prevalent in the early morning. If this condition is neglected it can lead to constriction of the tendon and may need surgical intervention. Injections may cure early lesions but must not be aimed into the tendon. Achilles tendinopathy and paratenonitis can be extremely debilitating for the athlete if not managed correctly. Treatment often requires lower limb biomechanical correction and benefits from a heel lift, progressive eccentric strengthening, stretching, electrotherapy, relative rest and functional rehabilitation. The prognosis for this injury will improve with early diagnosis and intervention, however complete resolution may require 3–6 months of treatment strategies. Adequate rehabilitation is the key to recovery and surgical intervention is indicated only if conservative treatment fails.

Achilles tendon partial rupture

With repeated heavy loading, the tendon may form small lesions of varying degree. The athlete may feel the tendon 'snap' and has ensuing weakness of plantar flexion. Treatment is conservative and surgery should not be considered until rehabilitative efforts have failed for several months.

Achilles tendon total rupture

The patient has a history of a snapping sensation and has subsequent partial or total loss of foot plantar flexion and a gap between tissues. Treatment is controversial, but it is generally agreed that the ideal treatment is prompt surgical repair followed by immobilisation with plaster casting for several weeks (Lynch, 2004). Recent evidence suggests that early mobilisation and weight-bearing may improve functional outcome (Costa et al., 2003).

Achilles tendon bursitis

This condition presents as a tender, inflamed and hardened area at the top of the heel near the insertion of the tendon. It can be relieved by heel lift, padding the inflamed area, and stretching the back of shoes to reduce irritation. NSAIDs and corticosteroids may be helpful.

The ankle

Ankle sprain

Differential diagnosis and adequate rehabilitation is extremely important to ensure the necessary functional outcome, particularly in elite athletes. The immature skeleton of a child is susceptible to epiphyseal stress fractures. Immediate treatment consists of RICE methodology (see p. 114) and a stabilising brace (see Table 4.6) helps if the injury is past the acute phase.

Lateral ankle sprain: differential diagnosis

There are many structures commonly involved with this injury, including lateral ligaments, disruption to peroneal muscles, tendons or retinaculae, and bony injury to the shaft of the fibula or lateral malleolus. Particularly with athletes, peroneal tendinopathy and tenosynovitis is often evident as a chronic overuse injury and may be present with acute findings. With severe sprains there may be damage to the connective tissue between the tibia and fibula – this may be a syndesmosis sprain which may have serious implications for rehabilitation and an orthopaedic referral is most certainly required.

The ligament anatomy of the foot is shown in Figure 4.4.

Lateral ankle pain

This presentation is commonly associated with biomechanical dysfunction and is usually a peroneal tendinopathy or sinus tarsi.

Peroneal tendinopathy   This is the most common lateral overuse injury and is caused by excessive eversion and pronation such as in running on slopes, or excessive muscular action such as in dance.

Peroneal tenosynovitis   This condition can often be linked to an inversion ankle sprain or is a result of poor gait pattern and overuse. It commonly presents as swelling and tenderness on the lateral aspect of the ankle. Corticosteroid injections into the sheath may help, however they must not be overused.

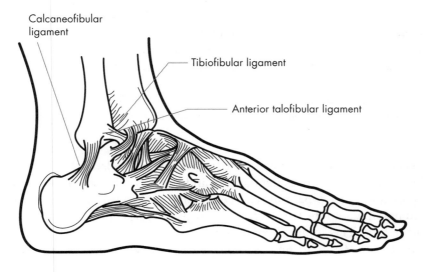

Calcaneofibular
ligament

Tibiofibular ligament

Anterior talofibular ligament

Figure 4.4 Anatomy of the foot ligaments (lateral view).

Peroneal nerve entrapment   Neural tension can cause associated referred symptoms. Peroneal nerve entrapment more commonly involves the superficial and deep peroneal nerves and tends to present as sensory disturbance over the dorsum of the foot. Superficial nerve entrapment may present as pain in the distal third of the leg and possibly with swelling. It is seen in a wide variety of athletes and is exacerbated by activity, particularly running.

Sinus tarsi   This injury is sometimes a complication of a major or deep sprain, or may result from overuse secondary to compromised bio-mechanics, such as excessive pronation of the heel. Pain symptoms are often more severe in the morning, although they may diminish with exercise.

Bursitis at the malleoli   Wearing tight boots or ice skates can cause enough pressure at the malleolus to lead to bursitis. Treatment is con-servative unless symptoms persist and excision may be required.

Medial ankle pain

Flexor hallucis longus tendinopathy   Patients complain of pain at the medial ankle, particularly when standing on forefoot or pushing off the great toe. This pathology is very common amongst ballet dancers.

An example of a flexor hallucis longus tendon split and its surgical debridement (cleaning and trimming) and repair is shown in Figures 4.5 to 4.7. If the injury had not been adequately diagnosed it could have led to a career-threatening rupture for this adolescent ballet dancer.

Tibialis posterior tendinopathy   This condition is often linked with excessive pronation and repeated movements that combine weight-bearing and eversion.

Posterior tibial nerve entrapment (tarsal tunnel syndrome)   This condition is often seen in ballet dancers and runners. The patient will often complain of sharp pain in the heel, medial malleolus, arch of the foot, and possibly into the toes. Occasionally parasthaesia presents on the sole of the foot. This injury is commonly aggravated by prolonged walking, running or standing, and is often associated with overuse linked to excessive pronation.

Medial calcaneal nerve entrapment   This condition presents as pain at the inferomedial aspect of the calcaneus, which often radiates into the arch. It is often linked to excessive pronation and aggravated by running.

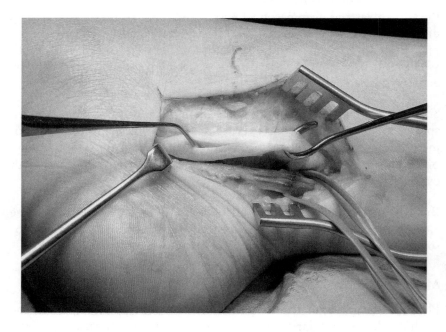

Figure 4.5 FHL tendon showing a split.

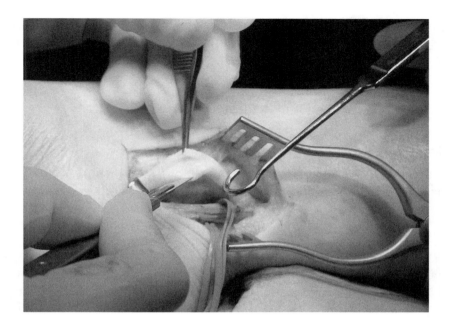

Figure 4.6 Debridement (cleaning and trimming) of the FHL tendon.

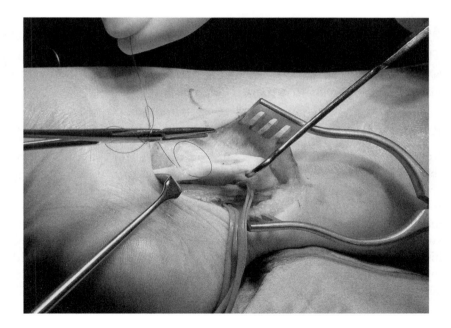

Figure 4.7 Repair of the FHL tendon injury.

Medial plantar nerve entrapment This pathology usually presents as pain in the midfoot region and is seen in middle-aged joggers. It is often associated with use of a new arch support.

Sural nerve entrapment This condition can occur secondary to recurrent ankle sprains and is most often found in runners.

Impingement syndromes

These conditions are generally considered overuse injuries, however they may be present after an acute ankle injury.

Anterior impingement

Repeated microtrauma to the ankle joint can give rise to anterior impingement, which is the formation of osteophytes and subsequent loose bodies within the joint. This condition is commonly seen in many sports involving repeated ankle movement. Management depends largely on symptoms but if conservative treatment is not effective then surgical excision is indicated.

Anterolateral impingement

This pathology can be caused by a major sprain or repeated minor sprains, resulting in a meniscoid lesion. Symptoms include pain and an intermittent catching sensation.

Posterior impingement syndrome

Repetitive forced plantar flexion can lead to posterior impingement of the ankle and can result in os trigonum and the formation of a talar spur. This condition is commonly seen in ballet dancers, gymnasts, footballers and athletes involved in jumping activities. Pain is evident locally with forced plantar flexion, and often presents with a little swelling. Treatment consists of relative rest, ice therapy, physiotherapy, biomechanical and technical correction, and NSAIDs. Corticosteroid injection may provide relief (see Chapter 5). If symptoms persist, surgical excision is indicated.

Serious ankle injury complications

Tibialis posterior dislocation

This is a comparatively rare injury that presents as moderate medial ankle pain and an inability to bear weight. It requires a surgical correction followed by immobilisation and 6 weeks of non-weight-bearing. Functional rehabilitation is crucial for a satisfactory outcome.

Tibialis posterior rupture

With this injury, pain is experienced along the posteromedial tibial border and down to the medial malleolus and navicular tuberosity. The patient is unable to raise the heel and may have a collapsed medial arch. Surgical repair is required.

Peroneal tendon dislocation

These tendons can become dislocated with forceful passive dorsiflexion, as the retinaculae allows the tendons to slip out of their groove. They can spontaneously relocate, however they remain susceptible to further injury and recurrent subluxation. Dislocation is treated surgically.

Post-traumatic synovitis

Persistent ankle pain related to synovitis is often experienced by athletes who have chronic mild ankle instability or return to training too quickly after injury. Treatment requires relevant rest, physiotherapy, NSAIDs, and possibly corticosteroids. Chronic instability may also be aided by taping or bracing (Spaulding *et al.*, 2003).

Complex regional pain syndrome (reflex sympathetic dystrophy)

The history of injury usually presents as a relapse of symptoms after an initial improvement. Symptoms include pain, swelling, changes in cutaneous temperature, and often discolouration, hypersensitivity and sweating.

Syndesmosis sprain

Severe ankle sprains may involve the connective issue between the distal tibia and fibula. The injury has potentially difficult rehabilitative implications and requires immediate investigation and management.

Foot problems and injuries

Stress fractures

These athletic overuse injuries are commonly found in the talus, medial malleolus, navicular, calcaneus, metatarsals and sesamoids. Pain associated with stress fracture of the talus is often reported on the postero-lateral aspect of the ankle and is seen more commonly in footballers and track and field athletes.

Heel spurs and plantar fasciitis

These are two distinct conditions and are not necessarily related, although abnormal biomechanics may give rise to either. Plantar fasciitis is an overuse injury near its attachment into the calcaneus. Fascial tightness can be a secondary problem for those who have been immobilised because of other injury. The patient usually complains of pain that is worst in the morning, with tenderness along the medial fascial border. X-ray may show a calcaneal spur, although they are not a causative pain factor (Lu *et al.*, 1996). Treatment includes gentle stretching of the plantar fascia (particularly in the morning before weight bearing) and calf muscles, massage, use of a heel cup, arch support and properly supportive shoes, taping, ultrasound, and NSAIDs. Corticosteroid injection may be helpful (see Chapter 5). Surgery may be required for chronic symptoms but not as a pain solution for a calcaneal spur (Lu *et al.*, 1996).

Calcaneal fat pad syndrome

This injury may be precipitated acutely by jumping or falling onto the heels from a height or chronically from poor heel cushioning or excessive heel strike. Treatment includes a heel cup, adequate footwear, taping, ultrasound and rest.

Metatarsophalangeal joint synovitis

This condition, commonly known as 'metatarsalgia', is caused by repetitive stress to the metatarsal heads and metatarsophalangeal (MTP) joints. It can affect the first to third MTP joints (second is the most common) and is related to uneven and excessive load distribution, particularly due to excessive pronation. Treatment requires midfoot support via padding and adequate shoes. NSAIDs and corticosteroids may be helpful (see Chapter 5).

First metatarsophalangeal joint sprain ('turf toe')

This is a common sporting injury, often caused by excessive forced dorsiflexion leading to sprain of the plantar capsule and ligament. Immediate treatment includes ice therapy, taping, NSAIDs, and minimal weight-bearing to allow the injury to settle into the sub-acute phase. Repeated injury can lead to long-term reduced range of movement.

Morton's 'neuroma'

This condition is a neural swelling secondary to compression and presents as pain radiating between the toes, usually the third and fourth, often accompanied by paraesthesia. Overpronation may lead to metatarsal hypermobility and neural impingement. Treatment consists of ice therapy, intrinsic muscle strengthening and padding to support the metatarsals. Orthoses for pronation correction and corticosteroids may be helpful. Surgical excision of the nerve is indicated if the symptoms persist.

Interdigital neuromas (metatarsalgia)

This condition usually presents as sharp or burning pain in the forefoot or plantar aspect, possibly radiating into the toes, with and without numbness or tingling sensations.

Adolescent conditions: the young athlete

The primary concern for the adolescent is the potential implication of growing bones and their susceptibility to injury, giving rise to avulsion fractures, metaphyseal fractures and growth plate fractures. Avulsion fractures occur more commonly at the attachment of tendons to bone, however in the adolescent ligamentous attachment can also be involved, such as in ACL injury. Ligamentous avulsion is generally treated surgically whereas it is rarely necessary for musculo-tendinous avulsion in the adolescent. Metaphyseal fractures that do not involve growth plates tend to heal within approximately 3 weeks when they involve the shaft of long bones. Epiphyseal fractures are potentially more troublesome. Growth plate fractures can disrupt the growth process and can cause major complications if the joint surface is involved. Orthopaedic investigation and referral is imperative.

Other orthopaedic considerations for the young athlete include:

- Shoulder pain: impingment secondary to instability.
- Elbow pain: Panner's disease, osteochondritis dissecans and apophysitis – often due to throwing sports or gymnastics.
- Wrist pain: scaphoid fracture or (rarely) Kienbock's disease (osteonecrosis).
- Back pain: Scheurmann's disease (bone disease affecting the spine).
- Hip pain: Perthes (a condition characterised by a temporary loss of blood supply to the hip. When the blood supply is diverted, the bone of the femoral head (the 'ball' of the 'ball and socket' joint of the hip) dies).
- Knee pain: Osgood–Schlatter disease (caused by the powerful thigh muscles pulling on the attachment point of the patellar tendon such as during sporting activities, ballet dancing and Highland and Irish dancing), Sinding–Larsen–Johansson disease (contusion and subsequent tendonitis in the proximal attachment of the patellar tendon), osteochondritis dissecans, pain referred from hip associated with slipped capital femoral epiphysis or Perthes' disease. A young athlete with a slipped capital femoral epiphysis may present with a painless limp. A bone scan may be necessary for evidence of pathology. Osgood–Schlatter and related Sinding–Larsen–Johannson disease are forms of epiphysitis or osteochondritis and tend to dissipate by the age of 16. They are exacerbated by violent movments such as kicking or jumping. Rest and physiotherapy may help and local corticosteroid injection may bring relief.
- Foot pain: Sever's disease (injury to the growing part of the heel), Kohler's disease (where the navicular bone in the foot undergoes avascular necrosis) or Freiberg's disease (a crushing type of osteochondritis of the second and/or third metatarsals).

The female athlete

There are three musculoskeletal injuries that may occur more frequently in females than males: ACL injuries, stress fractures and patellofemoral problems. The incidence of stress fractures is highest in amenorrheic females, possibly as a result of lower bone density (Tomten et al., 1998). The female's relatively larger angle from the centre of the hip joint to the centre of the knee may leave them susceptible to a variety of biomechanical issues such as patellofemoral pathology and overuse injuries.

Furthermore, females have a much higher predisposition to ACL rupture than males, which is partly attributed to joint laxity and limb alignment (Malinzak, 2001; Ireland, 2002).

The older athlete

Injuries, arthritis, and loss of tissue strength

Sportspeople who have had previous injuries to joints have an increased tendency to develop osteoarthritis. Injuries to joints that have sustained degenerative changes may give rise to disproportionately serious symptoms.

Furthermore, one of the hallmarks of aging, particularly in the elderly, is the associated reduction in muscle strength. Muscle tissue diminishes with age, with a loss of fibres and atrophic changes. Tendons, ligaments and cartilage also suffer from an inactive lifestyle, which has a detrimental effect on their ability to withstand forces and strains. However, these changes can regress and possibly be reversed with regular exercise (Porter *et al.*, 1995). Therefore, the older exerciser has an opportunity to develop stronger, more supple muscle and connective tissue despite degenerative changes.

Management of acute soft tissue injury

Inflammatory process

The inflammatory response is often excessive relative to the amount of soft tissue damage, and if it is not minimised and treated effectively, it can continue to delay healing and lead to loss of strength, flexibility and function. Early and appropriate treatment can significantly enhance the recovery process.

Repair process

As early as 12–24 hours after an injury, new scar tissue and blood vessels are incorporated; however, depending on the nature of the injury the repair process can take weeks or even months. Collagen fibres are laid down as part of the scarring process. It is important to introduce gentle pain-free movement as soon as possible to minimise pain, stiffness and weakness. Movements that gently stretch the scar tissue along the lines of force of the injured tissue will lead to a stronger and more flexible result.

Treatment principles of acute soft tissue injury: RICE to MICE

$$R(rest) + I(ice) + C(compress) + E(elevate) = RICE$$
$$M(movement) + I(ice) + C(compress) + E(elevate) = MICE$$

Rest

For acute lower limb injuries, the use of crutches and relevant support for non-weight-bearing is generally indicated for the first 48–72 hours. Accurate diagnosis is needed to determine when progression to partial and full weight-bearing is appropriate. Acute upper limb injuries are often aided by the use of a sling, strapping or splint as appropriate.

Ice therapy (cryotherapy)

Cryotherapy is particularly useful in the acute phase of an injury as it helps to bring about changes in peripheral circulation, decreases the local metabolic rate and provides anaesthesia (Swenson *et al.*, 1996; Thorsson, 2001). Common application methods for cryotherapy are summarised in Table 4.4.

Ice must never be applied to someone with diminished skin sensation or circulatory deficiency. Changes in tissue temperature depend on the method and duration of application (Swenson *et al.*, 1996). Muscular temperature change also depends on the depth of subcutaneous fat (MacAuley, 2001). Using intermittent applications for 10 minutes is advocated to allow the skin to return to normal while sustaining reduced muscle temperature (Karunakara *et al.*, 1999; MacAuley, 2001) and reducing blood flow by approximately 50% (Thorsson, 2001). This process should be repeated several times per day during the acute phase. Prolonged application at low temperatures may cause nerve injuries or

Table 4.4 Common application methods for cryotherapy

- Rubbing ice cubes over the injured area – care must be taken to stop before ice-burn.
- Bucket of ice water to immerse a hand or foot.
- Crushed ice or frozen food package placed on top of wet towel to avoid skin damage.
- Cold compress pack.
- Inflatable splints.
- Iced towels.
- Refrigerated gases.

frostbite – skin colour change evident of an erythema is a good general indication that the desired effects have been achieved. Both the duration of post-injury muscular bleeding and the relevant effects of ice therapy remain uncertain, however cryotherapy is often used beyond the acute phase to reduce secondary hypoxic injury (Thorsson, 2001). Considerations should be made for patients' susceptibility to injury following cryotherapy, due to subsequent impairment of motor and reflexive function for approximately 30 minutes (MacAuley, 2001).

Compression

Immediate application of compression is an essential part of emergency treatment of an injury (Swensen *et al*., 1996), and should be used throughout the inflammatory phase. An elasticated bandage can be used to cover the entire affected area (see Table 4.5 for guidelines on application). It is extremely important that patients are advised about the potential risks of applying elastic wraps to swelling injuries, and they should be advised to watch for signs of restricted circulation. Bandages should be wrapped loosely at night.

Elevation

As a general guideline, elevating the injured limb above the level of the heart helps to aid venous return. For lower limb injuries, an elevation table can be helpful to keep the injured area above the level of the groin.

RICE to MICE

General guidelines for movement: after 48 hours, movement replaces rest (MICE) but pain should be the guide. Constant pain should fade to

Table 4.5 Principles of elastic wrap application

- Always apply the wrap from distal to proximal, and centre the injury in the middle of the wrap.
- Apply the bandage 10 cm above and below the injured area and be careful to not wrap excessively tight.
- Never finish the wrap on the medial (inside) aspect of a limb.
- For sporting competitions, elastic wrap must be secured with elastic tape, not clips.
- Always check circulation after application.
- Never allow the athlete to wear a tight bandage overnight.
- Educate the user about home application (i.e. wash bandage frequently).

intermittent pain when the repair process is under way. It is very important not to push through intermittent pain aggressively as this will likely slow healing and possibly start the inflammatory process again. The movement should be performed once and may cause some discomfort but should not cause pain. Continue the movement a few times to assess the level of discomfort; if it is only at the end of the movement it should be safe to continue. However, if there is pain on repetition or constant pain after exercising then stop and RICE for another 24 hours and start again.

The diversity of soft tissue injury is extensive, and the injury should be assessed and diagnosed by an appropriately qualified healthcare professional.

Heat therapy

This is particularly helpful in the sub-acute phase of injury as it increases the local cutaneous circulation and metabolic rate for optimal healing. However, it should not be applied in the acute phase. Alternating successive cold and warm water baths with gentle movement is often an effective method of gently increasing the range of movement of a sub-acute injury.

Taping (strapping) and bracing: their role and relevance

Stabilising intervention can be used to facilitate an injured athlete's return to competition or to prevent injury. Both braces and adequate taping can limit movement at a sprained joint and provide support to the related or compromised muscle. It is widely held that the ability to sense or perceive the spatial position and movements of the body (known as 'proprioceptive feedback') is also enhanced and this in turn can benefit the athlete's performance (Beynnon et al., 2002; Ramsey et al., 2003). Taping is known for its loss of effectiveness after approximately 20 minutes of exercise, possibly due to mechanical failure.

Bracing and strapping are not substitutes for rehabilitative exercise, and must work in conjunction with other treatment principles. The guidance of a rehabilitative professional (Chartered Physiotherapist) is essential to achieve the necessary outcome.

Strapping is a highly skilled procedure and if done incorrectly can cause further damage.

Tape and wraps

Athletic tape is manufactured in various sizes and textures and can be elastic or non-elastic. The chosen tape will depend on the treatment aim, the preference of the practitioner or user, the anatomical site to be strapped, the nature of the injury, and the size of the patient. Both wraps and tape come in varying widths, and wraps come in lengths to accommodate large body areas such as the hip and trunk. Some people are skin-sensitive to tape and underwrap is often used for comfort and protection (see Figure 4.8). Hypoallergenic tape (i.e. Strappal Zinc Oxide) is an alternative. Sprays and dressings can be used to help fix the strapping in place.

Non-elastic tape and non-elastic wraps

Using non-elastic tape (i.e. Leukotape) restricts abnormal joint range-of-movement (ROM) and provides optimal joint support (i.e. to prevent excessive ankle inversion). It usually has a porous construction and can be found in varying widths and tensile strengths. Non-elastic cloth wraps can be used in combination with tape, or used independently as a cheaper alternative.

Elastic tape and elastic wraps

These are applied to body parts that require greater degrees of movement (i.e. hamstrings), and to support protective padding to the body (i.e. for contusion). Elastic wraps are especially useful when compression is needed for cryogenic treatment of an acute injury. Elastic wraps vary in quality, but unlike tape they can be reused. The more expensive wraps are often better value, as low-quality wraps can perform poorly with continued reapplication. Some elastic bandages are self-adhesive.

If the goal of using an elastic wrap is to minimise swelling, the wrap must start distal to the injury and wrap proximally towards the heart to increase return of fluid to the circulatory system. Elastic tape would compromise circulation in this case. Patients must be advised about the potential risks of applying elastic wraps to swelling injuries and the signs of restricted circulation. The injured joint should be elevated and wrapped loosely at night.

The key steps in the application of an elastic wrap are given in Table 4.5 and the process is illustrated in Figures 4.9 and 4.10. Whenever possible, the injury should be assessed and diagnosed by an appropriately trained person as quickly as possible.

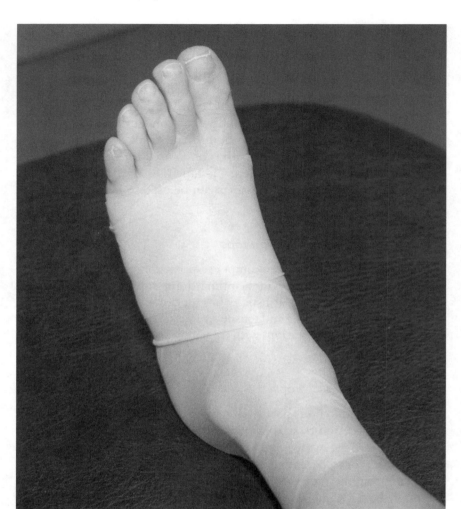

Figure 4.8 Underwrap.

Athletic braces, supports and stabilising aids

Athletes often brace joints with elastic bandages, neoprene sleeves or functional braces in the hope of reducing further injury and enhancing performance. Braces can be used to either supplement or replace athletic strapping, and can be cost-effective as they are reusable. However, functional braces can be very expensive, depending on the design and construction. For athletic purposes, the most commonly used braces are for the ankle, knee,

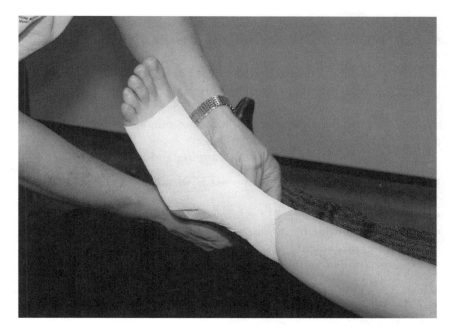

Figure 4.9 Applying elastic wrap to an injured ankle.

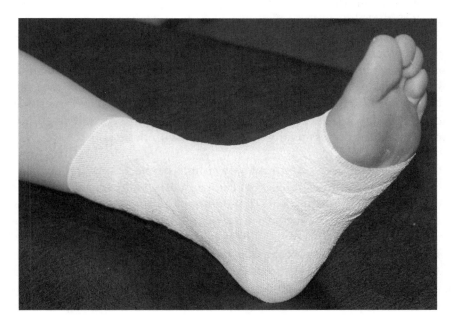

Figure 4.10 A well strapped ankle.

wrist, elbow and shoulder, and are used to support and prevent injury to unstable joints. The fit of a brace is extremely important to ensure its effectiveness and for this reason customised bracing is often used.

There is debate regarding the helpful or harmful effects of wearing braces to support joints or muscles (Birmingham *et al.*, 2002; Ramsey *et al.*, 2003; Spaulding *et al.*, 2003). It is imperative that athletes do not use these aids as an alternative to adequate rehabilitation or develop a psychological dependency on their usage.

In summary, the purposes of strapping and bracing are:

• support damaged connective tissue of unstable joints by limiting movement
• enhance proprioceptive feedback
• support injuries to the muscle-tendon units by compressing and limiting movement
• secure protective splints, pads, and dressings.

A mini-catalogue of common supports and braces is given in Table 4.6.

Figure 4.11 shows an orthopaedic walking brace. It is indicated for metatarsal fractures and severe sprains.

Considerations for regulation   To apply strapping effectively requires a great deal of skill and practice, as well as an understanding of the mechanism of injury and needs of the athlete. Some protective devices can injure other competitors, or give the user an unfair advantage. Furthermore, most governing athletic associations regulate the management of injuries during competition, such as the amount of restriction that can be provided for by bracing and strapping, and the types of materials that can be used. For these reasons, it is most important to consult an appropriate medical professional who is familiar with these issues.

Orthoses (orthotics)   Abnormal lower limb biomechanics can be aided by the use of orthoses to control compensatory and excessive subtalar or midtarsal movements. They should not be considered the only means of treatment for such excessive movement, nor do they change the structural abnormality (Nicolopoulos *et al.*, 2000). Other factors such as shoes, surfaces and muscle imbalance must be considered and addressed. Athletes often do not tolerate large degrees of orthotic foot control and should be observed running to measure the extent of abnormal movement. The key factors influencing the type of orthotic required are severity of abnormal motion, sporting activity, footwear and the weight of the patient.

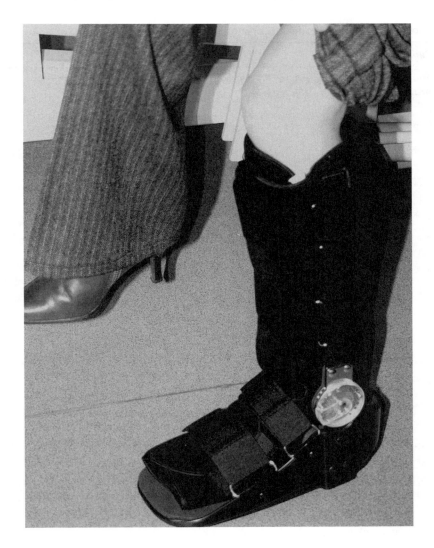

Figure 4.11 Orthopaedic walking brace.

- **Orthoses for over-pronating feet.** Orthotics may be flexible, semi-rigid or rigid. Trainers (running shoes) should have a good heel counter to control movement at the posterior foot, a support across the instep (saddle) to prevent excessive pronation, and a padded opening (collar) to support the ankle. The shoe must have adequate space for an insert.

Table 4.6 A mini-catalogue of common supports and braces

Supports/Braces	Proprietary products
Shoulder immobilising braces: provide support after dislocation	*Vulkan full and half shoulder brace* Thuasne Immo Shoulder
Supports	Vulkan Sports Shoulder: provides support Vulkan Neoprene Wrist Support: provides compression for light strains and swelling Vulkan Back Support: provides compression and warmth Vulkan Elasticated Back Support: includes rear compression strap Vulkan Back Brace: provides greater support for recovery from severe pain and injury. Additional supportive straps help limit unwanted twisting and bending movements Vulkan Elasticated Thigh Support: support and compression Vulkan Neoprene Thigh Support: warmth, compression and support Vulkan Knee Elasticated Support: for acute soft tissue injury management Vulkan Neoprene Knee Support: contoured, three-piece design that does not restrict movement Vulkan Neoprene Knee Free Support: has a patellar opening to help relieve patellar symptoms Vulkan Neoprene Stabilising Knee: helps provide stability Vulkan Patellar Knee Strap: provides compression and support for tendinopathy Vulkan Calf Support: provides compression to lower leg
Elasticated ankle supports: compression for small amounts of swelling	Vulkan Elasticated Ankle Vulkan Neoprene Ankle
Ankle braces	Aircast Standard Ankle Brace: for control of inversion/eversion related to moderate sprains Airsport Ankle Brace: designed for athletes or chronic sprains Swede O AnkleLok: for lateral instability Thuasne Silistab Malleo: for peroneal strains Thuasne Dynastab Ankle Brace: mild to moderate lateral ligament sprains

Table 4.6 *(Continued)*

Supports/Braces	Proprietary products
	Thuasne Ligaflex Ankle Brace: elasticated but helps maintain alignment of ankle. Useful for moderate sprains and chronic instability Thuasne Ankle Sport Strap: allows flexion and extension whilst inhibiting lateral movement
Tendinopathy compression braces	Aircast Tennis Elbow Band Aircast Achilles Wrap: intermittent compression that helps minimise swelling of tendinopathy Vulkan Tennis Elbow Strap: provides compression support Vulkan Tennis Elbow Brace: two-cuff brace with splint that provides support and braces forearm Vulkan Epi-Brace: provides compression support for epicondylitis Thuasne Anti-Epicondylitis Support
Wrist and thumb braces	Rehband Child's Wrist Brace Rehband Thumb Brace: preshaped plastic splint that braces CMC and MCP joints Rehband Thumboform: mouldable insert that can be customised and braces CMC and MCP joints Rehband Support: splint supports MCP and CMC joints Thuasne Thumb Brace: contains splint Thuasne Thumb Strap: prevents hyperextension
Knee braces	Vulkan Neoprene Hinged Knee: has hinges to further control stability Vulkan Functional Knee: brace allows altering of flexion angle for post-operative and instability

- **Preformed orthoses.** These provide conservative control and often give a good indication as to the tolerance of the patient to orthoses and potential benefit for injury management.
- **Casted orthoses.** These plaster orthoses can alter the mechanics significantly and the clinician should be acutely aware of these potential changes.

Prevention of soft tissue injury

The first step in the prevention of injury is to understand the likely predisposing causes, which can be divided loosely into intrinsic and extrinsic factors.

Predisposing intrinsic factors include:

- insufficient fitness training and preparation
- compromised fitness
- sudden increase in activity
- faulty or compromised technique
- muscle imbalance
- inadequate nutrition
- poor psychological preparation for performance
- skeletal structure and body type
- anatomical malalignment
- kinetic dysfunction
- fatigue

Intrinsic causes of injury are often strongly correlated; for instance, improper technique or compromised fitness can not only impede performance but can cause injury due to compromised biomechanics and inefficient effort. Finding a balance between pushing fitness levels and increased susceptibility to injury can be difficult for both unfit individuals and elite athletes, and should be guided by appropriate professionals. Furthermore, many injuries can be avoided or minimised with careful forethought and adequate preparation.

Predisposing extrinsic factors include:

- Environmental factors: training or performance surfaces (i.e. hard or uneven surface, wet pitch), hot/cold temperatures, wet weather, altitude changes.
- Equipment and kit: inadequate protection, poor fit, new equipment requiring adjustments and 'breaking-in'.
- Technical adjustments: in performance technique given by coaches.

Extrinsic factors are often difficult to manage, but need to be anticipated before accidents and ensuing injury. Extremes of temperature can lead to overheating, dehydration or hypothermia; skiers, climbers, distance runners and water-sports participants are at high risk of these concerns. The correct equipment for a given sport is essential to prevent accidents or injury and to enable optimal performance. The improper fit could impede performance and create another hazard for both the wearer and his/her competitors. Men and women often have different protection needs in sports that involve contact or projectiles (i.e. breast protection for women, groin protection for men). Children and teenagers who are still growing should be refitted regularly.

Preventative considerations for the athlete

Massage

Massage (with or without rubifacients) is often used before sports activity in the belief that it will prevent injury and improve recovery rate. The evidence for this is contradictory (see Chapter 6).

'Warming up' and 'cooling down'

'Warming up' is related to the initiation of biological processes that aid physical performance, and 'cooling down' refers to the safe return of exercise-stimulated biological functions to 'normal' resting levels. It is generally accepted that these processes can assist in injury prevention, reduction of muscle soreness, enhanced energy production and improved athletic performance (Bishop *et al.*, 2003; Jones *et al.*, 2003).

Warm-up

While a warm-up is generally considered necessary to optimise athletic capability, little is known about the related parameters of intensity, duration and recovery before performance (Bishop *et al.*, 2003; Jones *et al.*, 2003). As a result, warm-up procedures are usually based on the trial and error experience of the athlete or coach, rather than on scientific study.

Although the benefits of warming up are not fully understood, the aims are numerous. The principal aim is to increase the muscle temperature, thereby increasing the elasticity of muscle and connective tissue, and improving the speed, force and coordination of muscular contraction (Stewart *et al.*, 2003). Aided by the cardiovascular system and hormonal influence, this probably occurs as a result of an increased rate of muscular intracellular chemical reactions, increased conduction speed of nerve impulses, and reduced muscular viscosity via many physiological functions (Shellock *et al.*, 1985; Kato *et al.*, 2000; Gray *et al.*, 2002; Jones *et al.*, 2003). The benefit is likely to reflect the 'type' of warm-up utilised.

Furthermore, the 'proven' benefits of warm-up as related to injury prevention are also mostly anecdotal, although the associated benefits of improved coordination, proprioception, flexibility and reduced fatigue lends a very strong argument for utilising such practice to help avoid injury.

The benefits of warm-up are summarised in Table 4.7.

Principles and guidelines of warm-up   To maximise the potential benefits of active warm-up, specific methods and principles should be adhered to, such as:

* Warm-up should precede every training session or competition/performance.
* Intensity and duration of warm-up depends on the participant's level of fitness and the effects required. Athletes must be careful that the intensity of an active warm-up does not create fatigue.
* Warm-up exercises should progress from easy/simple to more difficult/complex, from large to small muscle groups, and should be selected to suit the individual's needs.
* Resting periods before training commences should not exceed 10 minutes.
* Environmental temperature and clothing must be considered to avoid body heat loss. Passive warm-up (i.e. hot shower) may be helpful in maintaining tissue temperature when an athlete is competing in cold weather (Bishop, 2003), however it does not elicit the same physiological responses from the body and hence does not confer the same benefits (Stanley *et al.*, 1994).

Elite athletes often warm up for an hour or longer. Regardless of duration, key aims must be met for a warm-up to be considered effective and can be broken down into three general stages:

Table 4.7 Benefits of warm-up

Warming up has been shown to have the following benefits:

* Protective effect on athletes with exercise-induced asthma to reduce post-exercise bronchorestriction (McKenzie *et al.*, 1994).
* Reduced DOMS (delayed-onset muscle soreness) (Rodenberg *et al.*, 1994).
* Increased anaerobic power and muscular strength (Rosenbaum *et al.*, 1995; Sen *et al.*, 1992; Stewart *et al.*, 2003).
* Improved flexibility and joint mobility (Ferris 1988).
* Improved gas exchange and buffering of metabolic by-products (Bishop, 2003; Black *et al.*, 1984; Kato *et al.*, 2000; Gray *et al.*, 2002; Jones *et al.*, 2003).
* Improved joint proprioception (Bartlett and Warren, 2002).

1. Activation of the cardiovascular system: this stage should last 5–10 minutes and progress from a slow jog to gentle running and stretching of large muscle groups.
2. Energy pathway stimulation and elevation of muscle temperature: this stage lasts for 10–15 minutes and involves higher-intensity cardiovascular work and the muscle-tendon units are stretched to full range. All muscle groups should be stretched and sweating should be moderate.
3. Specific soft tissue injury prevention: for another 5–10 minutes the individual should concentrate on those areas known to be tight or limited in range of movement. Oscillatory movements to loosen joints through full range of movement and sport-specific stretches and movement are utilised.

Cool-down

Cooling-down procedures have been likened to 'active recovery'. It allows a gradual slowing and balance of physiological processes after exercise, in order to help avoid muscle cramping, blood pooling and slow removal of waste products such as lactic acid (Takahashi *et al.*, 2002). Cool-down stages and procedures are in the reverse order to warm-up procedures.

Stretching

Research has not yet provided conclusive evidence regarding the benefits of stretching (Weldon and Hill, 2003; Thacker *et al.*, 2004). However, different types of stretching can seemingly produce varying results. Proprioceptive neuromuscular facilitation (PNF) techniques have been shown to produce superior hamstring flexibility to static stretching, when both were undertaken after exercise (Funk *et al.*, 2003). Furthermore, static stretching has been found to increase hamstring length for up to 24 hours regardless of prior warm-up exercise (de Weijer *et al.*, 2003). It has also been shown that the total stretching time within a day was more important than duration of a single stretch (Cipriani *et al.*, 2003). Tissue should be stretched to the point of tension or discomfort, but pain should be avoided, and as this is a largely subjective measure it should be approached cautiously. Extreme caution should be exercised in the case of tissues that are healing.

Flexibility

Flexibility refers to the general extensibility of tissues, principally peri-articular, in allowing physiological movement at a joint. It is generally agreed that flexibility is joint-specific and not uniform through any given individual and the strains placed on tissues related to particular activities are partly responsible for these differences (Alter, 1996). Long-term repetitive trauma can result in deformed tissues that exhibit reduced stability and efficiency.

Flexibility training is an important part of specificity training and injury prevention, and should be reflective of frequent movement patterns related to that sport. Therefore, functional flexibility is specific to the nature of the movement of a given athletic discipline, and takes into account factors such as speed, angle and range of movement. Static flexibility, however, does not necessitate movement through a joint's range.

The benefit of extensibility and joint mobility is dependent on its relevance to the discipline undertaken; not all athletes require extreme range of movement (ROM). Whether a lack of flexibility predisposes an athlete to injury is not quantified or proven. However, conventional wisdom suggests that 'short' muscle and connective tissue limits joint mobility and therefore can impede performance and increase the likeli-hood of injury.

Soft tissue extensibility and injury prevention

Joint flexibility requires stability provided by connective tissue and muscle to ensure that the joint is not compromised in any part of the range of movement.

An athlete would also be wise to be cautious about stretching weak muscle, as this may contribute further to joint instability. There is generally an optimal balance between flexibility and stability that will potentially prevent injury from overstretching tissues. This has import-ant implications for athletes as they must strengthen those body parts most likely to be stressed. Many elite athletes, such as gymnasts and ballet dancers, often have excessive joint ROM, known as laxity. Hyper-mobility is established by noting excessive ROM in many joints. This condition may be linked to chronic injury, elastin ratios in connective tissue, or hereditary conditions such as Ehlers–Danlos syndrome (Keer *et al.*, 2003).

General advice that may be offered to assist injury prevention is shown in Table 4.8.

Table 4.8 General advice for injury prevention

- Know your body's fitness level and understand your limitations.
- Assess the risks particular to your sport.
- Set realistic targets.
- Make sure you have adequate equipment – ask the experts.
- Do not 'train through pain' – get professional advice EARLY and adhere to advice.
- Do not train hard when you are ill.
- Familiarise with temperature, altitude, food, time shift (jet lag).
- Be sure to warm up and cool down with adequate stretching.

Overload training and overtraining

Training adaptation to overload requires specific recovery time. Overload training can be regarded as a positive process when the end result is adaptation and improved performance. However, overtraining without adequate recovery can cause a myriad of problems for the athlete and adversely affect performance (Fry *et al.*, 1991; McKenzie, 1999; Clow and Hucklebridge, 2001). Overtraining may lead to musculoskeletal injury and detrimental biomechanical adaptations (Kibler *et al.*, 1992). Screening throughout training cycles minimises the confusion of fatigue from overload training with that of overtraining (Fry *et al.*, 1991).

Recovery and fatigue

Many athletes suffer from acute fatigue occasionally, which may be defined as an inability to maintain a particular physical demand or rate of demand. This has significant implications for performance capability and injury prevention. Short-term fatigue can be caused by a depletion of muscle glycogen or phosphocreatine, decrease in blood glucose, dehydration, or a build-up of lactic acid. This sense of fatigue may itself affect coordination, which could lead to injury.

Many athletes are obsessive about training and feel guilty if they take a rest for even a single day. Closely spaced intensive workouts leave some muscles injured and depleted of glycogen while the remaining functioning fibres are subjected to more stress, which increases the likelihood of injury. Alternating workout intensities and targeted muscle groups can help prevent this type of injury (Kraemer *et al.*, 1998). It would be wise to suggest that one day of complete rest is included in a weekly training schedule.

Musculoskeletal injuries, psychological problems (Clow and Hucklebridge, 2001), neuroendocrine irregularities and immune system suppression can be chronic problems for athletes (Scott, 2002). Over-training is also a common cause of ongoing fatigue, whose clinical presentation is non-specific but common symptoms also include frequent illness and injury, emotional disturbances and a related decrease in performance (Kibler *et al.*, 1992; McKenzie, 1999; Scott, 2002).

To fully understand the decrease in performance levels due to chronic fatigue, the clinician must consider the interrelationship of the different systems possibly affected. It has been suggested that repeated non-physical stresses can lead to a dysfunction of the hypothalamic pituitary axis, and psychological testing may be the most helpful in revealing the early warning signs of this condition (McKenzie, 1999). It is also clinically important to consider the possibility of eating disorders or nutritional deficiency. Furthermore, recovery time due to overtraining can impede the training progress and compound the deconditioning process. This further emphasises the importance of a carefully monitored recovery process (Kenta and Hassmen, 1998).

Delayed-onset muscle soreness

Athletes commonly complain of muscle tenderness, pain and stiffness with movement – this is described as delayed-onset muscle soreness (DOMS) and can last for 1–5 days post-exercise. Pain can be quite severe and some research has suggested that DOMS is related to an acute inflammatory response (Smith, 1991). DOMS tends to be most prevalent when there has been a change in training parameters such as duration or frequency. This condition can not only disrupt training but can also cause compensatory alterations in motor patterns and technique, and thereby increase the risk of further injury and affect athletic performance (Armstrong, 1984; Cheung *et al.*, 2003).

Although treatment strategies remain uncertain, exercise appears to be the most effective means of alleviating pain during DOMS (Armstrong, 1984; Cheung *et al.*, 2003). However, a reduction of exercise intensity and duration is needed for 1–2 days after DOMS-inducing exercise (Cheung *et al.*, 2003). Particular care should be taken with eccentric exercises as they have been shown to induce micro-injury at a greater rate and severity than other muscular actions (Smith, 1991; Cheung *et al.*, 2003) (see also Chapter 6).

Muscle cramp

Analysis of the scientific literature has caused dispute over the definitive causes of cramp, and some researchers suggest muscle cramp is a result of sustained abnormal spinal reflex activity (Schwellnus *et al.*, 1997). Although preventative strategies are yet to be proven, cramp can often be immediately relieved by gently stretching the affected muscle (Bentley, 1996) (see also Chapter 6).

Sports injury and athletic rehabilitation

Although the athletic rehabilitative process will usually involve the relevant coach, manager, medical staff, parents, sports scientist, exercise physiologist, and psychologist, the physiotherapist is likely to make the initial injury assessment and direct referral to other practitioners as required. Throughout the rehabilitative process, the physiotherapist's role in clinical decision-making and coordination of clinical input will have a great bearing on the eventual outcome for the injured athlete.

Rehabilitation of an athlete must account for much more than the appropriate healing of the injured structures. Rehabilitation programmes involve a series of short- and long-term goals, which will depend on the nature of the injury, subsequent deconditioning, and related complications. Injured athletes are often very keen to return to their respective sport, however their enthusiasm can lead to them rushing their rehabilitation and ignoring their programme or need for rest. Progress is monitored and goals are reassessed on an ongoing basis, however it is of paramount importance not to disregard strict rehabilitative protocols. It is imperative that the athlete is 'retrained' and rehabilitated to fitness levels for optimal performance and secondary injury prevention.

Rehabilitative aims

It is crucial that the exercises and treatment are appropriate for the individual and the relevant stage of rehabilitation. Maintaining strength and joint range of movement are very important early objectives. Short-term aims for injury management largely involve correcting biomechanical and neuromuscular dysfunction, while minimising deconditioning of the athlete. Remodelling procedures such as stretching and manual mobilisation play a vital role in creating strong but flexible tissue, and returning the athlete to full function involves a multitude of therapies.

Neuromuscular, flexibility, cardiovascular and endurance training are adopted as quickly as possible and are often achieved through adopting alternative exercises and fitness regimes. Proprioceptive training may involve the use of a 'wobble' board (see Figure 4.13). The wobble board is probably one of the most widely used pieces of equipment for training core stability, balance and aiding in the rehabilitation of ankle and knee injuries. Hydrotherapy may also be useful in rehabilitation (see Figure 4.14).

Eventually issues such as speed, power, skill and endurance are addressed as part of the functional rehabilitative process specific to the

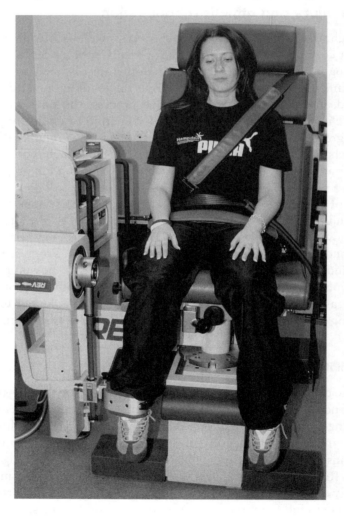

Figure 4.12 Isokinetic dynamometer.

demands of the individual athlete's sport. Muscle power and strength may be evaluated and monitored using an isokinetic dynamometer (see Figure 4.12).

Sport specificity and injury prevention

Injury prevention is an essential component of any exercise training programme, and certainly many acute and chronic injuries could be avoided. Performance enhancement and injury prevention necessitates

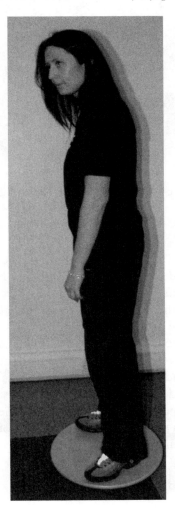

Figure 4.13 Wobble board.

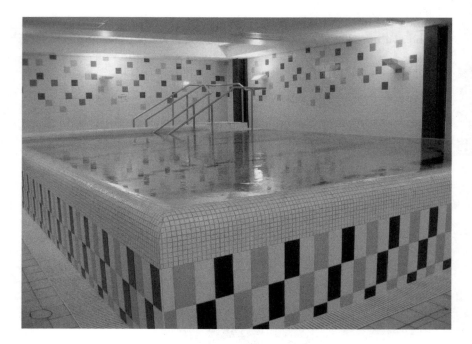

Figure 4.14 Hydrotherapy pool at the Scottish National Stadium, Hampden Park, Glasgow.

the coordination of training and conditioning specific to the demands of the sport and tailored to the individual athlete. Neuromusculoskeletal screenings, fitness tests and skill evaluations give the physiotherapist, exercise scientist and the performance coach the relevant information on how to best serve the athlete. Compromises in cardiovascular fitness, strength, proprioception, flexibility and stability can lead to fatigue and poor technique, and result in injury. The demands of different sports vary enormously, and specificity training helps to ensure that the principles of overload and adaptation meet those demands and elicit maximum performance. 'Prehabilitation' is the primary phase of rehabilitation and places the emphasis on injury prevention, education and related strengthening and conditioning.

Injury identification and management

The recognition of problems early or prior to the onset of injury is of vital importance in achieving the quickest recovery possible and to help avoid ensuing complications. Many athletes make the mistake of ignoring seemingly minor symptoms or letting 'nature run its course' when dealing with an injury and do not realise the potential implications. This in turn makes them very susceptible to reinjury or prolonged recovery, and compromises their performance capabilities. Secondary rehabilitation is geared towards minimising the damage incurred, which includes treatment, exercise modification, conditioning, etc. By tracking and effectively managing developing problems at this secondary stage, tertiary problems (indicated by rest, passive treatment, etc.), which have major implications for an athlete's fitness due to the rest required, can be avoided. Effective management in the secondary stage also helps in recognising injury trends, which can depend on the type of training regime they have been undertaking or other causative factors.

Furthermore, the importance of proper diagnosis and guidance through injury recovery by a trained professional cannot be overemphasised. Unfortunately, many elite and amateur athletes do not have ready access to relevant healthcare professionals and therefore differential diagnosis and adherence to rehabilitative programmes is often compromised. Chartered Physiotherapists are medical professionals trained in rehabilitative medicine, and many specialise in athletic rehabilitation. They will begin their treatment with assessment and diagnosis, and may offer manual treatment, biomechanical analysis, education, ultrasound, electrotherapy, laser therapy, hydrotherapy, strapping, orthopaedic devices, heat, cold, traction, etc. The length of time needed for physiotherapy depends on the severity and complexity of the injury. The Chartered Society of Physiotherapy (CSP) can provide advice and guidance regarding contacting an appropriate practitioner (www.csp.org.uk). Athletes should be encouraged to see a Chartered Physiotherapist specialising in sports medicine as soon as possible after an injury to ensure the most efficient and complete recovery. There is also a UK organisation known as the Association of Chartered Physiotherapists in Sports Medicine (ACPSM), who can be contacted at www.acpsm.org.uk.

Adherence to rehabilitation

Most research into patient compliance with injury rehabilitation has been focused on determining key issues categorised as personal or situational factors (see also Chapter 2). Although few conclusions can be drawn, specific patterns have been identified. Belief in the effectiveness of the treatment, pain tolerence, and support from others have been found to be statistically significant predictors of adherence to athletic rehabilitation programs (Duda *et al.*, 1989; Byerly *et al.*, 1994). Although making an athlete aware of the potential implications of poor adherence (i.e. reinjury) may enhance patient compliance (Taylor and May, 1996), practitioners using threat or fear as a motivator may harm the relationship with the athlete.

Most authorities agree that given the potential range of psychological, emotional and behavioural changes often associated with injury rehabilitation, a holistic approach is often best (Friedman and Litt, 1987; Fisher, 1999; Schindler and Zimmerman, 1999). Principally, the quality of interaction between the athlete and the therapist, the rehabilitative setting, the self-confidence of the athlete, and the therapist's ability to determine the needs of the athlete are central to compliance and adherence to rehabilitation (Fisher, 1990).

Financial aspects of rehabilitation

Rehabilitation can be neglected by many athletes because of the costs involved, and for many the problem is compounded by loss of earnings while they are not participating because of injury. Financial loss and restriction from sport can often have a significant psychological impact on the sportsperson. Athletes' injuries must be addressed promptly, and hence waiting lists within public health systems are often problematic for them. Even those with health insurance coverage must usually visit their GP initially for referral, and often the coverage is very limited for physiotherapy outpatient care. Practitioners often have to subsidise fees to accommodate low-income earners but they also have a responsibility to be careful about financial decisions. With increasing reliance on the private sector of health care to address these concerns, the athlete is often faced with a financial and professional crisis.

References

Ageberg E (2002). Consequences of a ligament injury on neuromuscular function and relevance to rehabilitation – using the anterior cruciate ligament as model. *J Electromyogr Kinesiol* 12: 205–212.
Almekinders L C, Weinhold P S, Maffulli N (2003). Compression etiology in tendinopathy. *Clin Sports Med* 22: 703–710.
Alter M J (1996). *Science of Flexibility*, 2nd edn. Champaign, IL: Human Kinetics.
Armstrong R B (1984). Mechanisms of exercise-induced delayed onset muscular soreness: a brief review. *Med Sci Sports Exerc* 16: 529–538.

Bartlett M J, Warren P J (2002). Effect of warming up on knee proprioception before sporting activity. *Br J Sports Med* 36: 132–134.

Bentley S (1996). Exercise-induced muscle cramp. Proposed mechanisms and management. *Sports Med* 21: 409–420.

Beynnon B D, Good L, Risberg M A (2002). The effect of bracing on proprioception of knees with anterior cruciate ligament injury. *J Orthop Sports Phys Ther* 32: 11–15.

Birmingham T B, Kramer J F, Kirkley A (2002). Effect of a functional brace on knee flexion and extension strength after anterior cruciate ligament reconstruction. *Arch Phys Med Rehabil* 83: 1472–1475.

Bishop D (2003). Warm up II: performance changes following active warm up and how to structure the warm up. *Sports Med* 33: 483–498.

Black A, Ribiero J P, Bochese M A (1984). Effects of previous exercise on the ventilatory determination of the aerobic threshold. *Eur J Appl Physiol* 52: 315–319.

Bonfim T R, Paccola C A J, Barela J A (2003). Proprioceptive and behaviour impairments in individuals with anterior cruciate ligament reconstructed knees. *Arch Phys Med Rehabil* 84: 1217–1223.

Bruckner P (1993). Sports medicine in Australia. *Med J Aust* 158: 511–512.

Byerly P N, Worrell T, Gahimer J, *et al.* (1994). Rehabilitation compliance in an athletic training environment. *J Athletic Train* 29: 352–355.

Cheung K, Hume P, Maxwell L (2003). Delayed onset muscle soreness: treatment strategies and performance factors. *Sports Med* 33: 145–164.

Cipriani D, Abel B, Pirrwitz D (2003). A comparison of two stretching protocols on hip range of motion: implications for total daily stretch duration. *J Strength Cond Res* 17: 274–278.

Clow A, Hucklebridge F (2001). The impact of psychological stress on immune function in the athletic population. *Exerc Immunol Rev* 7: 5–17.

Costa M L, Shepstone L, Darrah C, *et al.* (2003). Immediate full-weight-bearing mobilization for repaired Achilles tendon ruptures: a pilot study. *Injury* 34: 874–876.

DeWeijer V C, Gorniak G C, Shamus E (2003). The effect of static stretch and warm-up exercise on hamstring length over the course of 24 hours. *J Orthop Sports Phys Ther* 33: 727–733.

Duda J L, Smart A E, Tappe M L (1989). Predictors of adherence in the rehabilitation of athletic injuries: an application of personal investment theory. *J Sport Exerc Psychol* 11: 367–381.

Dye S F (1996). The knee as a biologic transmission with an envelope of function. *Clin Orthop* 325: 10–18.

Feinberg J H, Nadler S F, Krivickas L S (1997). Peripheral nerve injuries in the athlete. *Sports Med* 24: 385–408.

Ferris M F (1998). Warm-up, flexibility, and exercise. *Scott J Phys Ed* 16: 8–11.

Fisher A C (1990). Adherence to sports injury rehabilitation programmes. *Sports Med* 9: 151–158.

Fisher A C (1999). Counselling for improved rehabilitation adherence. In: Ray R, Wiese-Bjornstal D M, eds. *Counselling in Sports Medicine*. Champagne, IL: Human Kinetics, 275–292.

Francis A, Thomas R de W M, McGregor A (2001). Anterior cruciate ligament rupture: reconstruction surgery and rehabilitation. A nation-wide survey of current practice. *Knee* 8: 13–18.

Friedman I M, Litt I F (1987). Adolescents' compliance with therapeutic regimes: psychological and social aspects and intervention. *J Adolesc Health Care* 8: 52–67.

Fry R W, Morton A R, Keast D (1991). Overtraining in athletes. An update. *Sports Med* 12: 32–65.

Funk D C, Swank A M, Mikla B M, *et al.* (2003). Impact of prior exercise on hamstring flexibility: a comparison of proprioceptive neuromuscular facilitation and static stretching. *J Strength Cond Res* 17: 489–492.

Gray S C, Devito G, Nimmo M A (2002). Effect of active warm-up on metabolism prior to and during intense dynamic exercise. *Med Sci Sports Exerc* 34: 2091–2096.

Ireland M L (2002). The female ACL: why is it more prone to injury? *Orthop Clin North Am* 33: 637–651.

Jarvinen T A, Kaariainen M, Jarvinen M, *et al.* (2000). Muscle strain injuries. *Curr Opin Rheumatol* 12: 155–161.

Jones A M, Koppo K, Burnley M (2003). Effects of prior exercise on metabolic and gas exchange responses to exercise. *Sports Med* 33: 949–971.

Karmani S, Ember T (2004). The anterior cruciate ligament – II. *Curr Orthop* 18: 49–57.

Karunakara R G, Lephart S M, Pincivero D M (1999). Changes in forearm blood flow during single and intermittent cold application. *J Orthop Sports Phys Ther* 29: 177–80.

Kato Y, Ikata T, Takai H, *et al.* (2000). Effects of specific warm-up at various intensities on energy metabolism during subsequent exercise. *J Sports Med Phys Fitness* 40: 126–130.

Keer R, Graham R, eds (2003). *Hypermobility Syndrome Recognition and Management for Physiotherapists*. London: Butterworth Heinemann.

Khan K M, Cook J L, Kannus P, *et al.* (2002). Time to abandon the "tendonitis" myth. *BMJ* 324: 627–628.

Kibler W B, Chandler T J, Stracener E S (1992). Musculoskeletal adaptations and injuries due to overtraining. *Exerc Sport Sci Rev* 20: 99–126.

Kraemer W J, Duncan N D, Volek J S (1998). Resistance training and elite athletes: adaptations and program considerations. *J Orthop Sports Phys Ther* 28: 110–119.

Lorei M P, Hershman E B (1993). Peripheral nerve injuries in athletes. Treatment and prevention. *Sports Med* 16: 130–147.

Lu H, Gu G, Zhu S (1996). [Heel pain and calcaneal spurs]. *Chung Hua Wai Ko Tsa Chih* 34: 294–296.

Lynch R M (2004). Achilles tendon rupture: surgical versus non-surgical treatment. *Accident Emergency Nursing* 12: 149–158.

Malinzak R A, Colby S M, Kirkendall D T, *et al.* (2001). A comparison of knee joint motion patterns between men and women in selected athletic tasks. *Clin Biomech* 16: 438–445.

MacAuley D C (2001). Ice therapy: how good is the evidence? *Int J Sports Med* 22: 379–384.

McKenzie D C (1999). Markers of excessive exercise. *Can J Appl Physiol* 24: 66–73.

McKenzie D C, McLuckie S L, Stirling D R (1994). The protective effects of continuous and interval exercise in athletes with exercised-induced asthma. *Med Sci Sports Exerc* 26: 951–956.

Muhle C, Ahn J M, Yeh L, *et al.* (1999). Iliotibial band friction syndrome: MR imaging findings in 16 patients and MR arthrographic study of six cadaveric knees. *Radiology* 212: 103–110.

Nicholas S J, Tyler T F (2002). Adductor muscle strains in sport. *Sports Med* 32: 339–344.

Nicolopoulos C S, Scott B W, Giannoudis P V (2000). Biomechanical basis of foot orthotic prescription. *Curr Orthopaed* 14: 464–469.

Perlmutter G S, Apruzzese W (1998). Axillary nerve injuries in contact sports: recommendations for treatment and rehabilitation. *Sports Med* 26: 351–361.

Porter M M, Vandervoort A A, Lexell J (1995). Aging of human muscle: structure, function, and adaptability. *Scand J Med Sci Sports* 5: 129–142.

Ramsey D K, Wretenberg P F, Lamontagne M, *et al.* (2003). Electromyographic and biomechanic analysis of anterior cruciate ligament deficiency and functional knee bracing. *Clin Biomech* 18: 28–34.

Rodenberg J B, Steenbeck D, Schiereck P, *et al.* (1994). Warm-up, stretching and massage diminish harmful effects of eccentric exercise. *Int J Sports Med* 15: 414–419.

Rosenbaum D, Hennig E M (1995). The influence of stretching and warm-up exercises on Achilles tendon reflex activity. *J Sports Sci* 13: 481–490.

Schindler Zimmerman T (1999). Using family systems theory to counsel the injured athlete. In: Ray R, Wiese-Bjornstal D M, eds. *Counselling in Sports Medicine.* Champagne, IL: Human Kinetics, 111–126.

Schwellnus M P, Derman E W, Noakes T D (1997). Aetiology of skeletal muscle 'cramps' during exercise: a novel hypothesis. *J Sports Sci* 15: 277–285.

Scott W A (2002). Maximizing performance and the prevention of injuries in competitive athletes. *Curr Sports Med Rep* 1: 184–190.

Sen C, Grucza R, Pekkarinen H, *et al.* (1992). Anaerobic power response to simulated warm-up procedures for skiers. *Biol Sport* 9: 103–108.

Shellock F G, Prentice W E (1985). Warming-up and stretching for improved physical performance and prevention of sports-related injuries. *Sports Med* 2: 267–278.

Smith L L (1991). Acute inflammation: the underlying mechanism in delayed onset muscle soreness? *Med Sci Sports Exerc* 23: 542–551.

Spaulding S J, Livingston L A, Hartsell H D (2003). The influence of external orthotic support on the adaptive gait characteristics of individuals with chronically unstable ankles. *Gait Posture* 17: 152–158.

Stanley D C, Kraemer W J, Howard R L, *et al.* (1994). The effects of hot water immersion on muscle strength. *J Strength Cond Res* 8: 134–138.

Sternbach G (1999). The carpal tunnel syndrome. *J Emerg Med* 17: 519–523.

Stewart D, Macaluso A, De Vito G (2003). The effect of an active warm-up on surface EMG and muscle performance in healthy humans. *Eur J Appl Physiol* 89: 509–513.

Swenson C, Sward L, Karlsson J (1996). Cryotherapy in sports medicine. *Scand J Med Sci Sports* 6: 193–200.

Takahashi T, Okada A, Hayano J, *et al.* (2002). Influence of cool-down exercise on autonomic control of heart rate during recovery from dynamic exercise. *Front Med Biol Eng* 11: 249–259.

Thacker S B, Gilchrist J, Stroup D F, *et al.* (2004). The impact of stretching on sports injury risk: a systematic review of the literature. *Med Sci Sports Exerc* 36: 371–378.

Thorsson O (2001). [Cold therapy of athletic injuries. Current literature review] *Lakartidningen* 98: 1512–1513.

Tomten S E, Falch J A, Birkeland K I, *et al.* (1998). Bone mineral density and menstrual irregularities. A comparative study on cortical and trabecular bone structures in runners with alleged normal eating behaviour. *Int J Sports Med* 19: 92–97.

Further reading

Alter, M J (1998). *Sport Stretch*. Leeds: Human Kinetics.

Alfredson H, Lorentzon R (2000). Chronic Achilles tendinosis: recommendations for treatment and prevention. *Sports Med* 29: 135–146.

Baechle T R (2000). *Essentials of Strength Training and Conditioning*. Leeds: Human Kinetics.

Bare A A, Haddad S L (2001). Tenosynovitis of the posterior tibial tendon. *Foot Ankle Clin* 6: 37–66.

Bartold S J (1997). Conservative management of plantar fasciitis. *Sport Health* 10: 17–28.

Bartold S J (2001). Biomechanical problems of the lower limb. In: Marfuli N, Chan K M, McDonald R, *et al.*, eds. *Sports Medicine for Specific Ages and Abilities*. Edinburgh: Churchill Livingstone, 425–435.

Beynnon B D, Ryder S H, Konradsen L, *et al.* (1999). The effect of anterior cruciate ligament trauma and bracing on knee proprioception. *Am J Sports Med* 27: 150–155.

Borsa P A, Lephart S M, Irrgang J J, *et al.* (1997). The effects of joint position and direction of joint motion on proprioceptive sensibility in anterior cruciate ligament-deficient athletes. *Am J Sports Med* 25: 336–340.

Bradshaw C, McCrory P, Bell S, *et al.* (1997). Obturator Nerve Entrapment. A cause of groin pain in athletes. *Am J Sports Med* 25: 402–408.

Cochrane D J (2004). Alternating hot and cold water immersion for athlete recovery: a review. *Phys Ther Sport* 5: 26–32.

Cornwall M W, McPoil T G (1999). Plantar fasciitis; etiology and treatment. *J Orthopaed Sports Phys Ther* 29: 756–760.

Corrigan J P, Cashman W F, Brady M P (1992). Proprioception in the cruciate deficient knee. *J Bone Joint Surg* 74: 247–250.

Daum W J (1995). The sacroiliac joint: an underappreciated pain generator. *Am J Orthop* 24: 475–478.

DeMaio M, Payne R, Mangine R E, *et al.* (1993). Plantar fasciitis. *Orthopaedics* 16: 1153–1162.

De Paulis F, Cacchio A, Michelini O, *et al.* (1998). Sports injuries in the pelvis and hip: diagnostic imaging. *Eur J Radiol* 27: S49–S59.

DonTigny R L (1979). Dysfunction of the sacroiliac joint and its treatment. *J Ortho Sports Phys Ther* 1: 23–35.

DonTigny R L (1985). Function and pathomechanics of the sacroiliac joint. A review. *Phys Ther* 65: 35–44.

Fomby E W, Mellion M B (1997). Identifying and treating myofascial pain syndrome. *The Physician and Sports Medicine* 25: 67–75.

Fry R W, Morton A R, Keast D (1992). Periodisation and the prevention of over-training. *Can J Sport Sci* Sep 17: 241–248.

Gilmore J (1998). Groin pain in the soccer athlete: fact, fiction, and treatment. *Clin Sports Med* 17: 787–793.

Hackney R G (1997). The sports hernia. *Sports Med Arthroscop Rev* 5: 320–325.

Harris J, Elbourn J (2001). *Warming Up and Cooling Down*. Leeds: Human Kinetics.

Harvey G, Bell S (1999). Obturator neuropathy. An anatomic perspective. *Clin Orthop* 363: 203–211.

Hertel J, Denegar C R, Buckley W E, *et al.* (2001). Effect of rearfoot orthotics on postural sway after lateral ankle sprain. *Arch Phys Med Rehabil* 82: 1000–1003.

Holmich P, Uhrskou P, Ulnits L, *et al.* (1999). Effectiveness of active physical training as treatment for longstanding adductor-related groin pain in athletes: ran-domised trial. *Lancet* 353: 439–443.

Kentta G, Hassmen P (1998). Overtraining and recovery. A conceptual model. *Sports Med* Jul 26: 1–16.

Kibler W B, Chandler T J. (1994). Sport-specific conditioning. *Am J Sports Med* 22: 424–432.

Kogler G F, Solomonidis S E, Poole J P (1996). Biomechanics of longitudinal arch support mechanisms in foot orthoses and their affect on plantar aponeurosis strain. *Clin Biomechanics* 11: 243–252.

Kosmahl E M, Kosmahl H E (1987). Painful plantar heel, plantar fasciitis and cal-caneal spur: etiology and treatment. *J Orthop Sports Phys Ther* 9: 14–17.

Koutedakis Y, Sharp N C. (1998). Seasonal variations of injury and overtraining in elite athletes. *Clin J Sport Med* Jan 8: 18–21.

Leach R E, Seavey M S, Salter D K (1996). Results of surgery in athletes with plantar fasciitis. *Foot and Ankle* 7: 156–161.

Martin R L, Irrgang J J, Conti S F (1998). Outcome study of subjects with inser-tional plantar fasciitis. *Foot Ankle Inter* 19: 803–811.

McCrory J L, Martin D F, *et al.* (1999). Etiologic factors associated with Achilles tendinitis in runners. *Med Sci Sports Exerc* 31: 1374–1381.

Mellion M B (1991). Common cycling injuries. Management and prevention. *Sports Med* 11: 52–70.

Minoyama O, Uchiyama E, Iwaso, H *et al.* (2002). Two cases of peroneus brevis tendon tear. *Br J Sports Med* 36: 65–66.

Mozes M, Papa M Z, Zweig A *et al.* (1985). Iliopsoas injury in soccer players. *Br J Sports Med* 19: 168–170.

Nicholls R A (2004). Intra-articular disorders of the hip in athletes. *Phys Ther Sport* 5: 17–25.

O'Brien M, Delaney M (1997). The anatomy of the hip and groin. *Sports Med Arthroscop Rev* 5: 252–267.

Paish W (1998). *The Complete Manual of Sports Science*. London: A & C Black.

Pearson P (1998). *Safe and Effective Exercise*. Marlborough: Crowood Press.

Pecina M M, Bojanic I (1993). *Overuse injuries of the musculoskeletal system.* Boston: CRC Press.

Risberg M A, Lewek M, Snyder-Mackler L (2004). A systematic review of evidence for anterior cruciate ligament rehabilitation: how much and what type? *Phys Ther Sport* 5: 125–145.

Roberts C P, Palmer S, Vince A and Deliss L J (2001). Dynamised cast management of Achilles tendon ruptures. *Injury* 32: 423–426.

Roberts D, Fridén T, Zätterström R, *et al.* (1999). Proprioception in people with anterior cruciate ligament-deficient knees: comparison of symptomatic and asymptomatic patients. *J Orthop Sports Phys Ther* 29: 587–594.

Schepsis A A, Jones H, Haas A L (2002). Achilles tendon disorders in athletes. *Am J Sports Med* 30: 287–305.

Seligman D A, Dawson D R (2003). Customized heel pads and soft orthotics to treat heel pain and plantar fasciitis. *Arch Phys Med Rehabil* 84: 1564–1567.

Snyder A C (1998). Overtraining and glycogen depletion hypothesis. *Med Sci Sports Exerc* 30: 1146–1150.

Spetch L A, Kolt G S (2001). Adherence to sport injury rehabilitation: implications for sports medicine providers and researchers. *Phys Ther Sport* 2: 80–90.

Taylor A H, May S (1996). Threat and coping appraisal as determinants of compliance with sports injury rehabilitation: an application of protection motivation theory. *J Sports Sci* 14: 471–482.

Touliopolous S, Hershman E B (1999). Lower leg pain. Diagnosis and treatment of compartment syndromes and other pain syndromes of the leg. *Sports Med* 27: 193–204.

Weldon S M, Hill R H (2003). The efficacy of stretching for prevention of exercise-related injury: a systematic review of the literature. *Man Ther* 8: 141–150.

Wilmore J, Costill D (1999). *Physiology of Sport and Exercise*, 2nd edn. Leeds: Human Kinetics.

Useful addresses

Chartered Society of Physiotherapy
14 Bedford Row
London WC1R 4ED
Tel: +44 (0)20 7306 6666
http://www.csp.org.uk

Association of Chartered Physiotherapists in Sports Medicine
5 Ewden House
12 Holyrood Avenue
Lodge Moor
Sheffield S10 4NW
Tel: +44 (0)114 230 5665
http://www.acpsm.org

5

Pharmacotherapy for soft tissue injury

Mark C Stuart

Introduction

Even in athletes with the most efficient training programmes, a near-perfect diet, and state-of-the-art equipment and footwear, injury is still almost a fundamental certainty. Pharmacotherapy can effectively complement physical treatment, with anti-inflammatory drugs being most commonly used for soft tissue injury (see Chapter 4).

The pharmacy is very often the first port of call for athletes with injuries, which may range from a minor graze caused by a fall on the field, to serious musculoskeletal injury including ligament rupture and broken bones. Pharmacists should be able to recognise the signs and symptoms of sports and exercise related injuries, understand the pharmacology of suitable drug treatments, and recognise more serious symptoms of conditions that require referral.

The effect of other drugs on performance should also be considered when treating sportspeople. For example, tendon inflammation and rupture may occur with quinolone antibiotics such as ciprofloxacin. These reactions have been observed particularly in older patients and in those treated concurrently with corticosteroids. Treatment with such drugs should be reviewed at the first sign of pain or inflammation.

Most soft tissue injuries will heal completely given sufficient time, with most people recovering to full previous functional ability. Particularly with professional athletes, the time to recovery can be a critical factor in the athlete's continued performance and even career prospects. For some athletes, pharmacotherapy may be one way to accelerate the natural timescale of recovery.

Performance continuation in sport

In sports medicine, the ethical boundary between the use of pharmacotherapy for the treatment of injury and the use of drugs to enhance performance is often debated.

Amendments to the list of prohibited substances reflect changing opinions on drug use for performance continuation, and the practical and necessary pharmacological treatment requirements of athletes. Local anaesthetics were removed from the banned list in January 2004 and codeine was removed in 1993. One of the original reasons for the inclusion was an attempt to protect athletes from the risk of further injury, which may occur if these drugs are used to enable exertion past natural pain limits.

With the constant pressures on athletes to maintain a high level of performance, athletes may be tempted to use anti-inflammatory and analgesic drugs for the purposes of performance continuation. The result is often aggravation or worsening of an existing sports injury. An understanding that many athletes seek medical treatment solely to enable continued competition, possibly against rational therapeutic recommendations, is necessary so that the pharmacist can offer a realistic approach to the best therapy. However, pharmacists are also in an ideal position to educate on the safe and effective use of drug therapy and to influence and facilitate a healthy change in attitude.

In contrast to the sometimes inappropriate use of drugs for performance continuation, and because most injuries do better with correct exercise rather than absolute rest, anti-inflammatory and analgesic drugs may be prescribed to enable the sportsperson to engage in exercise as a form of rehabilitation. Particularly during the later stages of healing, inflammation can have a negative influence on tissue repair. The use of NSAIDs to reduce inflammation to enable exercise during rehabilitation may assist the restoration of normal muscle function, which may consequently act to prevent further injury.

The pharmacist has a professional duty to provide advice on the best possible pharmacological treatment and to advise on appropriate non-drug measures to ensure optimum recovery. However, it is easy to understand how the pressure and determination to win can sometimes over-ride the athlete's commitment to such rational medical treatment. An athlete's ambitious and sometimes reckless desire to win can provide a challenging obstacle to treatment for the healthcare professional.

Acute and chronic injuries

Acute injuries are commonly caused in sport by collision, fall, twist or sudden impact, where pain is immediately felt. Most commonly, tears and sprains of the ligament and muscles are the consequence of such injuries, demanding immediate medical attention. Repeated and escalating musculoskeletal pain can also be an indicator of the development of a significant injury, which also requires prompt attention. Anti-inflammatory drugs are used to reduce the inflammatory response in these injuries, with oral NSAIDs most frequently used for this purpose.

Chronic soft tissue injury, for example tendonitis, can start as mild pain without imposing any physical limitations. Chronic inflammation is often treated through rest, physical therapy and NSAIDs. Local corticosteroid injections are also sometimes used for such injuries. Compared to NSAIDs, corticosteroid drugs are associated with a more pronounced and lasting anti-inflammatory effect, but their use can impair the healing response and they are subject to a number of side-effects.

Non-steroidal anti-inflammatory drugs

Non-steroidal anti-inflammatory drugs (NSAIDs) are one of the most widely used classes of drugs to treat soft tissue, musculoskeletal and joint conditions associated with sporting injury. Their primary use is in pain reduction and inflammation control, demonstrating advantages over other analgesia used for musculoskeletal problems because of this dual effect. In addition, they have an antipyretic effect and are also used for a variety of other conditions such as headache, menstrual cramps and arthritis. NSAIDs are available in a number of dosage forms including oral, topical, rectal, intravenous and intramuscular, with the oral and topical route being most frequently used for sports injuries.

Unlike most NSAIDs, aspirin is a salicylate, but is the prototype of this group and often the drug to which other anti-inflammatory agents are compared. However, about 15% of patients show intolerance to aspirin (Mycek *et al.*, 1997). Of all the NSAIDs available, aspirin probably carries the greatest risk of serious adverse reactions and its use as an analgesic is declining.

The healing of an acute soft tissue injury where there is an inflammatory response may be slightly faster with the use of NSAIDs than without them. Inflammation is certainly better controlled with their use, however most patients will usually recover from the acute condition irrespective of taking NSAIDs (Kannus, 2000).

A short course (3–5 days) of ibuprofen may improve recovery from minor injuries such as ankle sprains. In severe or acute conditions in adults, it can be advantageous to increase the dosage of ibuprofen until the acute phase is brought under control, provided that the total daily dose does not exceed 2400 mg, given in divided doses. If inflammatory symptoms can be reduced in the early stages of recovery, quicker progression into remedial exercise programmes can occur (Sperryn, 1983).

NSAIDs are used in the treatment of injury due to overuse and are beneficial in treating patients with more chronic overuse injury symptoms to assist compliance with rehabilitation. Both oral and topical NSAIDs have been shown to be effective in lateral elbow pain (tennis elbow); resting the elbow and taking NSAIDs in the early stage of the condition is likely to be beneficial. These drugs are often the first-line therapy and are used in the early stages of the disease at the point where many cases show spontaneous resolution (Mellor, 2003).

Treatment for post-exercise muscle stiffness may include NSAIDs, which can offer highly effective relief from the uncomfortable symptoms. Muscle stiffness can present a day or two after heavy or unfamiliar training or over-exertion, and is often more troublesome for the older sportsperson. Over-the-counter (OTC) NSAIDs such as ibuprofen can be recommended for short-term relief of symptoms; however longer-term strategies should be considered, such as a review of training techniques and training intensity. Post-exercise ache and stiffness can often be prevented by a stretching programme before and after exercise. Additionally, muscle relaxants such as diazepam are occasionally used for short-term relief of muscle stiffness due to over-exercise (Sperryn, 1983).

Arthritis can be a common problem among both amateur and elite athletes and can present at a relatively young age, with the major joints including the knee, hip, shoulder and elbow most commonly affected. Shoulder pain, decreased range of movement and mechanical symptoms often present in athletes with arthritis. NSAIDs are used in the treatment of these symptoms. A common problem in athletes is shoulder arthritis secondary to injury. Athletes typically at risk are those involved in sports with an overhead arm movement and weightlifters.

Although effective in the treatment of pain and stiffness of soft tissue injury, NSAIDs also have the potential to mask the symptoms associated with sports injury and may enable the athlete to continue with a normal training schedule. Athletes should be made aware of the risk of further injury if NSAIDs are used for performance continuation during the recovery period (Renström, 1996). However, compared to centrally acting drugs such as the opiates, NSAIDs are less likely to increase the risk of significant sudden injury.

Mechanism of action

The anti-inflammatory effects of NSAIDs are primarily due to the inhibition of prostaglandin synthesis. They inhibit the cyclo-oxygenase enzyme, which in turn inhibits the conversion of arachidonic acid to cyclic endoperoxides. This results in a reduced production of prostaglandins including PGE_2 and prostacyclin (Figure 5.1).

Prostaglandins contribute to the development of symptoms during an inflammatory response, which may include an increased sensitivity to pain, erythema and exudation. Other inflammatory mediators also work synergistically with prostaglandins to produce this response.

The inhibition of prostaglandins by NSAIDs and consequent reduction in inflammation leads to a reduction in pain, less heat around the area, decreased swelling and improved flexibility. Mobility and strength of joint movement also improve when the inflammation is reduced. Unlike corticosteroids, NSAIDs do not inhibit fibroblast or macrophage activity (Curwin, 1996).

Two isoforms of the cyclo-oxygenase enzyme have been identified: cyclo-oxygenase-1 (COX-1) and cyclo-oxygenase-2 (COX-2). Each has a different function; COX-1 is involved in the physiological function of the platelets, gastrointestinal tract and kidney, whereas COX-2 is induced at sites of inflammation.

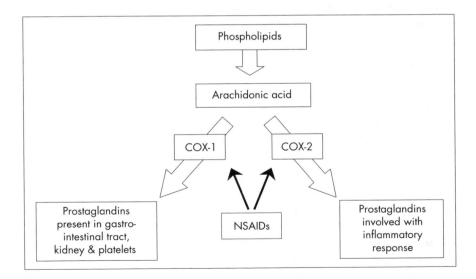

Figure 5.1 Effect of NSAIDs on cyclo-oxygenase and prostaglandin synthesis.

COX-1-mediated prostaglandins have a gastroprotective action by preventing gastric acid secretion and maintaining the gastric mucosal barrier. Suppression of COX-1-mediated prostaglandins by NSAIDs may lead to gastrointestinal effects such as dyspepsia, epigastric pain, indigestion, heartburn, nausea and vomiting. The most desirable and specific pharmacological situation for musculoskeletal injury in terms of such drugs would be the use of an agent that selectively inhibited COX-2, but was a weaker inhibitor of COX-1. This would effectively reduce inflammation, but minimise gastrointestinal side-effects. The inhibitory effect of NSAIDs on each of these isoforms of cyclo-oxygenase varies between drugs.

NSAIDs are weak acids and are therefore attracted to cells present within acid environments such as the stomach, kidney, and injured and inflamed joints. The attraction to the joints is responsible for the therapeutic effect, whereas the stomach and kidney are the sites where toxicity occurs.

Bioavailability

The bioavailability of NSAIDs after oral administration is usually very high, with the exception of diclofenac with only 54% bioavailability, and aspirin with 70% bioavailability. It is usually recommended that NSAIDs are taken with a meal in order to reduce direct gastric irritation. Although this may delay the absorption time of the drug, the extent of absorption is generally not affected.

The effect of half-life

NSAIDs are most effective when steady-state plasma concentrations are reached in the body. However, pain responds much faster to NSAIDs than inflammation, with analgesic effects noticeable before a steady-state plasma concentration occurs. Pain relief starts soon after the first dose and full analgesic effect occurs within a week. Steady-state concentrations are achieved within a few days of taking NSAIDs with a short half-life, but take longer for those with a greater half-life. Full anti-inflammatory effects may not be seen for up to 3 weeks.

It takes about a week for piroxicam, with a longer half-life of 30 to 50 hours, to accumulate to 90% of its steady-state value. In contrast naproxen, with a half-life of around 14 hours, will accumulate about 2 days after the first dose. The use of longer-acting NSAIDs may be a preferred option for patients with continuous pain, but of the non-selective NSAIDs, those with a short half-life are less likely to cause serious upper gastrointestinal bleeding when used at recommended doses (Table 5.1).

Loading doses are sometimes used for NSAIDs with longer half-lives in order to achieve high plasma concentrations more quickly. The fact that NSAIDs can take days to reach a steady-state plasma concentration illustrates the importance of taking these drugs regularly for the best therapeutic response and to maximise the anti-inflammatory effect.

Table 5.1 Properties of NSAIDs

Drug	Cox selectivity	Daily dose	Half-life (hours)	Route(s)
Aceclofenac	COX-1, COX-2	2	4	Oral
Acemetacin	COX-1, COX-2	1	1.5–5	Oral
Aspirin	COX-1, COX-2	3–4	0.25	Oral
Azapropazone	COX-1, COX-2	2–4	15	Oral
Benorilate	COX-1, COX-2	2–3	0.25–3	Oral
Celecoxib	COX-2	1–2	4–15	Oral
Dexketoprofen	COX-1, COX-2	4–6	1.5	Oral
Diclofenac	COX-1, COX-2	2–3	1–2	Oral, rectal, topical, IM, IV
Diflunisal	COX-1, COX-2	2–3	5–20	Oral
Etodolac	COX-2	1–2	7	Oral
Etoricoxib	COX-2	1	22	Oral
Fenbufen	COX-1, COX-2	2	11	Oral
Fenoprofen	COX-1, COX-2	3–4	1–2	Oral
Flurbiprofen	COX-1, COX-2	2–6	3–4	Oral, rectal
Ibuprofen	COX-1, COX-2	3–4	2–2.5	Oral, topical
Indometacin	COX-1, COX-2	2–4	4.5–6	Oral, rectal
Ketoprofen	COX-1, COX-2	2–4	1.5–2	Oral, rectal, topical, IM
Ketorolac	COX-1, COX-2	4–6	4–6	IM, IV, oral
Mefenamic acid	COX-1, COX-2	3	3–4	Oral
Meloxicam	COX-2 (also COX-1 at higher dose)	1	20	Oral, rectal
Nabumetone	COX-1, COX-2	1–2	26	Oral
Naproxen	COX-1, COX-2	2	12–15	Oral
Parecoxib	COX-2	1–2	3.5–4	IM, IV
Piroxicam	COX-1, COX-2	1–2	30–50	Oral, rectal, topical, IM
Sulindac	COX-1, COX-2	2	7	Oral
Tenoxicam	COX-1, COX-2	1	60	Oral, IM, IV
Tiaprofenic acid	COX-1, COX-2	2–3	2–3	Oral
Valdecoxib	COX-2	1	8–11	Oral

Adverse effects of NSAIDs

In the UK, around 25 million prescriptions for NSAIDs are dispensed annually. There are more reports of adverse effects from NSAIDs than from any other drugs, with typically around a quarter of all adverse drug-reaction reports relating to this class (Day *et al.*, 2000).

Side-effects of NSAIDs occur in 20–30% of people taking these drugs regularly and include upper gastrointestinal problems – mainly dyspepsia, heartburn and, less commonly, nausea. Inhibition of prostaglandin synthesis is partly responsible for the side-effects caused by NSAIDs, although the drugs also directly irritate the gastrointestinal mucosa, further contributing to the risk of peptic erosions and ulcers. Direct gastric irritation may be partially reduced by using enteric-coated, modified-release or rapidly dissolving dosage forms.

The elderly are at even greater risk of experiencing side-effects. Gastric ulcers and more serious bleeding from the gastrointestinal tract are more common in elderly patients and those with a previous history of peptic ulcer or bleeding. Concomitant administration of cortico-steroids and increasing doses of NSAIDs can also contribute to a greater risk of adverse effects.

Some NSAIDs can be given by intravenous or intramuscular injection, for example diclofenac, ketorolac, parecoxib and tenoxicam. These may be used when the oral route is unsuitable or after surgery. Intramuscular injection of NSAIDs is associated with considerable pain at the injection site and should therefore be avoided where possible (Jones and Gautam, 2004).

There is a clear relationship between increasing daily doses and the risk of upper gastrointestinal bleeding or perforation. However, side-effects of NSAIDs are not necessarily uniform across the class; for example, indometacin and naproxen may produce gastrointestinal side-effects in one patient, but diclofenac may not.

Of seven non-selective NSAIDs, azapropazone is associated with the highest risk of upper gastrointestinal side-effects; piroxicam, keto-profen, indometacin, naproxen and diclofenac are considered to have intermediate risk of upper gastrointestinal side-effects; ibuprofen has the lowest risk.

Currently, two evidence-based methods are used to prevent gastro-intestinal side-effects associated with NSAIDs: the use of gastroprotec-tive agents concomitantly with non-selective NSAIDs, and the prescribing of selective inhibitors of COX-2, which generally have a lower incidence of gastrointestinal side-effects, further reducing the need for concomitant prophylactic therapy. Synthetic prostaglandin replacement therapy (misoprostol), and the use of proton pump inhibitors such as omeprazole, has been shown to reduce the incidence of NSAID-induced gastrointestinal side-effects. H_2-receptor antagonists such as ranitidine also protect against NSAID-associated gastric and duodenal ulcers.

Although less common than gastrointestinal side-effects, dizziness and drowsiness are also reported with NSAIDs. Athletes competing in sports where this may put them at risk of accidental injury, such as high-speed or motor sports should be warned about the possibility of such effects.

In general, patients should be prescribed NSAIDs at the lowest effective dose, for the shortest period of time, to minimise the risk of gastrointestinal and other adverse effects.

Selective COX-2 inhibitor drugs in sport

Drugs that selectively inhibit COX-2 include celecoxib, etoricoxib, parecoxib and valdecoxib. These drugs are often preferred because they cause fewer gastrointestinal side-effects than non-selective NSAIDs, which inhibit the effects of both COX-1 and COX-2. These drugs improve pain treatment options in patients at high risk of gastrointestinal side-effects, including the elderly, those with a history of peptic ulcers, or those at increased risk of bleeding, as COX-2 inhibitors do not affect platelets.

In general, selective COX-2 inhibitors are better tolerated than non-selective NSAIDs, with the benefit seemingly greater with respect to gastric ulcers (CCOHTA, 2004). However, use of these drugs does not completely eliminate the risk of ulcer complications in high-risk individuals (MacRae et al., 2004a). On the basis of cost-effectiveness the use of selective COX-2 inhibitors may not be justified in low-risk patients (MacRae et al., 2004b).

Reports from trials lasting 6 months show that COX-2 inhibitors are associated with a lower incidence of gastrointestinal adverse events than non-selective NSAIDs. However this may not be the case for patients taking COX-2 inhibitors for longer periods, where it has been suggested that the risk of ulcer-related complications increases (Jüni et al., 2002). Two trials following participants for 1 year or more did not report a significant difference in frequency of perforation, ulceration or bleeding between non-selective NSAIDs and the selective COX-2 inhibitors rofecoxib or etodolac (De Vries, 2002).

Similar to non-selective NSAIDs, the efficacy of COX-2 selective drugs reaches a plateau with increasing doses, where further dose increases may have little effect on the anti-inflammatory action of these drugs (Mauskop, 2003). It is also unclear whether the co-administration of a selective COX-2 inhibitor with a gastroprotective agent such as prostaglandin analogue, H_2-receptor antagonist, or protein pump inhibitor, significantly improves safety over the use of a selective COX-2 inhibitor alone (CCOHTA, 2004).

Parecoxib is a selective COX-2 inhibitor available for use as an intravenous or intramuscular injection. It is used for the short-term management of acute post-operative pain.

Until September 2004, rofecoxib was the only oral COX-2 inhibitor licensed in the UK for acute pain and was often used to treat pain and inflammation associated with sports injuries. The drug was withdrawn globally by the manufacturer (MSD) following the results of a study to determine the effects of 3 years of treatment with rofecoxib on the recurrence of neoplastic polyps of the large bowel in patients with a history of colorectal adenoma. The results indicated an increased risk of thrombotic events including myocardial infarction and stroke compared to placebo following long-term use. On the basis of these data, the drug was withdrawn and all clinical trials involving the drug were stopped (Medicines and Healthcare products Regulatory Agency, 2004a).

Data from one clinical trial for celecoxib has also shown an increased risk of heart attack, stroke and death compared to placebo (Medicines and Healthcare products Regulatory Agency, 2004b). Another study has shown that the use of parecoxib and valdecoxib after coronary artery bypass grafting was associated with an increased incidence of cardiovascular events including myocardial infarction, cardiac arrest, stroke and pulmonary embolism (Nussmeier *et al.*, 2005). Consequently, the cardiovascular safety of all COX-2 inhibitors is currently being closely examined and the future of this class of drugs remains uncertain.

Other selective COX-2 inhibitors are not licensed in the UK for pain associated with musculoskeletal injury, although they are still sometimes prescribed by specialists outside their licence, for intermittent use by athletes who develop pain and inflammation related to sprains and strains from recreational sport (Andrews, 2000). Long-term use of selective COX-2 inhibitors would not usually be anticipated with most acute sports injuries.

Selecting NSAIDs

Systematic reviews have found no important differences in beneficial effect between different NSAIDs. However, varying toxicities relating to increasing doses have been identified. Toxicity profiles for different NSAIDs are often unique and relate to the nature of the NSAID itself (Gøtzsche, 2003).

Selection may be based on a patient's previous reaction to NSAIDs, the preferred dosing frequency, safety or tolerance of individual drugs. The cost of treatment and patient concordance also need to be considered. For example, an athlete with a hectic training schedule may prefer a once-daily, slow-release diclofenac tablet rather than taking a lower dose three times daily. Particular attention is needed when prescribing for the elderly, those with low body weight, and patients with cardiac, renal or liver impairment. A reduction in dose or the use of an alternative treatment may need to be considered in these patients.

During drug treatment, doses should be adjusted according to the clinical response and the lowest dose to achieve the required response should be used. However, before switching from one NSAID to another after an unsatisfactory response, it should be established that the dosage and frequency of administration was sufficient. It should be borne in mind that anti-inflammatory activity often requires a week or more to become effectively established.

Around 60% of patients will be responsive to any NSAID; those who do not respond may respond to another, however switching to another NSAID will not always solve the problem. Similarly, doubling the dose of an NSAID may lead to only a small and possibly clinically insignificant increase in effect (Gøtzsche, 2003). However, if adverse reactions such as dyspepsia occur, switching to a different NSAID can sometimes be a solution in alleviating some side-effects.

When pain is severe, it is inappropriate to keep trying various NSAIDs, as they have an upper limit of effectiveness for severe pain. In this situation the use of adjuvant analgesia or a different class of analgesic drug should be considered (Gøtzsche, 2003).

Asthma

All NSAIDs, including those used topically, are contraindicated in patients who have previously developed signs of asthma, urticaria, rhinitis or angioedema following the administration of any NSAID, including aspirin. Although uncommon, NSAIDs can precipitate an acute asthma attack and potentially lethal bronchospasm in susceptible individuals. Patients who have well-controlled asthma and have taken NSAIDs previously without problems are unlikely to be affected, however extreme caution should be exercised when first initiating NSAID therapy in patients with a history of asthma. Deterioration in the peak expiratory flow rate after starting NSAID therapy is an indicator that NSAID treatment should be discontinued.

In those susceptible to exercise-induced asthma, particular care should be taken when recommending NSAIDs, as asthmatic individuals may be sensitive to more than one trigger factor (Armstrong and Chester, 2004).

Rational NSAID prescribing

The properties of NSAIDs are summarised in Table 5.1. When reviewing anti-inflammatory pharmacotherapy for the sportsperson, the following questions may be helpful in rationalising NSAID treatment (MacRae *et al.*, 2004a):

- Does the patient still need the NSAID?
- Could the pain and inflammation be managed with non-pharmacological treatments?
- Is the patient on the lowest effective dose, and the safest type of anti-inflammatory drug possible?
- Does the patient know the risk of taking NSAIDs for extended periods of time?
- Is the patient getting the rest required for optimal recovery from the injury?
- Is the patient using the medication to enable inappropriate performance continuation?
- Does the patient need a gastroprotective agent?

Counselling for patients taking oral NSAIDs

Patients taking oral NSAIDs should be advised to:

- take oral preparations after food
- report symptoms of indigestion
- report symptoms of allergy such as wheezing or rash immediately
- be aware that NSAIDs may cause dizziness, and exercise caution if driving, or continuing sporting competition
- swallow modified-release preparations whole

• avoid concomitant use of antacids with modified-release oral NSAIDs

When recommending NSAIDs for pain or inflammation, patients should be encouraged to use the lowest possible dose of the drug, as most serious side-effects are dose-related (Prescott, 1998).

Topical NSAIDs

Like oral NSAIDs, topical NSAIDs are also used in the relief of pain and inflammation caused by soft tissue injury, sprains, strains and trauma. Over 5 million prescriptions are dispensed, and around £30 million are spent annually on prescribing topical NSAIDs in England alone (National Prescribing Centre, 1997).

Several trials have shown topical NSAIDs to be more effective than placebo in acute and chronic conditions (Gøtzsche, 2003). However, there is insufficient evidence to rank the preparations in terms of efficacy between different NSAIDs or doses (National Prescribing Centre, 1997), but differences in toxicity relating to increasing doses have been observed (Gøtzsche, 2003). The benefit of topical agents over oral simple analgesic preparations has not yet been demonstrated (Randall and Neil, 2003).

Topically applied NSAIDs penetrate the skin and result in therapeutically significant concentrations in underlying inflamed soft tissues, joints and synovial fluid. Despite evidence suggesting that topical NSAIDs diffuse through the skin to directly penetrate soft tissue, it is thought that topical NSAIDs may enter the synovial joint mainly via the systemic circulation. To support this theory, small trials have shown equal drug concentrations in both knees after application of topical NSAIDs to a single knee (National Prescribing Centre, 1997). It has also been argued that the physical rubbing action and the rubifacient effect of topical NSAIDs contribute to their efficacy.

After topical administration of diclofenac, about 6% of the applied drug is absorbed, resulting in plasma concentrations of diclofenac that are 100 times lower than after oral administration. Synovial fluid concentrations are also lower, but concentrations in meniscus or cartilage are 4–7 times higher than after oral administration (Bandolier, 2004). The low plasma concentration that results from the use of topical diclofenac and other topical NSAIDs are unlikely to be sufficient to cause the systemic side-effects generally associated with oral NSAID use. Studies indicate minimal risk of gastrointestinal adverse reactions with topical NSAIDs (National Prescribing Centre, 1997).

Topical NSAIDs cause few side-effects and are relatively safe. Side-effects may include local skin reactions (dermatitis, pruritis or erythema), and photosensitivity reactions, which usually resolve on discontinuation of treatment. Systemic effects including asthma and bronchospasm have only rarely been reported after application of large amounts of topical NSAIDs.

Topical NSAIDs should not be applied to open wounds or broken skin. For maximum efficacy the preparation should be massaged into the skin until completely absorbed.

There are unlikely to be any additional benefits to be gained by using topical NSAIDs as an adjunct to oral NSAID therapy. If treatment with oral NSAIDs is not therapeutically adequate, the drug, dose and frequency of oral administration should be reviewed rather than incorporating a topical NSAID into the treatment. Topical NSAIDs as sole therapy may be useful if the patient cannot tolerate oral NSAIDs.

Many topical NSAID preparations are available over-the-counter, which may be recommended by pharmacists for sports injuries. Examples are given in Table 5.2.

Table 5.2 Examples of OTC topical NSAIDs in the UK

Drug(s)	Proprietary name
Diclofenac diethylammonium 1.16%	Voltarol Emulgel P
Ibuprofen 5%	Care Ibuprofen Gel
	Cuprofen Gel
	Ibuleve Gel
	Ibuleve Mousse
	Ibuleve Spray
	Ibutop Ralgex Ibuprofen Gel
	Mentholatum Ibuprofen Gel
	Nurofen Muscular Pain Relief Gel
	Proflex Pain Relief
	Radian B Ibuprofen Gel
Ibuprofen 5% + Levomenthol 3%	Deep Relief
Ibuprofen 10%	Ibuleve Maximum Strength Gel
	Nurofen Gel Maximum Strength
Ketoprofen 2.5%	Oruvail
Piroxicam 0.5%	Feldene P Gel

Opioid analgesic drugs for sports injury

Opioid analgesic drugs are sometimes used in the treatment of moderate to severe pain associated with sports injuries. They are most frequently used for pain associated with an acute injury, for short-term relief immediately after the injury has occurred. For the treatment of mild to moderate pain in sports injury, drugs other than opioid analgesics are often preferred, with NSAIDs having the advantage of an additional anti-inflammatory action.

Opioid drugs exert their analgesic action by acting predominantly on the μ opioid receptors found throughout the brain and spinal cord. This results in inhibition of nociceptive pathways in the brain, the dorsal horn of the spinal cord, and peripheral terminals of nociceptive afferent neurons. The consequential response is analgesia, euphoria, pupil constriction, constipation and drowsiness, with respiratory depression and hypotension at higher doses.

A limiting factor of opioid use is the development of side-effects. Tolerance to side-effects and pain relief can also develop with opioid drugs with repeated use. The development of tolerance to an opioid usually presents as a shorter duration of action. Cross-tolerance between opioids is often incomplete, so switching to a different opioid can sometimes reduce the need for a dose increase.

There are reports of opioid analgesic abuse amongst athletes, particularly by those also abusing anabolic steroids (British Medical Association, 2002). Nalbuphine hydrochloride abuse is relatively common among weightlifters because of its reputation as an anti-catabolic agent (Lenehan, 2003). Opioid analgesics may be taken by the athlete to alleviate training-related pain in muscles and joints, enabling them to continue training or competing despite the presence of injury. In this situation the athlete is more susceptible to new injury and more likely to exacerbate existing injuries. Opioid drugs are also abused by weightlifters and other athletes to alleviate the pain of pre-competition fasting and to reduce anxiety before competition. Physical and psychological addiction with serious withdrawal problems in athletes abusing these drugs has been reported (British Medical Association, 2002).

Athletes taking opioid analgesics may also have a competitive advantage because of reduced pain, and therefore an increased ability to exert themselves further. For these reasons, the use of many of the strong opioid analgesics is prohibited in sport and tested for during competition time.

Conversely, many of the opioid analgesic drugs have side-effects that could impair the performance of an athlete, which need to be taken into careful account when recommending these drugs to those still competing or training. Side-effects of opioid analgesic drugs commonly include nausea, vomiting, constipation and drowsiness; with high doses of opioids causing respiratory depression. Doses that may have the potential to cause drowsiness or visual disturbance could put the athlete, and the other competitors, at risk of accidental injury. At higher doses, reaction time may be impaired and may be disadvantageous to competitors in sports where reaction speed is crucial, for example table tennis, football and clay pigeon shooting. NSAIDs may be a suitable alternative for athletes who continue to compete in sports where the risk of adverse effects of opioid drugs must be avoided.

According to the WADA list of prohibited substances (see Chapter 8), the use of the following opioid drugs during sporting competition is prohibited: buprenorphine, dextromoramide, diamorphine (heroin), hydromorphone, methadone, morphine, oxycodone, oxymorphone, pentazocine and pethidine (World Anti-Doping Agency, 2005a). Because each of these drugs might be tested for in the athlete's urine, the intake of their precursors could also lead to a positive result.

Codeine was removed from the Prohibited List by the IOC in 1993 and so can be used for the treatment of pain in athletes. However, one of the metabolites of codeine is morphine, which creates difficulties in testing for the use of morphine alone. For this reason the WADA continues to monitor the morphine/codeine urine ratio as part of the Monitoring Program to detect patterns of codeine and morphine abuse in sport (World Anti-Doping Agency, 2005b).

A selection of less potent opioid analgesic drugs remain permitted in sport during competition and out of competition, and are often used for the short-term treatment of pain associated with sporting injury (Table 5.3). The use of tramadol for moderate to severe pain associated with sports injury has increased because of its reduced opioid side-effect profile.

Muscle relaxants are sometimes used in combination with opioid analgesic drugs in situations where pain control and a reduction in muscle spasm are required. Such a combination might be used to control pain and muscle spasm when a dislocated anterior shoulder is being replaced (Rubinovich, 1996). In this setting, higher doses of the drugs may be used compared with the doses used to just control the pain of such an injury, and because both classes of drugs have the ability to induce apnoea and respiratory depression, artificial ventilation should be accessible.

Table 5.3 Examples of opioid analgesics permitted in sport

Drug	Adult dose (oral)
Codeine phosphate	30–60 mg every 4 hours as required (maximum 240 mg daily)
Dextropropoxyphene	60 mg every 6–8 hours as required
Dihydrocodeine tartrate	30 mg every 4–6 hours as required
Meptazinol	200 mg every 3–6 hours as required
Tramadol hydrochloride	50–100 mg not more often than every 4 hours (total daily dose of more than 400 mg is not usually required)

Using opioid analgesic drugs with NSAIDs

NSAIDs have a ceiling effect, where the level of pain relief fails to increase past a certain point. Opioid analgesic drugs may provide additional pain relief past this point.

Because opioid drugs and NSAIDs have different mechanisms of action, their synergistic effect when used in combination can sometimes enable a reduction of the opioid dose for some patients. This may be desirable for a sportsperson whose performance might be impaired by the sedative, or other CNS depressant effects of opioids. Because many of the stronger opioids are prohibited in sport, the combination of a permitted opioid such as tramadol, codeine or dihydrocodeine with an NSAID may be an effective option for athletes who are registered for testing by doping-control authorities.

There is limited evidence on the efficacy of low doses of opioids (e.g. 8 mg codeine or 10 mg dihydrocodeine) when combined with simple analgesics such as aspirin or paracetamol, compared with the use of aspirin or paracetamol alone. Such combinations are common in OTC analgesic preparations. It is better to recommend individual drugs initially, then use combination products once pain control is achieved; thereby minimising potential side-effects from the unnecessary use of opioid analgesics (Randall and Neil, 2003).

Corticosteroid drugs for sports injury

Corticosteroids are the most potent anti-inflammatory drugs. Unlike androgenic anabolic steroids, corticosteroids do not possess anabolic activity. They are widely used in the treatment of soft tissue injuries, with good results in chronic injury where physiotherapy has failed (Sperryn, 1983). They can be given by intra-articular injection to relieve pain and to increase mobility in inflammatory joint conditions. Smaller amounts can be injected directly into soft tissues to reduce inflammation in conditions such as tennis elbow, or compression neuropathies. If pain and injury results in the immobilisation of a joint, then secondary stiffness and soft tissue fibrosis can result, particularly for the shoulders. Early treatment using corticosteroids can be effective for this. Corticosteroid injections should generally be avoided in injury caused by overuse because of the risk of necrosis (Renström, 1996).

Corticosteroids act by suppressing the tissue's inflammatory response to injury and have catabolic (tissue breakdown) effects. It is thought that the effectiveness of corticosteroids is a result of the suppression of inflammation while the injury heals. They are sometimes used for chronic injuries to provide anti-inflammatory cover, thus enabling chronic fibrous adhesions to be torn, creating an acute condition that may heal more effectively.

Corticosteroid injections are particularly effective when used for specific, localised inflammation present where the muscles, tendons and ligaments attach to the dense connective tissue that covers the bone at the articular surfaces (Table 5.4). These areas are described as musculo-periosteal (e.g. tennis elbow), tendo-periosteal (e.g. tendon insertions at the heel or wrist) and musculo-tendinous (e.g. calf). Corticosteroid injections are also used for chronic ligament sprains and tenosynovitis.

Corticosteroid injections may help to break the pain cycle, but patients should be warned about inflicting further injury by continuing to compete during the subsequent pain-free period (Mellor, 2003). Injury flare-up after corticosteroid injections can occur, with about 1 in 5 patients experiencing an increase in pain for up to a couple of days after injection, followed by rapid improvement. Corticosteroid injections usually provide fast relief, but recurrence of the pain after several weeks is not uncommon and repeated treatment may be necessary. Corticosteroid injections should be combined with reduced physical activity for 5–10 days (Sperryn, 1995).

Systemic side-effects after administration of corticosteroid injections in the doses used for sporting injuries are minimal and are not often a problem in fit athletes, but as with systemic corticosteroid administration, undesirable effects including adrenal suppression and weakness may be experienced. Steroid-induced euphoria is a side-effect of systemic corticosteroids that could be a danger to an injured athlete due to the fact that they feel better than they really are, and may continue to train or compete despite the presence of injury.

Intra-articular injection of corticosteroids has been associated with an increased risk of inflammatory response in the joint, particularly in response to bacterial infection. If any infection is present, corticosteroid injections should not be given as they can mask the signs of infection. Local injection into a previously infected joint should also be avoided. Suppression of both the inflammatory response and the immune function can increase susceptibility to infection, and so stringent aseptic procedures must be used when injecting corticosteroid drugs.

Tendon rupture has been reported after corticosteroids have been injected into tendons. Corticosteroids may have a negative effect on the structure of tensile-strength muscles, tendons and ligaments, predisposing them to rupture (Kannus, 2000). In tendonitis, injections should be made into the tendon sheath and not directly into the tendon. Injections such as this around a tendon may be a satisfactory way of avoiding surgery, but it is essential to know why the injury occurred and to correct the predisposing factors before resorting to injections. Because of the absence of a true tendon sheath, the Achilles tendon should not be injected because of the risk of rupture.

If tendons are injected with corticosteroids, force applied to the tendon should be reduced for 10–14 days and the injury rested, followed by gradual loading starting about 2 weeks later (Curwin, 1996). Repeated corticosteroid injections into a tendon are likely to result in substantial mechanical disruption and should be avoided.

Corticosteroids should not be injected into unstable joints because even though the inflammation will be reduced, the injured joint capsule and the surrounding ligaments may not be able to withstand full weight-bearing load. Depending on the type of joint and dose of drug, intra-articular injections of corticosteroids may affect the hyaline cartilage, making it highly desirable to limit the number of injections into each joint.

Corticosteroid injections are often combined with a local

Table 5.4 Examples of corticosteroids used for local injection

Drug	UK Proprietary name
Dexamethasone sodium phosphate	Decadron
Hydrocortisone acetate	Hydrocortistab
Methylprednisolone acetate	Depo-Medrone
Methylprednisolone acetate + lidocaine hydrochloride	Depo-Medrone with Lidocaine
Prednisolone acetate	Deltastab
Triamcinolone acetonide	Adcortyl Intra-articular/Intradermal
Triamcinolone acetonide	Kenalog Intra-articular/Intramuscular

anaesthetic. The local anaesthetic eases the local pain immediately, indicating to the doctor that the precise area has been infiltrated with the anti-inflammatory corticosteroid.

According to the 2005 WADA list of prohibited substances, the use of glucocorticosteroids (corticosteroids) is prohibited in athletes when administered orally, rectally, or by intravenous or intramuscular injection. The use of these drugs by any other route, such as intra-articular, requires notification to the relevant sporting authority. A therapeutic use exemption (TUE) form may have to be completed by the prescribing doctor to verify the drug is being used for a legitimate reason by the athlete (World Anti-Doping Agency, 2005a) (see also Chapter 8).

Local anaesthetics for sports injury

Local anaesthetics are occasionally used to relieve some forms of pain associated with musculoskeletal injury. They are also used topically for painful skin conditions, and in combination with corticosteroid injections in the treatment of some sports injuries.

Local anaesthetics cause a temporary and reversible blockage to conduction along nerve fibres. They act primarily by impairing the function of the sodium channels in the axon membranes of nerve tissue, blocking the transmission of the action potential along the nerve. The effect of local anaesthetic agents is dose-dependent; an increase in the dose of a local anaesthetic produces a faster onset and a longer duration of pain block (Rosenberg, 2000). The injection of a local anaesthetic close to a sensory nerve or plexus produces a nerve block – lidocaine is often used for this purpose.

Lidocaine is the most versatile and most frequently used local anaesthetic agent as a result of its rapid onset of action, potency and moderate duration of action. It is the drug of choice for short procedures, but to prolong its duration of action and enhance its systemic safety, it is often used in conjunction with a vasoconstrictor such as adrenaline (epinephrine). Except for surface anaesthesia, lidocaine solutions should not usually exceed 1% in strength.

Local anaesthetics such as lidocaine are sometimes used to inject muscle trigger points, which are distinct hypersensitive spots of a harder than normal consistency, located in skeletal muscle. They can produce local pain and often accompany chronic musculoskeletal disorders. Trigger points can be caused by acute or repetitive trauma. Injection of these points with local anaesthetics is an effective way to provide prompt relief of symptoms (Alvarez and Rockwell, 2003).

Direct mechanical stimulus to the trigger point seems to give symptomatic relief equal to that of treatment with various types of injected medication (Garvey *et al.*, 1989). However, myofascial trigger point injection with 0.5% lidocaine is recommended over the use of no injectable drug at all, because lidocaine reduces the intensity and duration of post-injection soreness compared with that produced by dry-needling (Hong, 1994).

Local anaesthetics including lidocaine are sometimes used for pain relief associated with bursitis in shoulder injuries. However, in the presence of a rotator cuff tear, which can be detected by ultrasound and MRI, abduction strength and pain will not improve after injection of lidocaine (Albright, 2004). Combinations of a corticosteroid with lidocaine are also sometimes injected into the shoulder bursa for the treatment of shoulder tendonitis and bursitis. Patients should refrain from vigorous activities for about 2 weeks following such treatment.

Restrictions regarding the use of local anaesthetic drugs in athletes were removed from the WADA list of prohibited substances in January 2004, with the exception of cocaine, which remains prohibited because of its stimulant effect. Nevertheless, local anaesthetics still have the potential for misuse by athletes by masking the pain associated with injury, to enable them to continue training or competing. As well as the questionable ethics of this practice, the athlete may be at greater risk of exacerbating the existing injury.

Skeletal-muscle relaxants for sports injury

Skeletal-muscle relaxants can be used to manage acute pain caused by muscle spasm, which may be a symptom of musculoskeletal injury, commonly lower back or neck pain. A short course (up to a few weeks) of a benzodiazepine may help significantly (Mauskop, 2003). Diazepam is one of the most commonly prescribed benzodiazepine drugs for this purpose, however all of the benzodiazepines have muscle-relaxant properties. The dosage of benzodiazepines as muscle relaxants are similar to those used to treat anxiety.

Muscle relaxants can be effective for some neuropathic pain syndromes and neuralgias, as well as muscle spasm. Baclofen, dantrolene and tizanidine are mostly used for chronic pain conditions. If additional relief is required for acute lower back pain after NSAIDs or weak opioid combination preparations such as co-dydramol have been tried, a short course of diazepam or baclofen may be considered (Royal College of General Practitioners, 2003).

Carisoprodol and methocarbamol are both licensed for short-term treatment, as an adjunct to the symptomatic treatment of acute musculoskeletal disorders associated with painful muscle spasm. The mode of action of these drugs has not been clearly identified, but is thought to be due to CNS depression, as they have no direct action on the contractile mechanism of striated muscle. Both these drugs can cause drowsiness and the clinical efficacy is not well established.

Topical rubifacients for sports injury

Rubifacients are found in many topical preparations marketed for sports injuries. They work by counter-irritation, causing skin irritation, increased blood flow to the skin surface, redness, heat, and a feeling of warmth when applied topically to the skin surrounding soft tissue injuries. In producing this surface stimulation, relief from deep-seated or superficial pain can be obtained to some extent. They may provide comfort to injuries involving the muscles, tendons, joints and non-articular musculoskeletal conditions.

The effect of rubifacients is thought to be due to the activation of Aβ-fibres, which modulate pain signals transmitted by C-fibres to the dorsal horn of the spinal cord. This prevents pain signals reaching the brain. The action of rubbing the skin also results in the activation of Aβ-fibres and may thus enhance the analgesic effect of rubifacients. The pressure created by massaging is thought to help disperse local mediators of pain in the tissues.

Rubifacients can be used as adjuvants to oral analgesic therapy, support bandages, rest, ice and compression, and may be useful in patients who cannot tolerate oral analgesics (Mason *et al.*, 2004a). They are often used in combination with massage therapy (see Chapter 6), with the rubbing action also contributing to the local heat and rubifacient effect. Depending on the type of compounds used, either a 'warm' or 'cold' sensation can be produced after topical administration. Topical rubifacients should only be applied to unbroken skin and can be applied two or three times daily.

Examples of rubefacients currently available in the UK are set out in Table 5.5.

Rubifacients with a 'warming' effect

Salicylate compounds are the most common substances used as topical rubifacients. They are often combined with menthol for a strong and

Table 5.5 Examples of OTC topical rubifacients available in the UK

Product	Ingredient(s)
Balmosa	Camphor 4% Menthol 2% Methyl salicylate 4% Capsicum oleoresin (capsicin) 0.035%
Chymol Emollient Balm	Eucalyptus oil 1.2% Terpineol 4% Methyl salicylate 0.8% Phenol 2.4%
Deep Freeze Cold Gel	Menthol 2%
Deep Freeze Spray	Menthol 2% N-Pentane 40%
Deep Heat Spray	Methyl salicylate 1% Methyl nicotinate 1.6% Ethyl salicylate 5% 2-Hydroxyethyl salicylate 5%
Deep Heat Maximum Strength	Menthol 8% Methyl salicylate 30%
Deep Heat Rub	Turpentine oil 1.47% Eucalyptus oil 1.97% Menthol 5.91% Methyl salicylate 12.8%
Dubam Cream	Methyl salicylate 20% Menthol 2% Cineole (eucalyptol) 1%
Dubalm Cream	Ethyl nicotinate 1% Methyl nicotinate 1% Benzyl nicotinate 1% Glycol salicylate 2% Capsicum oleoresin 0.01%
Elliman's Universal Embrocation	Turpentine oil 35.41% Acetic acid (33%) 10.37%
Lloyd's Cream	Diethylamine salicylate 10%
Movelat Relief Gel/Cream	Mucopolysaccharide polysulphate 0.2% Salicylic acid 2%
PR Heat Spray	Camphor 0.62% Methyl salicylate 1.25% Ethyl nicotinate 1.1%

(Continued)

Table 5.5 *(Continued)*

Product	Ingredient(s)
Radian B Heat Spray	Camphor 0.6% Menthol 1.4% Methyl salicylate 0.6% Aspirin 0.6%
Radian B Muscle Lotion	Camphor 0.6% Menthol 1.4% Salicylic acid 0.54% Ammonium salicylate 1%
Radian B Muscle Rub	Camphor 1.43% Menthol 2.54% Methyl salicylate 0.42% Capsicum oleoresin 0.005%
Ralgex Cream	Glycol monosalicylate 10% Methyl nicotinate 1% Capsicum oleoresin (capsicin) 0.12%
Ralgex Freeze Spray	Isopentane 67.77% Methoxymethane 14.41% Glycol monosalicylate 10%
Ralgex Heat Spray	Glycol monosalicylate 6% Methyl nicotinate 1.6%
Ralgex Stick	Menthol 6.19% Methyl salicylate 0.6% Glycol salicylate 3.01% Ethyl salicylate 3.01% Capsicum oleoresin (capsicin) 1.96%
Tiger Balm Red – extra strength	Camphor 11% Menthol 10% Cajuput oil 7% Clove oil 5%
Tiger Balm White – regular strength	Camphor 11% Menthol 8% Cajuput oil 13% Clove oil 1.5%
Transvasin Heat Rub	Ethyl nicotinate 2% Hexyl nicotinate 2% Tetrahydrofurfuryl salicylate 14%
Transvasin Heat Spray	2-Hydroxyethyl salicylate 5% Diethylamine salicylate 5% Methyl nicotinate 1%

distinctive smell and are used for the relief of musculoskeletal, joint, soft tissue and rheumatic pain. Salicylate compounds include methyl salicylate, ethyl salicylate, diethylamine salicylate, glycol salicylate, salicylamide, ammonium salicylate, glycol monosalicylate and thurfyl salicylate.

Salicylate compounds can be absorbed through the skin and so should be used with caution in those at risk of salicylate sensitivity. The amount of salicylate penetrating the skin is increased by exercise, heat, broken skin, or covering the area with a bandage. Methyl salicylate is metabolised to salicylic acid in the dermal and subcutaneous tissues after topical application, but the exact mechanism of action of topical salicylates is still unclear (Cross *et al.*, 1997).

Efficacy estimates for rubifacients are unreliable because of the lack of good clinical trials. Information from three double-blind placebo-controlled trials with a total of 182 patients with acute pain, and six double-blind placebo-controlled trials with a total of 429 patients with chronic pain, demonstrated that topical salicylate is significantly better than placebo. However, other larger trials have shown no significant effect between salicylate and placebo (Mason *et al.*, 2004b).

Nicotinate compounds are present in some topical analgesic preparations and serve a similar purpose to salicylate compounds. Examples include ethyl nicotinate, hexyl nicotinate and methyl nicotinate. Mucopolysaccharide polysulphate is also a compound with rubifacient effects used in topical OTC preparations.

Many essential oils act as counter-irritants and have been used for centuries for the relief of symptoms of musculoskeletal injuries. Compounds available in OTC preparations include mustard oil, turpentine oil and cajuput oil. Other essential oils used in complementary therapies for their rubifacient properties include birch, black pepper, eucalyptus, juniper and rosemary (see Chapter 6).

Camphor acts as a rubifacient with a mild analgesic effect and is an ingredient of some liniments. Camphor liniment (camphorated oil) has been withdrawn from the market in the UK and the USA because of its potential toxicity. For this reason, the concentration of camphor in topical preparations in the USA must not exceed 11%. Camphor has been used as a counter-irritant in conditions such as fibrositis and neuralgia.

Rubifacients with a 'cooling' effect

In contrast to the previous compounds, some substances produce a cooling effect when applied to the skin. Menthol and levomenthol produce a cold sensation by dilating the blood vessels, which is followed by a mild analgesic effect.

Volatile agents including isopropyl alcohol, N-pentane, isopentane, ethyl chloride and halogenated hydrocarbon propellants are often found in OTC aerosol sprays marketed for musculoskeletal injury. As these compounds evaporate from the skin they produce an extreme cold sensation and have a numbing effect on the surface tissue.

Capsicum

Compounds derived from capsicum are used topically for a range of painful conditions including osteoarthritis and rheumatoid arthritis. These substances are what give chilli peppers their 'hot' taste and include capsaicin, capsicin, capsaicinoids and capsicum oleoresin. Preparations containing these are less commonly used for pain associated with acute sports injuries, as the therapeutic response may not be achieved until after 1–4 weeks.

Unlike other rubifacients, capsaicinoid compounds do not have a vasodilatory effect. They cause counter-irritation by acting on vanilloid receptors to cause a depletion of the neurotransmitter, substance-P. This results in reduced pain-signal transmission from the injured area.

Capsaicin has moderate to poor efficacy in the treatment of chronic musculoskeletal or neuropathic pain. Products containing capsaicin may be useful as treatment, or as adjunct therapy in those unresponsive or intolerant to other treatments (Mason et al., 2004a). Capsaicin preparations are only available on prescription in the UK.

Adverse effects from topical rubifacients are rare (2%) in studies of acute pain, and are poorly reported in patients with chronic pain. Most trials on rubifacients have been for periods of only up to 4 weeks, so more information is needed about long-term efficacy and adverse events (Mason et al., 2004b). Adverse reactions most commonly include skin irritation at the site of application.

Studies on the comparative effect of counter-irritants on skin blood flow have shown that methyl salicylate formulations achieve a greater increase in skin blood flow than camphor and menthol. All three substances produce a dose-related increase in skin blood flow in human volunteers (Kulkarni and Saraf, 1999).

Drugs for bruising

Bruising occurs when blood vessels under the skin rupture and blood escapes into the surrounding tissue causing discolouration. Bruises are a common occurrence in sports as a result of forceful, blunt impact, perhaps due to collision with another competitor or sporting equipment such as a fast-flying ball. The initial pink or red colour of a bruise is due to the colour of haemoglobin, which gradually changes to a bluish hue, and then greenish-yellow colour as the haemoglobin is broken down and absorbed.

The extent of bruising can be disproportionate to the apparent injury and the pain associated with it. Sometimes a minor bump results in an impressive bruise when, in contrast, a more forceful blow can leave nothing to show for the pain of the injury.

Bruising often accompanies fractures as a result of local soft tissue haemorrhage. However, with an indirect force, minimal soft tissue injury may occur at the site of a fracture, and so bruising may not be evident. A suspected fracture should not be dismissed because of absence of bruising. Underlying soft tissue injury should always be treated as a priority in injuries where bruising is present.

A number of topical products containing heparin derivatives (heparinoids) are licensed for the relief of superficial bruising and haematoma (Table 5.6). Heparinoids are absorbed transdermally and have anticoagulant, thrombolytic and anti-exudatory activity, however there is limited evidence for the effectiveness of these preparations. First aid measures such as rest, elevation of the affected limb, ice and compression should be used before considering the use of heparinoid preparations.

Because of the anticoagulant effect of heparinoids, they should not be applied to broken skin, or to open or infected injuries. Side-effects with these preparations are very rare, but erythema and hypersensitivity reactions have been reported. Comfrey ointment is a herbal preparation also used for the topical treatment of bruising (see Chapter 6). OTC preparations for bruising are summarised in Table 5.6.

Table 5.6 OTC preparations for bruising available in the UK

Trade name	Drug	Application frequency
Hirudoid Cream/Gel	Heparinoid 0.3%	Apply up to 4 times daily
Lasonil	Heparinoid 'Bayer' 5000 HDB-U 0.8%	Apply 2–3 times daily

OTC analgesics

Paracetamol is an OTC drug frequently used for mild to moderate pain associated with sports injuries. Compared to NSAIDs and aspirin, it is less irritating to the stomach and side-effects are relatively rare, but it has no demonstrable anti-inflammatory activity. Paracetamol may be a useful analgesic for patients where NSAIDs or aspirin are unsuitable, such as those with a history of peptic ulceration.

A number of OTC combination products for analgesia contain caffeine as an ingredient, but there is little evidence to support claims that it enhances the effect of other analgesics (Randall and Neil, 2003). Caffeine was removed from the WADA list of prohibited substances in January 2004. Before this, caffeine in analgesic preparations could have contributed to an unacceptable urine caffeine level in athletes also taking other sources of caffeine. Although no longer banned, the WADA will continue to monitor caffeine in order to detect patterns of drug misuse in sport. Some examples of analgesics used for pain control are given in Table 5.7.

New treatments

There are a number of new substances and techniques being used by sport and exercise medicine specialists, but more research is needed to demonstrate their effectiveness in treating sports injuries.

Prolotherapy is a technique that involves repeatedly injecting a weakened or damaged ligament with a sclerosant. This is often an irritant solution containing phenol, dextrose and glycerol mixed with a local anaesthetic. A small amount of the solution is injected into the ligament, close to where it attaches to the bone. This causes localised inflammation, which increases the blood supply to the area and stimulates collagen production and tissue repair. Each ligament is injected 3–4 times at weekly intervals. This technique has been used for patients with lower back pain, to strengthen the ligaments and reduce pain, and has also been used in the ankle and shoulder regions. There is conflicting evidence regarding the efficacy of sclerosant injections and these substances are not licensed in the UK for this use.

A number of growth factors play a role in muscle regeneration following muscle injury. New techniques are in development whereby autologous conditioned serum is injected locally around an injured muscle. The serum is produced from whole blood that has been chemically stimulated to produce a higher concentration of growth factors.

Table 5.7 OTC analgesics available from pharmacies in the UK

Drug	Proprietory brand
Paracetamol	Anadin Paracetamol Calpol Disprol Hedex Medinol Panadol
Paracetamol + Caffeine	Hedex Extra Panadol Extra
Paracetamol + Codeine	Panadol Ultra Paracodol
Paracetamol + Codeine + Caffeine	Solpadeine Veganin
Paracetamol + Codeine + Caffeine + Doxylamine	Syndol
Paracetamol + Codeine + Caffeine + Diphenhydramine	Propain
Paracetamol + Dihydrocodeine	Paramol
Ibuprofen	Advil Anadin Ibuprofen Care Ibuprofen Tablets Cuprofen Ibuprofen Hedex Ibuprofen Nurofen
Ibuprofen + Codeine	Nurofen Plus Solpaflex
Aspirin	Aspro Clear Disprin
Aspirin + Codeine	Codis 500
Aspirin + Paracetamol	Disprin Extra
Aspirin + Paracetamol + Caffeine	Alka-Seltzer XS Anadin Extra Anadin Extra Soluble Tablets
Aspirin + Caffeine	Anadin Phensic Original

Research has shown that local injection of autologous conditioned serum is a promising approach to reduce the time to recovery from muscle strains (Wright-Carpenter *et al.*, 2004).

Although costly, the use of guided injections is becoming more common among medical specialists. Imaging using ultrasound, X-ray or CT can now be used to ensure the accurate placement of injections used in the treatment of sports injuries.

Role of pharmacists in sport

Pharmacists can be involved in the management of drug therapy for chronic and long-term conditions encountered by athletes. They have an important role in monitoring the effectiveness of the therapy, side-effects and the clinical progress of the patient. Hospital orthopaedic ward pharmacists may encounter more severe sports injuries requiring post-operative pharmacotherapy management. In whatever setting, pharmacists must ensure the best clinical outcome is reached in the shortest time, using optimal drug treatment.

Patients presenting to the pharmacy with soft tissue injury caused by sport should always be questioned as to what sport they play. The type of sport may be a factor in recommending some drugs. As discussed, the drowsy side-effects of opioid analgesics or other drugs may put an athlete who intends to continue with competition at risk of further accidental injury.

Pharmacists are in the ideal position to monitor an athlete's medication with respect to the WADA list of prohibited substances. When dispensing drugs that may have restrictions in sport, such as corticosteroids or opioid analgesic drugs, pharmacists should always question the patient about their involvement in sport. The knowledge that an athlete is registered with a drug-testing authority may enable the pharmacist to advise on the notification procedures required, as a TUE form may be necessary (see Chapter 8). Such advice could potentially save an unsuspecting athlete's career should they test positive for a drug used for legitimate therapeutic use, but have failed to inform the relevant authorities that they are taking it.

Pharmacists should be aware that the athlete may be taking other drugs, including those used for performance enhancement, when advising on therapeutic drug use for sporting injury. For example, the abuse of anabolic-androgenic steroids such as testosterone-derived drugs has been associated with an increased risk of developing tendon injury (Curwin, 1996). The concomitant use of locally injected corticosteroids, which have a similar risk of tendon rupture when injected into tendons, might be reconsidered in such patients.

The monitoring of pain control, side-effects and interactions between individual drugs is an important role for the pharmacist.

Although many minor injuries can be treated using the resources available in community pharmacies, referral of patients to appropriate practitioners should always be considered for those with more serious injuries.

References

Andrews J R (2000). Current concepts in sports medicine: the use of COX-2 specific inhibitors and the emerging trends in arthroscopic surgery. *Orthopedics* 23(7 Suppl): S769–S772.

Albright J (2004). Specific injuries by anatomic location: shoulder. Virtual Hospital, University of Iowa. http://www.vh.org/adult/provider/orthopaedics/sports injuries/shoulder.html (accessed 19 August 2005).

Alvarez D J, Rockwell P G (2003). Trigger points: diagnosis and management. *Am Fam Physician* 67: 32.

Armstrong D J, Chester N (2004). IOC regulations in relation to drugs used in the treatment of respiratory tract disorders. In: Mottram D R, ed. *Drugs in Sport*, 3rd edn. London: Routledge, 102–137.

Bandolier (2004). Topical NSAIDs: plasma and tissue concentrations. http://www.jr2.ox.ac.uk/bandolier/booth/painpag/topical/topkin.html (accessed 19 July 2005).

British Medical Association (2002). *Drugs in Sport: The Pressure to Perform*. London: BMJ Books.

Canadian Co-ordinating Office for Health Technology Assessment (2004). *Gastro-duodenal Ulcers Associated with the Use of Non-steroidal Anti-inflammatory Drugs: A Systematic Review of Preventive Pharmacological Interventions*. Ottawa, Canada: CCOHTA.

Cross S E, Anderson C, Thompson M J, Roberts M C (1997). Is there tissue penetration after application of topical salicylate formulations? *Lancet* 350: 636.

Curwin S L (1996). The aetiology and treatment of tendinitis. In: Harries M, Williams C, Stanish W D, Micheli L J, eds. *Oxford Textbook of Sports Medicine*. New York: Oxford University Press, 512–528.

Day R, Quinn D, Williams K, *et al.* (2000). Rheumatic disorders. In: Carruthers S G, Hoffman B B, Melmon K L, Nierenberg D W, eds. *Melmon and Morrelli's Clinical Pharmacology*, 4th edn. New York: McGraw-Hill, 645–702.

De Vries C (2002). COX-II inhibitors versus non-steroidal anti-inflammatory drugs in rheumatoid and osteoarthritis patients: gastrointestinal effects. *STEER* 2(8): 3–12.

Garvey T A, Marks M R, Wiesel S W (1989). A prospective, randomized, double-blind evaluation of trigger-point injection therapy for low-back pain. *Spine* 14: 962–964.

Gøtzsche (2003) Non-steroidal anti-inflammatory drugs. In: Godlee F, ed. *Clinical Evidence*. London: BMJ Publishing Group, 1393–1401.

Hong C Z (1994). Lidocaine injection versus dry needling to myofascial trigger point. The importance of the local twitch response. *Am J Phys Med Rehabil* 73: 256–263.

Jones O, Gautam N (2004). *The Hands-On Guide to Practical Prescribing*. Oxford: Blackwell.

Jüni P, Rutjes A W S, Dieppe P A (2002). Are selective COX-2 inhibitors superior to traditional non steroidal anti-inflammatory drugs? *BMJ* 324: 1287–1288.

Kannus P (2000). Nature, prevention, and management of injury. In: Harries M, McLatchie G, Williams C, *et al.*, eds. *ABC of Sports Medicine*, 2nd edn. London: BMJ Books, 2000: 1–6.

Kulkarni K, Saraf M N (1999). Comparative assessment of the effect of counter irritants on skin blood flow by Doppler flowmetry. *Indian Drugs* 36: 301–306.

Lenehan P. (2003). *Anabolic Steroids and Other Performance Enhancing Drugs*. London: Taylor & Francis.

MacRae F, MacKenzie L, McColl K, Williams D (2004a). Strategies against NSAID-induced gastrointestinal side-effects: part 1. *Pharm J* 272: 187–189.

MacRae F, MacKenzie L, McColl K, Williams D (2004b). How to change NSAID prescribing. *Pharm J* 272: 249–252.

Mason L, Moore R A, Derry S, *et al.* (2004a). Systematic review of topical capsaicin for the treatment of chronic pain. *BMJ* 328: 991.

Mason L, Moore R A, Edwards J E, *et al.* (2004b). Systematic review of efficacy of topical rubifacients containing salicylates for the treatment of acute and chronic pain. *BMJ* 328: 995.

Mauskop A (2003). Symptomatic care pending diagnosis. In: Rakel R E, Bope E T, eds. *Conn's Current Therapy*. Philadelphia, PA: Elsevier Science, 1–11.

Medicines and Healthcare products Regulatory Agency (2004a). Immediate withdrawal of rofecoxib (Vioxx/VioxxAcute). http://www.mhra.gov.uk/news/vioxx. pdf (accessed 22 August 2005).

Medicines and Healthcare products Regulatory Agency (2004b). New data on cardiovascular risk with celecoxib (Celebrex). http://medicines.mhra.gov.uk/ourwork/monitorsafequalmed/safetymessages/celecoxib_171204.pdf (accessed 22 August 2005).

Mellor S (2003). Treatment of tennis elbow: the evidence. *BMJ* 327: 330.

Mycek M J, Harvey R A, Champe P C (1997). *Lippincott's Illustrated Reviews: Pharmacology*. Philadelphia, PA: Lippincott-Raven, 401–413.

National Prescribing Centre (1997). Topical non-steroidal anti-inflammatory drugs: an update. *MeReC Bulletin* 8: 29–32.

Nussmeier N A, Whelton A A, Brown M T, *et al.* (2005). Complications of the COX-2 inhibitors parecoxib and valdecoxib after cardiac surgery. *N Engl J Med* 352: 1081–1091.

Prescott L F (1998). Current status of issues concerning the safety of over-the-counter analgesics and non-steroidal anti-inflammatory drugs. In: Rainsford K D, Powanda M C, eds. *Safety and Efficacy of Non-Prescription (OTC) Analgesics and NSAIDs*. Boston, MA: Kluwer Academic Publishers, 1–10.

Randall M, Neil K (2003). *Disease Management*. London: Pharmaceutical Press.

Renström A F H (1996). An introduction to chronic overuse injuries. In: Harries M, Williams C, Stanish W D, Micheli L J, eds. *Oxford Textbook of Sports Medicine*. New York: Oxford University Press, 531–545.

Rosenberg P (2000). *Local and Regional Anaesthesia*. London: BMJ Books.

Royal College of General Practitioners (2003). Guidelines for the management of acute low back pain. *Guidelines* 21: 331–332.

Rubinovich R M (1996). Glenohumeral instability. In: Harries M, Williams C, Stanish W D, Micheli L J, eds. *Oxford Textbook of Sports Medicine*. New York: Oxford University Press, 440–442.

Sperryn P N (1983). *Sport and Medicine*. London: Butterworths.

Sperryn P N (1995). *The Sports Medicine Handbook*. London: The Medical News Tribune Group.

World Anti-Doping Agency (2005a). *The World Anti-Doping Code. The 2005 Prohibited List. International Standard*. http://www.wada-ama.org/rtecontent/document/list_2005.pdf (accessed 22 August 2005).

World Anti-Doping Agency (2005b). *The 2005 Monitoring Program. International Standard*. http://www.wada-ama.org/rtecontent/document/Monitoring_Program_2005.pdf (accessed 22 August 2005).

Wright-Carpenter T, Klein P, Schaferhoff P, *et al.* (2004). Treatment of muscle injuries by local administration of autologous conditioned serum: a pilot study on sportsmen with muscle strains. *Int J Sports Med* 25: 588–593.

Further reading

Abbott Laboratories Ltd (2002). *Brufen 400 mg Tablets – Summary of Product Characteristics*.

Bayer plc (2003). *Ciproxin 500 mg Tablets – Summary of Product Characteristics*.

Bayer plc (2000). *Lasonil – Patient Information Leaflet*.

Bayer plc (2001). *Lasonil – Summary of Product Characteristics*.

Carlson C R, Okeson J P, Falace D A, *et al.* (1993). Reduction of pain and EMG activity in the masseter region by trapezius trigger point injection. *Pain* 55: 397–400.

Davis P (1999). *Aromatherapy, An A–Z*. Saffron Walden: The C W Daniel Company Ltd.

Dermal Laboratories Ltd (2002). *Ibugel Forte 10% – Summary of Product Characteristics*.

Eastwood D (1998). Breaks without bruises. *BMJ* 317: 1095–1096.

Forest Laboratories UK Ltd (2000). *Carisoma Tablets – Summary of Product Characteristics*.

Grahame-Smith D G, Aroson J K (2002). *Oxford Textbook of Clinical Pharmacology and Drug Therapy*, 3rd edn. Oxford: Oxford University Press.

Grant R (1992). *Which Medicine?* London: Consumers' Association and Hodder & Stoughton.

Martin E A, ed. (2003). *Oxford Concise Colour Medical Dictionary*, 3rd edn. Oxford: Oxford University Press.

Martin M, Yates W N (1998). *Therapeutic Medications in Sports Medicine*. Baltimore, MD: Lippincott, Williams & Wilkins.

Mehta D K, ed. (2005). *British National Formulary*, 50th edn. London: British Medical Association, Royal Pharmaceutical Society.

Merck Sharp & Dohme Ltd (2003). *Vioxx Acute 25 mg and 50 mg Tablets – Summary of Product Characteristics*.

Novartis Pharmaceuticals Ltd (2001). *Voltarol Emugel – Summary of Product Characteristics*.

Pharmacia Ltd (2001). *Depo-Medrone with Lidocaine – Summary of Product Characteristics*.

Proprietary Association of Great Britain (2002). *OTC Directory for the Pharmacy 2002/2003*. London: Proprietary Association of Great Britain.

Rossi S, ed. (2003). *Australian Medicines Handbook*. Adelaide: The Royal Australian College of General Practitioners, Australian Society of Clinical and Experimental Pharmacologists and Toxicologists, Pharmaceutical Society of Australia.

Sankyo Pharma UK Ltd (2000). *Hirudoid Cream – Summary of Product Characteristics*.

Shire Pharmaceuticals Ltd (2003). *Robaxin 750 – Summary of Product Characteristics*.

6

Complementary and alternative medicine in sport

Steven B Kayne and Mark C Stuart

Introduction

The term 'complementary and alternative' is used to describe over 700 different traditional and non-orthodox treatments and diagnostic methods. A distinction is often made between 'complementary and alternative medicine', which involves the use of medicines and other products (e.g. herbalism and homeopathy), and 'complementary and alternative therapies', which rely mainly on a procedural technique (e.g. acupuncture and chiropractic). In this chapter the term complementary and alternative medicine (CAM) will be used to refer to both groups.

Research has shown that more people are likely to seek advice about CAM from pharmacists than from all other healthcare professionals combined (Alton and Kayne, 1992). This chapter aims to provide the pharmacist with the fundamental principles of a range of available treatments. Qualified practitioners or specialist texts (see end of chapter) should be consulted for more extensive information about each discipline.

Reasons athletes choose CAM

The holistic concept

A therapeutic link between these widely differing disciplines may not be immediately obvious. They are grouped together by virtue of the fact that they are all said to be 'holistic', a term that was first explained by Cicero (106–43 BC) in the following way:

> A careful prescriber before he attempts to administer a remedy to a patient must investigate not only the malady of the person he wishes to cure, but also his habits when in health, and his physical condition.

In holistic treatment, interventions are tailored to the requirements of the individual in his or her own particular environment, taking into account the person's lifestyle, individual circumstances and any symptoms prompting the consultation. The holistic nature of the complementary disciplines often appeals to sportspeople, where the individual demands of the sport, the specific nature of sporting injury, and the sometimes unique lifestyle are taken into consideration during treatment.

There is a modern tendency to skip the holistic approach when using complementary and alternative treatments. An example of this is the use of a remedy that deals with a specific local problem rather than treating the body as a whole. This has been fuelled partly by the increasing availability of OTC products labelled for use in specific conditions. This makes it easier for the untrained seller and buyer alike, but complementary therapists argue that this approach goes against the holistic principles of complementary practice. On the other hand, this approach makes complementary treatments more accessible, and enables a greater number of people to experience their benefits. However, long-term chronic conditions do need to be treated by qualified practitioners.

Perception of safety

Many people choose CAM over conventional therapies believing that it is totally safe in all respects. In fact, some therapies are potentially dangerous, having risks associated with toxicity or injury.

Potential risks also exist when conditions are misdiagnosed or are treated incorrectly. Lack of formal regulation in some disciplines and limited education and experience of some practitioners can result in individuals practising outside their limits of competence, creating serious safety concerns. Injury resulting from inappropriate or unskilled manipulation, particularly cervical manipulation (Powell et al., 1993) and lumbar-spine manipulation have been reported (Halderman and Rubinstein, 1992; Assendelft et al., 1996; Triano and Shultz, 1997). Incorrect and inappropriate self-prescribing of complementary medicines can also pose a significant risk.

Effectiveness

For many sportspeople the rationale for the use of CAM is based on information passed on by word of mouth and other circumstantial evidence from case studies or individual experiences.

There is no doubt that the reputation of CAM suffers through an inability to provide robust scientific evidence to support the apparent benefits. Where research is available, the methodology is often of poor quality and inconsistencies between different studies make overall evaluation difficult. Regardless of this fact there is still a significant demand for these treatments, particularly for insomnia and anxiety, for which there are a limited number of orthodox OTC products available.

Complementary medicines, supplements, and doping control

One of the difficulties in treating athletes is the fact that if registered for drug testing they can be tested both during competition and out of competition. Recent studies have shown that an alarming percentage of supplements sold over the counter contain ingredients not listed on the label that could lead to a doping offence (see Chapter 8). This may be attributed to poor manufacturing techniques or even deliberate addition of a banned substance such as an anabolic agent to enhance the effects of the product. Some herbal medicines may also contain prohibited substances as constituents. For example, *Ephedra sinica* contains ephedrine as a constituent, which is prohibited. Athletes who are registered for drug testing should use nutritional and herbal supplements with caution in light of these reports. When recommending herbal complementary treatments for athletes, healthcare professionals should always check if the athlete is registered for drug testing, as this may affect the choice of treatment considered. Homeopathic remedies are less of a concern because of the extreme dilutions involved.

Types of CAM

Acupuncture

Acupuncture is a system of healing that has been practised in China and other Far Eastern countries for thousands of years. Although often described as a means of pain relief, it is in fact used to treat people with a wide range of illnesses. Its focus is on improving the overall wellbeing of the patient, rather than the isolated treatment of specific symptoms. According to traditional Chinese philosophy, our health is dependent on the body's motivating energy – known as Qi – moving in a smooth and balanced way through a series of meridians (channels) beneath the skin. Qi consists of equal and opposite qualities – Yin and Yang – and when these become unbalanced, illness may result. By inserting fine needles into the channels of energy (known as 'needling') at specific points on the body (Figure 6.1), an acupuncturist can stimulate the body's own healing response and help restore its natural balance. The flow of Qi can be disturbed by a number of factors. These include emotional states such as anxiety, stress, anger, fear or grief, poor nutrition, weather conditions, hereditary factors, infections, poisons and trauma. The principal aim of acupuncture in treating the whole person is to restore the equilibrium between the physical, emotional and spiritual aspects of the individual.

Although many people have benefited from acupuncture over hundreds of years, many healthcare professionals remain unconvinced of the effectiveness of this treatment. The lack of satisfactory placebo-controlled randomised trials makes it difficult to show whether needling is an important part of the method, or whether the improvement felt by the patient is due to the therapeutic setting and psychological or placebo effect.

Cautious approval of some applications of acupuncture was given by the US National Institute of Health consensus development meeting in 1997 (Marwick, 1997). A number of randomised controlled trials have been conducted providing results that, with a few notable exceptions, are inconclusive.

The adverse effects that may be attributed to acupuncture include infection during needling, trauma and triggering of asthma. Some patients complain of nausea or headaches after treatment.

Chiropractic

Chiropractors specialise in the diagnosis, treatment and prevention of biomechanical disorders of the musculoskeletal system, particularly those involving the spine and the consequent effect on the nervous system. Procedures used during chiropractic treatment may include gentle massage, ultrasonic treatment and adjustment (Freeman and Lawlis, 2001). The chiropractic adjustment or manipulation of joints in the spine or extraspinal regions involves the practitioner placing their hand on the appropriate contact point, followed by repositioning of the joint by delivering a short, sharp thrust. Chiropractors use different parts of the hand to direct the thrust, depending on the joint being adjusted. During treatment the patient may feel tension in the muscles and ligaments and hear a popping sound. A typical course of treatment for an uncomplicated case may involve six sessions over a period of 2–3 weeks.

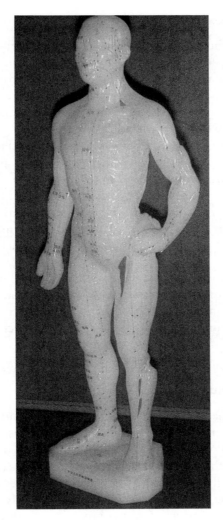

Figure 6.1 Acupuncture doll showing needle points.

Dabbs and Lauretti (1995) conducted a literature review to compare the risk of complication from NSAIDs with the risk associated with cervical manipulation. They concluded that cervical manipulation for neck pain was several hundred times safer than the use of NSAIDs. Severe complications, including death, have been reported with chiropractic treatment, but the incidence of adverse reactions is relatively low when the treatment is performed by trained practitioners (Terrett, 1996).

Essential oils (aromatherapy)

The word aromatherapy was first used in the early 1980s to describe the use of fragrant essential oils to affect or alter a person's mood or behaviour. Essential oils are fragrant and highly volatile aromatic compounds generated by plants through photosynthesis. They are chemically highly complex and contain a hundred or more constituents, many of which are present in very low concentrations.

Adverse effects of essential oils are usually associated with inappropriate or prolonged use of high concentrations by people with acute hepatic or renal problems. Local skin reactions have also been reported with topical use. Some essential oils contain potentially toxic chemicals and these products should always be used with caution and according to the manufacturer's instructions. Essential oils should not be applied to the skin without dilution in a suitable carrier oil such as olive, almond or wheatgerm oil.

Most of the available toxicity data relates to the ingestion of essential oils. Reports of oral administration of large quantities of essential oils are uncommon, but toxicity data is often based on accidental or intentional ingestion. There are reports in the UK of child fatalities after oral ingestion of large doses of peppermint oil.

Flower remedy therapy

Flower remedy therapy involves treating mental and emotional components of disease rather than the physical symptoms. The remedies are derived from the flowering parts of plants and there are several variants produced around the world. In the UK, Bach remedies (Nelson-Bach) are used widely, but others such as Australian bush flower remedies are also becoming popular. Evidence of effectiveness is largely anecdotal. There are no documented reports of adverse reactions to flower remedies.

Herbalism

Herbalism is the practice of using medicines of botanical origin to treat disease. A European Directive defines a herbal medicine as 'a substance or combination of substances presented for treating or preventing disease or with a view to making a medical diagnosis or to restoring, correcting or modifying physiological functions' (EC Directive, 1965).

The quantity and quality of research varies greatly with herbal medicines. Some herbs such as St John's Wort have been extensively studied using both *in vivo* (animal and human) and *in vitro* studies. Other medicines rely on folk tradition to govern their usage, due to a lack of specific scientific evidence relating to them.

Of all the complementary therapies that pharmacists are most likely to recommend, herbal medicines pose the greatest safety concerns. Some herbal preparations can be potentially dangerous, even in therapeutic doses (Barnes *et al.*, 2002) and so a good knowledge of these products is essential when advising patients.

Homeopathy

Homeopathy was promoted during the second half of the 18th and early 19th centuries by Christian Samuel Hahnemann, a German physician.

Homeopathic products are traditionally called 'remedies' and are described by an abbreviation of the Latin name together with an indication of the potency (strength). They are prepared according to methods specified in various homeopathic pharmacopoeias. All the remedies have a 'drug picture'. This is a written survey of the symptoms noted when the drug was given to healthy volunteers – a process known as 'proving the drug'. Drug pictures may also contain symptoms derived from observations of toxological effects arising from therapeutic, deliberate or accidental administration (Belon, 1995). The drug pictures are collected together in books known as materia medica, many of which are now available in convenient electronic formats.

The aim of homeopathic treatment is to stimulate a person's own capacity to heal. It involves the administration of a highly diluted form of a remedy whose drug picture closely matches the main symptoms of disease exhibited by the patient. This principle is known as the 'Law of Similars'.

As a general guide, for injuries, homeopathic medicines in solid or liquid dose forms may initially be given in potency 30c (i.e. a 1 in 100 serial dilution 30 times) every 2 hours for six doses and then three times daily for 7–10 days. Chronic conditions may be treated twice daily with the 6c potency for up to 6 weeks before review. Topical forms include creams, gels, ointments, lotions and mother tinctures. Mother tinctures are the strongest form of homeopathic remedy. They are generally used topically although some can be diluted and taken orally.

The use of homeopathic medicines in the treatment of sports-related injuries and illnesses has a number of important advantages over conventional preparations. They can be effective, quick-acting, cheap and, above all, do not interfere with any subsequent therapy. Because there is no proven unfair competitive advantage to be gained from taking homeopathic medicines, or any demonstrable risk to an athlete's heath, the medicines are not prohibited or restricted by the WADA.

Robust scientific evidence of efficacy for homeopathic interventions is generally lacking; the rationale for using homeopathy is based on circumstantial observation over almost 200 years. Shang *et al.* (2005) compared the treatment effects in homeopathy and conventional medicine. The Swiss researchers concluded that the clinical effect of homeopathy was a placebo effect. Protagonists of homeopathy questioned the findings but the *Lancet* thought them to be of such quality as to signify the 'end of homeopathy' (Anon, 2005).

Because of the use of minute – in some cases infinitesimal – amounts of medicine the risk of toxicity from orally administered homeopathic remedies is extremely low. The main safety issue is associated with choosing the wrong remedy, resulting in a lack of effective treatment. Although safe, treatment can be slow and not all conditions respond to homeopathy. For example, mineral and vitamin deficiencies and hormonal imbalance may require administration of material doses.

Although herbal and homeopathic remedies may be derived from similar source materials and have similar names, they are quite different products and are generally used to treat different conditions.

Massage

Although remedial massage has its own methods and procedures, at its simplest it may be considered as being the age-old rubbing response to a painful stimulus.

Massage is the systematic manipulation of body tissues, performed primarily (but not exclusively) with the hands for therapeutic effect on the nervous and muscular systems and on systemic circulation. The primary characteristics of massage are touch and movement. It may be performed in association with another therapy or alone. Treatment often involves several different techniques and may last between 15 and 90 minutes (Zollman and Vickers, 2000).

Massage has always maintained a high profile in sport and is an important part of an athlete's preparation. Statistics from the Great Britain team at the Atlanta Olympics in 1996 revealed that massage formed 47% of all treatments to athletes from all sports. The demand for massage at the Olympics in Albertville (1992) and Barcelona (1992) was also significant. It is claimed that massage can reduce recovery time, minimise injury, and improve body movement and fluidity (Angus,

2001). Different sports or even different disciplines within the same sport require a different massage regime. Massage is also used on horses and other animals involved in sport.

Despite the popularity of massage, it is difficult to obtain a consensus on its benefit from the literature, because of the wide range of techniques employed and the outcome measures chosen (Callaghan, 1993).

Osteopathy

Osteopathy is based primarily on the manual diagnosis and treatment of impaired function resulting from loss of movement. Osteopathic treatment is based on manual techniques that are used to adjust and correct mechanical problems in the whole body. The osteopath does not prescribe any medicines or employ any invasive techniques (injections, surgery, etc.), although in the USA the scope of treatment is often wider.

When a sportsperson consults an osteopath, the posture and condition of muscles, ligaments and tendons of all joints from head to toe are examined. The strength and flexibility of these tissues indicates how well they are adapted to the individual and the chosen sport.

Reflexology

Reflexology is based on a theory that maps out the reflexes on the feet and hands to all the organs and the rest of the body. It involves the application of pressure to reflex areas of the hands or feet to produce specific effects in other parts of the body. Reflexologists do not seek to diagnose medical conditions, nor do they prescribe medicines, although the topical use of oils or herbal preparations is often recommended (Wolfe, 1999). Dietary advice may also be given during a reflexology consultation.

A treatment session lasts around 40 minutes; the effects of a treatment may last up to a week. The need for further treatment will vary according to the severity of the condition and the patient.

Botting (1997) mentions a number of trials in her review of the literature on the effectiveness of reflexology in treating stress-related conditions (anxiety, migraine), back pain, gastrointestinal complaints and arthritis, splitting the evidence into 'anecdotal' and 'scientific'. They add up to more than a mere impression that reflexology is of benefit, but do not provide firm evidence for the effectiveness of this therapy.

Relaxation

Relaxation and other psychological interventions (e.g. meditation and visualisation) are used in sport, particularly at elite levels.

Yoga

Yoga involves postures, breathing exercises and meditation and is aimed at improving mental and physical functioning. Yoga and sport are often seen in opposition, by nature of the quiet approach in yoga compared to the competitiveness of sport. Some practitioners understand yoga in terms of traditional Indian medicine, with the postures improving the flow of 'prana' energy around the body. Others see yoga in more conventional terms of muscle stretching and mental relaxation with an ability to improve vitality (Wood, 1993).

Commonly practised yoga methods are 'pranayama' (controlled deep breathing), 'asanas' (physical postures) and 'dhyana' (meditation), mixed in varying proportions with differing philosophic ideas. Yoga is used by gymnasts and weight trainers to improve body form and balance.

Sports-related conditions commonly treated with CAM

Abrasions and cuts

Many natural therapies, including the application of honey, larval therapy, aromatherapy, herbal medicine, homeopathy, nutrition, and mind-body-spirit techniques, demonstrate potential benefit in the management of acute and chronic wounds (Leach, 2004).

Essential oils

Tea tree oil   Tea tree oil (*Melaleuca alternifolia*) is native to the east coast of Australia and has well documented antiseptic properties. The primary constituent, terpinen-4-ol, is active against numerous pathogenic bacteria and fungi but seems to spare normal skin flora. Other constituents, including alpha-terpineol and linalool, may also contribute to its antimicrobial activity.

Tea tree oil can be applied to cuts and abrasions to prevent and inhibit infection. It is generally well tolerated topically, however adverse reactions including local irritation, inflammation, contact dermatitis and allergic reactions have been reported.

Herbalism

Aloe vera   The sap of the bush *Aloe vera* has traditionally been used by the American Indians for its healing properties. It can be applied topically to reduce inflammation, assist with pain relief and promote the healing of cuts and grazes.

A glycoprotein fraction (G1G1M1DI2) has been isolated and is believed to be involved in the wound-healing effect of *Aloe vera* via cell proliferation and migration. This isolated glycoprotein has been shown to accelerate wound healing in human keratinocytes and enhance wound healing by day 8 after injury in mice (Choi *et al.*, 2001).

The fresh sap can be squeezed from a cut branch of the *Aloe vera* plant and applied directly to the wound. The plant is commonly available in most garden centres and is easily grown indoors, providing a handy natural first-aid remedy. Ready-prepared *Aloe vera* preparations containing 99.5–100% strengths can be purchased from most pharmacies and health food stores and can provide a convenient alternative.

Echinacea   Echinacea (*Echinacea angustifolia*, *Echinacea purpurea*) may act to stimulate the function of the immune system and is used both topically and orally in conditions where infection is involved. Echinacea can be applied topically to assist in the healing of cuts and abrasions. The expressed juice of fresh flowering *Echinacea purpurea* applied topically on local tissues inhibits hyaluronidase, which helps to stimulate wound healing (Blumenthal *et al.*, 2000). An ointment made from freshly pressed juice, or a tincture, can be applied three or more times daily to cuts and abrasions.

Homeopathy

Several remedies may be used orally for abrasions and wounds. Superficial wounds may be swabbed with calendula (or hypericum and calendula) lotion made by diluting mother tincture with freshly boiled and cooled water.

Infected wounds respond to hepar sulph (when symptoms are better in wet weather and for the application of warmth) or sulphur (when symptoms are better in dry weather, but worse for warmth in bed). If the lacerations are deep then staphysagria should be considered. Ledum is indicated for injuries caused by spiked running shoes. These four remedies are all given orally.

Anxiety, excitement and stress

Acupuncture

A study of the effect of acupuncture treatment on the physical well-being of elite female football players during a competition period provided evidence to support the effectiveness of acupuncture for the mental well-being of athletes during competition (Akimoto *et al.*, 2003).

Essential oils

Various proprietary blends of essential oils are available to assist with anxiety before competition. Lavender and geranium are common ingredients.

Flower remedy therapy

There is a combination of five Bach flower remedies known as Five Flower Remedy or Rescue Remedy. It was so named for its stabilising and calming effect on the emotions during a crisis. The remedy comprises cherry plum (for fear of not being able to cope mentally), clematis (for unconsciousness or the 'detached' sensations that often accompany trauma), impatiens (for impatience, agitation), rock rose (for terror), and Star of Bethlehem (for the after-effects of shock). This remedy is often used to allay anxiety before competition or after competition in place of arnica, where the mental symptoms resulting from exhaustion or failure are more evident than the physical. Four drops of Rescue Remedy should be diluted in a small glass of water and sipped at frequent intervals until relief is obtained. It can also be used as drops placed directly under the tongue.

Herbalism

Herbal remedies for anxiety include St John's Wort (*Hypericum perforatum*) and Asian ginseng (*Panax ginseng*). Hops (*Humulus lupulus*) and scullcap (*Scutellaria baicalensis*) may be used to treat insomnia.

Homeopathy

Anxiety and excitement can affect performance in competitive sport. They may also lead to diarrhoea and insomnia. In such circumstances argent nit or aconite may be effective. Gelsemium have been suggested to relieve anxiety before a boxing match (de Schepper, 1994). Insomnia may be treated with coffea or passiflora, and diarrhoea (associated with anxiety) with arsenicum album.

Massage

A psychological evaluation of pre-event massage was undertaken in 10 healthy men (Boone *et al.*, 1991). Each subject was assigned to a group receiving massage or a group receiving no massage before undertaking 10 minutes of submaximal exercise. Various parameters were measured, including VO_2 (the amount of oxygen a person uses in 1 minute per kg of body weight) and cardiac output. No difference in performance was detected between the two groups. The very low numbers of subjects would be a major criticism of the study. The difficulty of eliminating bias in the placebo group, who obviously knew they were not receiving treatment, is always a potential problem in this type of study.

There is also other evidence from randomised clinical trials that massage can reduce anxiety in the short term (Field *et al.*, 1992).

Relaxation

Relaxation techniques are normally used in sport for the purpose of improving the rate of recovery or enhancing performance by improving the handling of anxiety pressures.

Reflexology

Patients have reported an improvement in their ability to relax following reflexology (Shaw, 1987). Other reported benefits have included a pleasant warming sensation to the injured area and improved sleep patterns.

Blisters

Blisters caused by footwear (walking boots or training shoes) or by equipment friction (tennis racquets or golf clubs) can be a problem, especially at the start of the season when the equipment is new and the skin is soft.

Essential oils

For blisters caused by rubbing of new or poorly fitting shoes, St John's wort oil or tea tree oil diluted in olive oil may be applied twice daily and combined with an assessment of footwear.

Herbalism

The following external herbal treatments provide soothing relief and may help to heal the blister:

- Apply calendula ointment on an opened blister. Aloe vera gel is also excellent for drying and healing an open blister.
- Apply crushed fresh dandelion leaves or dandelion juice.
- Add an antiseptic thyme infusion to the bath water or foot bath.

Homeopathy

The combination of calendula and hypericum (often called Hypercal) may be applied locally, as a tincture or cream. Causticum can be given orally twice daily if the blisters are burning. The blisters should be covered with a non-adhesive sterile dressing. Blisters caused by burns respond to cantharis and urtica.

Bruises

Essential oils

Essential oils of fennel, hyssop or lavender may help to reduce the symptoms of bruising. They can be applied in an ice-cold compress soon after the bruising has occurred, or applied diluted to 3 drops in 5 mL of a carrier oil such as almond or sesame oil. In the later stages, when the bruise turns green or yellowish, rosemary essential oil can be used. It can be diluted in a carrier oil and gently applied to the bruised area to help increase circulation and may assist in dispersing the blood into the surrounding tissues.

Herbalism

Arnica   Herbal arnica (*Arnica montana*) is used topically and is a popular treatment for bruising, with a number of commercial creams available from pharmacies and health food stores. Arnica has pain-relieving properties, particularly with the pain associated with bruises and haematomas, and is claimed to promote re-absorption of blood into the surrounding tissues. Its main constituents are helanalin and dihydrohelanalin.

One method of treating bruising is to use 30 mL of arnica tincture to about 500 mL of cold water, applied to the bruise as a wet compress several times per day. This also has a soothing action and may help with tenderness and other symptoms.

Skin reactions including allergy to arnica are rare, but are more frequent when compared with most plants. A skin-patch test should always be done before general application of products containing the herb. Arnica should be discontinued immediately if signs of local irritation occur.

Arnica should not be taken internally as it can irritate mucous membranes and is cardiotoxic. If swallowed, arnica can cause nausea, vomiting, severe hypertension, tachycardia, palpitations and shortness of breath. Coma and fatalities have been reported following consumption of herbal arnica.

Herbal arnica ointments and creams often contain 20–25% of a 1:10 tincture. They are also made using a 5–25% v/v tincture or fluid extract. Products containing arnica should only be applied to unbroken skin.

Bromelain   Bromelain is the enzyme complex extracted from pineapple (*Ananas comosus*). A dose of 125–450 mg (usually 250 mg) taken three times daily between meals can be used internally for the treatment of bruising (see also page 192). Several studies have demonstrated the advantages of using bromelain for bruising. Among those for sports injuries, one study in boxers showed that 58 of 74 athletes taking bromelain after a fight recovered from bruising after 4 days. Only 10 of the 72 boxers in the control group had complete healing in the same period (Blonstein, 1960).

Horse chestnut   Horse chestnut (*Aesculus hippocastanum*) has been used for centuries for conditions relating to venous and other circulatory conditions. Topical preparations containing extracts of horse chestnut have been used to reduce bruising, inflammation associated with sprains and strains, and for the symptomatic treatment of chronic venous insufficiency. However the mechanism of action is still unclear. The active ingredient of horse chestnut is aescin, which, using 2% preparations, has been shown to be more effective than placebo in the resolution of experimentally-induced bruising (Calabrese and Preston, 1993).

Sweet clover Ointment containing sweet clover (*Melilotus alba*) has been used for the symptomatic treatment of bruising. There is also some evidence to suggest that sweet clover aids wound healing. The herb contains coumarins, and may interfere with warfarin therapy (Heck *et al.*, 2000), so should be used with caution. If sweet clover is left to ferment, dicoumarol is produced, which is a potent anticoagulant and inhibitor of vitamin K. Such forms of sweet clover should therefore be avoided by those also taking anticoagulant drugs.

Topically, creams and ointments containing 3–5 mg/g of coumarin have been used for bruising. A poultice for bruises and wounds can be made by wrapping fresh sweet clover in linen, soaked with hot water and placed on the affected area.

Witch hazel Witch hazel (*Hamamelis virginiana*) is claimed to possess anti-haemorrhagic and anti-inflammatory properties and may be applied to bruised and inflamed tissue.

Homeopathy

Homeopathic arnica is often claimed to relieve pain and bruising effectively. It has been suggested that the 10M potency taken orally is to be preferred to the more usual 30c potency, which is more appropriate in acute cases. The remedy is also available in topical formulations. There is little robust scientific evidence to support the use of homeopathic arnica (see below).

There are a number of other homeopathic remedies used for bruising. Acid sulph is indicated when the skin is hot and the bruise is black and blue and *Bellis perennis* is indicated where a deep, intense pain is present and the injury is sensitive to the touch. Bellis is claimed to be specifically indicated for women who have been bruised on the breast.

There is a German product called Traumeel S that can be applied topically with gentle massage for swelling and bruising. It is also available as drops for internal use and contains more than 14 different homeopathic medicines. The product has been the subject of a number of clinical trials (Lussignoli *et al.*, 1999) and is an example of the complex OTC products for sports use marketed in continental Europe and the USA.

Colds and influenza, sore throat

Essential oils

Eucalyptus, lavender, menthol and tea tree may all be used either singly or in combination as an inhalation. A number of convenient proprietary products such as 'Karvol' or 'Vick' are available.

Herbalism

Echinacea is an extremely popular remedy for colds and 'flu and may be used prophylactically during the winter months and to treat the condition. Elderflower, garlic and goldenseal (*Hydrastis*) are also used.

Homeopathy

Aconite (first signs of cold), gelsemium (colds and 'flu) and belladonna (sore throat) are the main remedies. In each case they may be taken three or four times a day for the first 2 days (30c potency) then two or three times daily for a further 5–7 days.

Calendula mother tincture may be diluted with warm water (5 drops to a tumbler) and used as a gargle.

Coughs

Essential oils

Options here include inhalation with oil of lavender and chest massage with eucalyptus and thyme.

Herbalism

Coltsfoot, horehound (*Marrubium vulgare*), liquorice, mullein (*Verbascum*), thyme (*Thymus vulgaris*) and wild cherry bark (*Prunus serotina*) are all used to treat coughs.

Homeopathy

There are many homeopathic remedies indicated for different types of cough in the repertories, including bryonia (productive), phosphorus (dry and tickly) and spongia (dry, 'barking', croupy cough). Bryonia linctus is available as a proprietary brand and provides a useful option.

Eye injuries

Homeopathy

Providing the pain is relieved by cold applications, ledum given orally every 2–4 hours is almost specific for a black eye. If there is no relief from cold applications, then staphysagria should be given. Arnica and symphytum are also appropriate remedies to consider.

Swimmers are susceptible to a number of eye conditions that may respond to calendula or euphrasia (also known as eyebright) eyedrops. At the time of writing, homeopathic eyedrops are only available on a medical prescription but this situation may well change.

Fractured bones

Herbal

Comfrey   Comfrey (*Symphytum officinale*) has traditionally been used internally to assist the healing of fractures and broken bones, hence its alternative name, 'knitbone'. However, comfrey contains pyrrolizidine alkaloids, which have been associated with hepatotoxicity and carcinogenic effects when the herb is taken internally, and so it should never be used in this way.

Topical preparations are safe to use and are believed to also assist with the healing process of damaged cartilage, bone and muscle. The fresh herb can be combined with olive oil and a little hot water to form a paste which is then placed in a linen cloth to be applied topically as a poultice. Obviously, this type of treatment is impractical if a plaster cast or supportive strapping is necessary (see below).

Gotu kola   Gotu kola (*Centella asiatica*) is used in Ayurvedic medicine and is said to strengthen bones and tendons. It may be taken orally to assist with the healing of fractured or broken bones. There is some evidence to suggest triterpenoid saponins, including asiaticoside and madecassoside, might promote healing by stimulating collagen and glycosaminoglycan synthesis (Jellin, 2003). A typical dose of gotu kola is 600 mg of dried leaves made into a tea and taken three times daily.

Homeopathy

Arnica may be given immediately to allay shock and reduce trauma. Homeopathic symphytum ('knitbone') is given once the fracture has been reset, and it may act deeply on the periosteum, and helping in the formation of new bone and cartilage, but this has never been proven. Calc phos is also used commonly for fractures.

Motion sickness

Essential oils

Ginger (inhale 2–3 drops from a handkerchief) and peppermint oil are both indicated for motion sickness. The latter may be inhaled or taken orally in water.

Herbalism

Ginger (*Zingiber officinale*) may prove effective.

Homeopathy

Cocculus is commonly used to treat motion sickness. Tabacum is claimed to be specific for sea sickness.

Soft tissue injuries

Essential oils

Many essential oils have a rubifacient effect, causing surface stimulation of the skin. Rubifacients may provide a degree of pain relief by modulating the transmission of pain signals.

Essential oils with rubifacient properties include rosemary (*Rosmarinus officinalis*), juniper (*Juniperus communis*), thyme (*Thymus vulgaris*), wintergreen (*Gaultheria procumbens*), eucalyptus (*Eucalyptus globus*), cajuput (*Melaleuca leucodendron*) and peppermint (*Mentha piperita*).

These oils can be diluted by using 3 drops of essential oil in 5 mL of a carrier oil such as sweet almond, grapeseed, wheatgerm or olive oil. The oils can also be incorporated into many cream bases such as aqueous cream, which can be a more convenient way to use them. The diluted oils can be applied topically several times a day and may be particularly soothing for muscle pain following over-exertion.

Juniper, chamomile and lavender may also help in relieving the symptoms of inflammation.

Herbalism

There are a number of herbal remedies that may be used to treat problems associated with soft tissue injuries, including the following.

Bromelain   Bromelain is a proteolytic enzyme extracted from the stem of the pineapple (*Ananas comosus*) with well-documented efficacy in many inflammatory conditions. It may reduce oedema, bruising, healing time and pain following various injuries and surgical procedures, and possibly decreases joint swelling and increases joint mobility. Although bromelain has not been studied directly in patients with sprains and strains, the anti-inflammatory properties of this compound suggest it may be beneficial in assisting recovery from such injuries.

The effects of bromelain are due to an enzyme constituent that causes release of a kinin, which stimulates the production of prostaglandin E1-like compounds. This may help with the inflammation, swelling and pain associated with traumatic sports injuries.

Bromelain should be avoided by patients taking anticoagulant drugs because it may theoretically increase their anticoagulant effects. Bromelain can also increase plasma and urine concentrations of tetracycline if taken concomitantly. Individuals allergic to pineapple should avoid taking this preparation because of the possible increased risk of an allergic reaction to bromelain.

A dose of 125–450 mg (usually 250 mg) of bromelain can be taken orally three times daily between meals for 8–10 days. When taken concomitantly with curcumin extract, bromelain may increase the absorption of curcumin as it does for other compounds.

Comfrey   Comfrey (*Symphytum officinale*) is used topically for its anti-inflammatory properties and has long been used for ulcers, wounds, bruises, sprains and fractures. The healing activity of comfrey is thought to be due to the allantoin it contains. It also contains rosmarinic acid, which may further contribute to its anti-inflammatory effects.

Although historically it was considered effective when taken orally, it has now been shown to be hepatotoxic and carcinogenic when taken internally, because of the pyrrolizidine alkaloid content. Percutaneous absorption of pyrrolizidine alkaloids present in comfrey is reported to be low (Barnes *et al.*, 2002).

Studies have shown that topical use of comfrey ointment may benefit sprains and strains associated with sporting injury. It has been shown to reduce muscle pain and ankle oedema and to increase ankle mobility in patients with acute ankle distortion (Kucera *et al.*, 2004).

Ointments and other external preparations are commonly made with 5–20% comfrey. A poultice made from comfrey leaves and stems can also be applied to the unbroken skin and may provide relief from the symptoms of muscle injury. Topical preparations should be used on unbroken skin for no more than 10 days, and for a total of no more than 4–6 weeks per year.

Devil's claw Devil's claw (*Harpagophytum procumbens*) is native to South Africa and has been used as an analgesic and anti-inflammatory herb for a variety of musculoskeletal problems, particularly for arthritic and rheumatic conditions. Strong evidence exists for the use of an aqueous Harpagophytum extract at a daily dose equivalent of 50 mg harpagoside in the treatment of acute exacerbations of chronic non-specific low back pain (Chrubasik *et al.*, 2002). It may therefore be beneficial for sports injuries where there are symptoms of lower back pain.

The active constituents of devil's claw are iridoid glycosides, including harpagoside, which is found predominantly in the roots and to a lesser extent in the leaves. It has not been demonstrated that harpagoside is the most important pharmacologically active compound.

It has been suggested that devil's claw does not affect arachidonic acid, cyclo-oxygenase or lipoxygenase pathways, and may be inactivated by stomach acid, therefore not orally active. However, some effectiveness has been demonstrated when extracts have been injected subcutaneously beside the knee joint as supportive therapy (Beckwith, 1998). Studies in animals and humans have shown mixed results using devil's claw in inflammatory musculoskeletal conditions including rheumatoid arthritis, but there are many anecdotal reports to support the use of this herb for inflammatory conditions.

Some evidence suggests that 60 mg of harpagoside daily may be effective for lower back pain and osteoarthritic pain of the knee and hip. In one study, patients taking a preparation containing harpagoside in conjunction with an NSAID for osteoarthritis appeared able to reduce the dose of NSAID needed for pain relief (Jellin, 2003).

Side effects reported after short-term use of devil's claw are minimal, but have included mild, transient gastrointestinal effects such as diarrhoea and flatulence.

Devil's claw should be taken cautiously by patients with cardiovascular conditions, as heart rate and blood pressure may be affected. It should also be taken with caution by diabetic patients because it may decrease blood glucose levels and have an additive effect with diabetic medication. Devil's claw may increase bile production so should be avoided by those with gallstones. It should also be avoided by those with peptic or duodenal ulcers, as an increase in gastric acid secretion may occur after taking this herb.

The usual dose is 1.0–4.5 g of the root daily; alternatively 1 mL of a 1:5, 25% ethanol tincture can be taken three times daily.

Feverfew   Feverfew (*Tanacetum parthenium*) has been used traditionally to treat a variety of musculoskeletal conditions including arthritis. The active components of feverfew are parthenolides, which inhibit the process of inflammation and may therefore relieve pain. Although its mechanism of action is not completely understood, it appears that it does not inhibit cyclo-oxygenation of arachidonic acid (see Fig. 5.1, p. 147), but rather may block thromboxane synthesis. It may have a different mechanism of action to the prostaglandin inhibition by salicylates.

There are conflicting reports about the effectiveness of feverfew for arthritis. One study showed that feverfew provided no additional benefits when added to existing NSAID treatment (Barnes *et al.*, 2002). Another study found that feverfew was more effective than NSAIDs in preventing the release of inflammatory substances (Mitchell, 2000).

The main use of feverfew today is for migraine headaches. Despite inconclusive evidence of the effectiveness of feverfew in arthritis, anecdotal reports of its benefits in rheumatoid arthritis may prompt further investigation.

Tumeric   Tumeric (*Curcuma longa*) has a warm, bitter taste and is used to flavour and colour curry powders and mustards. It is used orally and topically in Indian and Chinese medicine, for the relief of symptoms associated with inflammation in musculoskeletal conditions. Ointments and lotions containing an alcoholic extract of the tumeric root are used in traditional medicine to treat sprains. Although taken orally, tumeric is not absorbed very well.

The most potent constituent of tumeric is its yellow pigment, curcumin. Curcumin promotes the production of anti-inflammatory prostaglandins and has antioxidant properties. Preparations containing curcumin extracts can be obtained commercially. Sodium curcuminate is another potent product obtained from tumeric. This was produced in ancient times by making a poultice of tumeric and slaked lime and was used to treat sprains, muscular pains and inflamed joints.

The volatile oil fraction has been shown to possess anti-inflammatory activity in a variety of experimental models, where its effects have been shown to be comparable to hydrocortisone and phenylbutazone in acute inflammation, but only half as effective in chronic models (Murray and Pizzorno, 1998). Constituents with antihistamine activity found in tumeric are also believed to contribute to anti-inflammatory effects in the early stages of inflammation.

Tumeric is contraindicated in patients with stomach ulcers or hyperacidity disorders, and long-term use may cause gastric ulcers. It should be avoided by patients taking antiplatelet medication as there is a possibility that the effects of these drugs could be increased.

The powdered root of tumeric can be taken in a dose of 0.5–1.0 g several times daily between meals up to a total daily dose of 1.5–3.0 g. Alternatively, 10–15 drops of a 1:10 tincture can be taken two or three times daily. The oral dose of curcumin extract is 250–500 mg three times a day between meals.

Willow bark   Willow bark (*Salix alba* and other species) was originally used by the Chinese and the native Americans for its analgesic, anti-inflammatory, antirheumatic and antipyretic properties. It is still used for musculoskeletal conditions including lower-back pain and arthritis.

Constituents of willow bark are salicylates, including salicin, and condensed tannins. French and German scientists were the first to isolate salicin in 1828, which led to the creation of aspirin (acetylsalicylic acid) 10 years later by European chemists.

When taken orally, salicin is hydrolysed by the stomach acid to saligenin and glucose. Once absorbed, saligenin is probably converted to salicylic acid, however sub-therapeutic amounts of salicylic acid are produced. Studies have shown that neither isolated salicin nor salicylic acid alone are responsible for the anti-inflammatory effects of willow extracts. Other constituents within the bark are thought to also contribute to its effectiveness. One study showed that willow bark extracts, standardised to deliver 240 mg of the salicin constituent daily, are more effective than placebo in lower back pain, however it can take up to a week to obtain significant relief (Jellin, 2003).

Willow bark has minimal effects on platelet function compared to aspirin and other NSAIDs. It has been suggested that platelet function is not affected after willow bark consumption (Beckwith, 1998).

Gastointestinal side-effects are infrequent with willow bark compared to those of aspirin. Salicoside and other glycoside constituents in willow bark act to significantly reduce the gastrointestinal irritation caused by the salicylates present. Furthermore, salicin is not as irritating to the gastrointestinal tract as salicylic acid or aspirin because it lacks carboxylic acid and phenol functional groups. Other side-effects that have been reported include nausea, dizziness and rashes.

Because of the presence of salicylates in willow bark, it should be used with caution in those sensitive to salicylates or those already taking salicylate drugs. Individuals with known sensitivity to aspirin, asthma, peptic ulceration, diabetes, gout, haemophilia, kidney or liver disease should be warned about the possible risk of taking willow bark.

Doses of willow bark can vary depending on the dosage form used. A dose of 1–3 g of dried bark can be used to make a tea and taken 3–4 times daily; 1–3 mL of a 1:1 liquid extract can be taken 3–4 times daily. Standardised extracts providing a total daily dose of 120–240 mg of salicin have been used in clinical trials for back pain.

Homeopathy

In soft tissue injuries arnica is generally used first, and this may be supplemented by rhus tox (where there is tendonitis or stiffness that feels better with warmth and gentle movement, bryonia (where the condition improves with the application of cold and there is pain on any movement) or anacardium (no pain on any movement). Ruta is often given subsequently, but may also be used on its own for strained muscles.

It is possible to combine some of these remedies into one dose form as a combination remedy. Rhus tox and ruta is administered when the exact nature of the injury is unknown. The same combination is often successful in treating the lumbago and low back pain suffered by windsurfers and weightlifters. If there is a haematoma at the site of the sprain or strain, *Bellis perennis* (from the daisy) is appropriate.

Topical preparations of arnica or rhus tox in cream, gel or ointment formulation can be used by direct application, direct application under occlusive dressings or in combination with physical therapy, including massage and ultrasound.

Combinations of allopathic and homeopathic treatments are not unusual. There are also OTC massage balms available from one or two manufacturers. The use of injected homeopathic preparations including rhus tox has been reported for foot problems involving considerable stiffness in the morning (Subotnick, 1991).

'Tennis elbow' refers to a painful condition involving the detachment of muscular and tendinous fibres; 'golf elbow' is a similar type of injury. Both respond to argent met twice daily for 10 days. Ruta may also help. 'Runners knee' (chondromalacia) is a frequent complaint of joggers and may be treated with a variety of preparations including arnica, rhus tox, rhododendron and ruta in turn, together with orthodox manipulations, according to the severity of the condition. Apis is another possible remedy where there is oedema and inflammation.

Muscle cramps

A cramp is an intense, involuntary contraction of a muscle that usually occurs during or immediately after exercise. Cramps were traditionally thought to stem from fluid or electrolyte imbalances, but they are not always the reason. Cramps may occur following chronic muscle use by individuals, such as musicians, who are not sweating.

The soreness may continue to develop, reaching a peak 24–48 hours after exercise, when it is known as 'delayed onset muscle soreness' (DOMS). The condition usually subsides after 3–4 days but can interrupt training and therefore decrease performance.

Treatments for DOMS include drugs, herbal remedies, stretching, massage and nutritional supplements. Anti-inflammatory drugs and antioxidants also appear to be effective (Connolly *et al.*, 2003). Other conventional approaches such as ultrasound, stretching and massage (see below) appear variable (see also chapter 4).

Essential oils

Essential oils that may be of use in skeletal muscle spasm include black pepper, lavender, marjoram and rosemary. The oils themselves, along with the physical action of massage, may provide soothing relief from painful conditions associated with muscle cramps and spasm. Three drops of essential oil diluted in 5 mL of carrier oil can be gently massaged into the affected area when required.

Herbalism

Herbal remedies with antispasmodic and relaxant properties can be taken as a tea and may help relieve the symptoms associated with muscle cramps. Such herbs include chamomile flowers, lemon balm, hops, lavender and valerian. A herbal tea can be made by infusing a teaspoonful of one, or a combination, of these dried herbs in a cup of hot water and taken 3–4 times daily.

Homeopathy

Arnica   Arnica is one of the most widely used homeopathic remedies (Rutten, 2004). It is taken orally to treat both exhaustion immediately after exercise and DOMS. However, evidence of its effectiveness is mixed. Vickers *et al.* (1998) conducted a study to determine whether homeopathic arnica was more effective in reducing muscle soreness following long-distance running than a placebo. In a randomised, double-blind placebo-controlled trial, a total of 519 runners competing in a long-distance race and who anticipated suffering from DOMS took homeopathic arnica for 2 days after the race. Muscle soreness was measured in this period. Subjects completed a visual analogue scale and Likert scale of muscle soreness. The conclusion was that homeopathic arnica was ineffective for muscle soreness following long-distance running.

Tveiten and Bruset (2003) examined whether arnica had any effect on muscle soreness and cell damage after marathon running. The subjects were 82 marathon runners from two separate randomised, double-blind, placebo-controlled trials participating in the Oslo Marathon in 1990 and 1995. Five pills of arnica or placebo were given morning and evening, starting on the evening before the marathon and continuing until 3 days after the race. Muscle enzymes, electrolytes and creatinine were measured before and after the marathon. The runners assessed their muscular soreness on a visual analogue scale. Muscle soreness immediately after the marathon was lower in the arnica group than in the placebo group. However cell damage measured by the enzyme levels was similar in the arnica and the placebo groups. The authors concluded that these pooled results suggest that arnica D30 has a positive effect on muscle soreness after marathon running, but not on cell damage.

It has been suggested that positive responses to homeopathic arnica could be due to a number of factors. The methodology of many of the trials is flawed – the remedy has been used for inappropriate conditions or at the wrong dose levels – so no firm conclusion is possible. Other areas of inconsistency include the use of herbal (non-diluted) arnica, and the variable natural course of disease (Ernst, 2003). Ernst (2004) has claimed that the results of rigorous clinical trials collectively show that arnica is no better than placebo.

Strontium carb is a remedy that may help old strains associated with intermittent pains and swellings given night and morning for 10 days.

OTC products   The French product Sportenine, made by Boiron in tablet form, claims to 'improve stamina, promotes recovery, and reduces the risk of cramps, aches, pains, exhaustion, muscular fatigue due to prolonged physical effort'. In the USA, Hylands have two sport-related products, Arnisport and Bioplasma, for muscle soreness, together with a leg cramp product comprising a mixture of remedies including quinine in homeopathic dilution. Several OTC products exist in Australia and New Zealand. None of these products are currently licensed for sale in the UK.

Massage

Bale and James (1991) conducted a study in which nine athletes rested, warmed down with moderate exercise, or received massage for 17 minutes having completed a maximal run. DOMS was less pronounced in the massaged individuals, who also showed a more rapid decline in muscle lactate levels. This showed promising results in support of massage therapy, but the small sample size hampered its conclusiveness. Another study investigated the physiological and psychological effects of massage on DOMS and concluded that massage administered 2 hours after exercise-induced muscle injury did not improve hamstring function but did reduce the intensity of soreness (Hilbert *et al.*, 2003).

A study in which 20 female volunteers received electrical vibration massages for 40 minutes after maximal muscular activity showed that there appeared to be less loss of muscular strength after 1 and 3 days in the massaged thighs compared to a control group. However, in the upper limbs no such difference could be demonstrated (Eltze *et al.*, 1982). In another study, 12 male volunteers performed quadriceps contractions up to the point of exhaustion and were given percussive vibratory massage bouts lasting 4 minutes. This did not alter the degree of fatigue (Cafarelli and Flint, 1993).

Robertson *et al.* (2004) examined the effects of leg massage compared with passive recovery on lactate clearance, muscular power output and fatigue characteristics after repeated high-intensity cycling exercise under controlled conditions in nine males. No measurable physiological effects of leg massage compared with passive recovery were observed after high-intensity exercise. However, the authors concluded that the subsequent effect on fatigue index warranted further investigation.

In one study, six elite cyclists performed a simulated 4-day race. After each day the cyclists were either massaged for 20 minutes or given 30 minutes of placebo microwave. Serum muscle and liver enzymes were measured to detect muscle damage and recovery status. There were no significant differences between massage and placebo at any time during the study. It was concluded that post-event massage did not improve muscle recovery or improve performance (Drews *et al.*, 1991).

Massage is commonly assumed to enhance muscle recovery from intense exercise, principally because it speeds up the blood flow to muscles (Hemmings *et al.*, 2000). However, studies to date on blood flow have been inconsistent and sometimes contradictory.

A systematic review of seven studies on DOMS and massage found that most of the methodology described was seriously flawed (Ernst, 1998a). It was concluded that massage therapy may be a promising treatment and that further study was warranted.

Pain

Acupuncture

A controlled trial of acupuncture in 75 patients with knee pain suggested that it might be beneficial as a treatment for the condition. There is also evidence that acupuncture may be effective when used for back (Ernst and White, 1998) and neck pain (Ross *et al.*, 1999). A rigorous well-designed trial investigating the effect of treating athletes with shoulder injuries using acupuncture showed positive results (Kleinherz *et al.*, 1999).

Chiropractic

The literature contains a variety of chiropractic low back pain research studies including randomised clinical trials, comparative randomised clinical trials and meta-analytic reviews (Kaptchuk and Eisenberg, 1998).

The use of chiropractic in sports medicine is increasing. For example the New Zealand Olympic Team in Barcelona appointed a chiropractor and found his involvement to be beneficial (Hill, 1993).

There is significant chiropractic involvement in US professional football; 31% of NFL teams have been shown to use the services of a chiropractor to treat low back pain (61%), neck injury (31%) and headaches (8%) (Stump and Redwood, 2002).

The clinical management of recurrent shoulder instability in a professional hockey player by using chiropractic management and rehabilitation exercises has been described (Moreau and Moreau, 2001).

Chiropractic may also be used in the treatment of running injuries, providing the practitioner has a thorough understanding of the anatomy, biomechanics, motor patterns and kinetic chains of the lower limb, including the pelvis (Conway, 2001). By identifying the underlying dysfunction, the chiropractor can implement a multilevel treatment protocol that involves manipulative therapy, restoration of faulty biomechanics, strengthening of weakened muscle groups, and motor pattern re-education.

Chiropractic is contraindicated in certain vascular complications, arteriosclerosis, traumatic injuries and arthritis.

Homeopathy

A number of homeopathic remedies are available to alleviate back pain. Rhus tox seems to be more successful in patients whose movement is painful when they get out of bed but that improves with movement. Bryonia is more successful with people for whom movement of any sort all day is painful.

Massage

Several studies have compared massage with a control group for the treatment of back pain, with variable outcomes being reported (Hoehler *et al.*, 1981; Godfrey *et al.*, 1984). There appears to be little convincing evidence of the effectiveness of manipulation (Ernst, 1998b). However, one randomised clinical trial with four groups sought to compare the effectiveness of massage therapy with other interventions for the treatment of low back pain and showed that massage was more effective than some other interventions (Preyde, 2000).

Relaxation

Relaxation has been found beneficial in the treatment of chronic pain (Carroll and Seers, 1998).

Skin conditions

Athlete's foot (tinea pedis) can be a recurrent problem for athletes, particularly those training in warm climates. Risk of infection is greater in warm, moist environments such as around swimming pools, and changing and shower rooms where it is commonly spread. Keeping the feet dry is very important in preventing and fighting athlete's foot.

Scrumpox is commonly caused by the herpes simplex virus, which is acquired by those competing in close contact sports. It is highly infectious, spreading in droplets by direct contact. Impetigo and erysipelas are also blamed for this condition.

Essential oils

Tea tree oil   Tea tree oil has antiseptic and antifungal properties and is used in the treatment of athlete's foot (Tong *et al.*, 1992). Application of a 10% tea tree oil cream has been compared in efficacy to 1% tolnaftate cream for relieving symptoms of athlete's foot such as scaling, itching and burning. Tea tree oil is not effective at this strength in producing a cure for tinea pedis (Jellin *et al.*, 2003), but may prove more effective if applied undiluted. Essential oils of lavender, lemon or thyme can also be applied directly to unbroken skin on affected areas of the feet three times a day.

Herbalism

The compound known as ajoene, found in garlic, is an antifungal agent. In a group of 34 people using a 0.4% ajoene cream applied once per day, 79% of them saw complete clearing of athlete's foot after 1 week; the rest saw complete clearing within 2 weeks (Ledezma *et al.*, 1996). All participants remained cured 3 months later. Another trial found a 1% ajoene cream to be more effective than the orthodox topical drug terbinafine for treating athlete's foot (Ledezma *et al.*, 2000). Ajoene cream is not yet available commercially, but topical application of crushed, raw garlic may be a potential alternative application.

Tinctures of echinacea, goldenseal and myrrh can also be applied three times a day to assist with symptom and infection control of tinea. The application of such herbal products should be continued for a few days after the symptoms disappear to ensure that the fungal infection has been adequately treated.

Garden celandine (*Chelidonium majus*) juice has been used topically in the treatment of verrucae.

Homeopathy

Old-fashioned remedies for athlete's foot, such as Whitfield's ointment and potassium permanganate, may be augmented with remedies such as rhus tox, sepia, sulphur or tellurium.

Scrumpox responds to homeopathic rhus tox or apis.

Verrucae and warts may be treated orally twice or three times daily with either acid nitric or thuja. If the skin is not broken thuja may be applied topically as ointment or mother tincture. Both are usually applied sparingly once daily.

Performance-enhancing methods

Acupuncture

Although some of the mechanisms of acupuncture as it applies to pain relief have been studied, little is known about the positive and/or negative effects of this procedure on the physical performance parameters of healthy people, particularly highly-trained athletes. Preliminary studies of the effects of acupuncture on strength, aerobic conditioning, flexibility and sport performance seem to suggest that there could be potential benefit from this practice, although there is a requirement for the establishment of guidelines covering the use of acupuncture in the sports community (Pelham *et al.*, 2001).

Herbalism

In the quest to find energy for that extra hundredth of a second and the medal it may bring, sports persons are constantly seeking products to enhance performance. Word goes from mouth to mouth about some new discovery and it may be taken without too much thought for safety or even legality. Unfortunately these products are often obtained in countries of the developing world where quality control is non-existent and the possibility of adulteration with banned substances is high. Ginseng is a good example of the potential risks involved (Figure 6.2). At the Seoul Olympics in 1988, the British athlete Linford Christie narrowly escaped suspension when a drugs test following the 200-metre race revealed traces of the stimulant, pseudoephedrine. Brought before the IOC's Medical Commission, Christie claimed the banned substance was contained in powdered ginseng that he was taking to improve his general vitality.

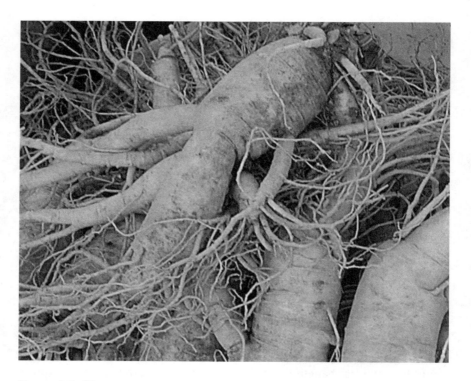

Figure 6.2 Ginseng root.

Herbs that are reported to have anabolic effects include yohimbine, wild yam, smilax and tribulus. Yohimbine (extracted from yohimbe bark or from the South American herb, quebracho) supposedly increases serum testosterone levels (presumably by increasing blood flow through the testes), thereby increasing muscle size and strength. Gamma oryzanol, which occurs in rice germs and rice bran, is also claimed to have anabolic effects. There is no evidence for these claims.

Ephedra sinica contains the prohibited substance ephedrine, which is a stimulant to the nervous system and cardiovascular system. It is used to accelerate fat loss and enhance energy. In one American survey it was found that ephedra was consumed at least once a week by 28% of visitors to a New York gym (Morrison *et al.*, 2004). There is no solid evidence that herbal ephedra can improve athletic performance, but the use of ephedrine-containing products can result in serious side-effects, including death (Coleman *et al.*, 2002).

Herbs such as ginseng, gingko biloba and gotu kola are included in some sports drinks designed to enhance performance (see Chapter 10).

Homeopathy

There is one anecdotal report in the literature of homeopathic arsenicum album being administered to the members of a boxing team in the Indian Military Academy with apparent success. Two unexpected wins were subsequently recorded (Negi, 1985).

Massage

Athletes often use massage before sports activities, but there is little evidence to show that it will enhance their performance. A whole range of liniments and rubs for use with accompanying massage are available. Many have the characteristic 'go faster' aroma of wintergreen, instantly recognisable in a typical changing room environment. Some of these products are rubifacients, containing constituents that are irritant to the skin (e.g. salicylates and capsicum) and causing dilation of superficial blood vessels, so creating a pleasant warm sensation. There is a risk of an allergic reaction to these chemicals.

The effects of pre-event massage, warm-up and stretching exercises on joints, range of movement and quadriceps and hamstring strength have been investigated (Wiktorsson-Moller *et al.*, 1983). The results showed that warm-up and stretching produced significant increases in all ranges of movement. The only other significant finding was that massage and warm-up, both separately and in combination, appeared to increase the range of movement on the calf. It was concluded that general warm-up and stretching are good techniques to increase flexibility, without the need for expensive equipment or operators.

Psychological interventions

The successful use of psychological interventions to improve performance in sport has been reported, but the validity of many studies has been questioned on the grounds of methodological inadequacies (Weinberg and Comar, 1994). Meditation may enhance competitive shooting performance through a calming effect and an ability to reduce hand tremor (Solberg *et al.*, 1996).

References

Akimoto T, Nakahori C, Aizawa K, *et al.* (2003). Acupuncture and responses of immunologic and endocrine markers during competition. *Med Sci Sports Exerc* 35: 1296–1302.

Alton S, Kayne S B (1992). A pilot study of the attitudes and awareness of homoeopathy shown by patients in three Manchester pharmacies. *Br Hom J* 81: 189–193.

Angus S (2001). Massage therapy for sprinters and runners. *Clin Podiatr Med Surg* 18: 329–336.

Anon (2005). The end of homeopathy (editorial). *Lancet* 336: 699.

Assendelft W, Bouter L, Knipschild P G (1996). Complications of spinal manipulation – a comprehensive review of the literature. *J Fam Pract* 42: 475–480.

Bale P, James H (1991). Massage, warmdown and rest as recuperative measures after short term intense exercise. *Physiother Sport* 13: 4–7.

Barnes J, Anderson L, Philipson J D (2002). *Herbal Medicines: A Guide for Healthcare Professionals*, 2nd edn. London: Pharmaceutical Press.

Beckwith J V (1998) Herbal medications and nutraceuticals used to treat rheumatoid or osteoarthritis. In: Miller L G, Murray W J, eds. *Herbal Medicinals: A Clinician's Guide*. Binghampton, NY: Pharmaceutical Products Press, 95–113.

Belon P (1995). Provings. Concept and methodology. *Br Hom J* 84: 213–217.

Blonstein J L (1960). Control of swelling in boxing injuries. *Practitioner* 185: 78.

Blumenthal M, Goldberg A, Brinkmann J, eds. *Herbal Medicine: Expanded Commission E Monographs*. Boston, MA: Integrative Medicine Communications.

Boone T, Cooper R, Thompson W R (1991). A psychological evaluation of the sports massage. *Athletic Training* 26: 51–54.

Botting D (1997). Review of literature on the effectiveness of reflexology. *Complement Ther Nursing Midwifery* 3: 123–130.

Cafarelli E, Flint F (1993). The role of massage in preparation for and recovery from exercise. *Physiother Sport* 16: 17–20.

Calabrese C, Preston P (1993). Report of the results of a double-blind, randomized, single-dose trial of a topical 2% escin gel versus placebo in the acute treatment of experimentally-induced hematoma in volunteers. *Planta Med* 59: 394–397.

Callaghan M J (1993). The role of massage in the management of the athlete. A review. *Br J Sports Med* 27: 28–33.

Carroll D, Seers K (1998). Relaxation for the relief of chronic pain: a systematic review. *J Adv Nurs* 27: 476–487.

Choi S W, Son B W, Son Y S, *et al.* (2001). The wound-healing effect of a glycoprotein fraction isolated from aloe vera. *Br J Dermatol* 145: 535–545.

Chrubasik S, Thanner J, Kunzel O, *et al.* (2002). Comparison of outcome measures during treatment with the proprietary Harpagophytum extract doloteffin in patients with pain in the lower back, knee or hip. *Phytomedicine* 9: 181–194.

Coleman E, Nelson-Steen S, Maughan R, *et al.* (2002). *Herbal Supplements and Sport Performance*. Gatorade Sports Science Institute. Sports Science Exchange Roundtable 50, Volume 13, No. 4 [available from http://www.gssiweb.com/reflib/refs/601/SSERT_50.cfm?pid=38&CFID=605699&CFTOKEN=92944192].

Connolly D A, Sayers S P, McHugh M P (2003). Treatment and prevention of delayed onset muscle soreness. *J Strength Cond Res* 17: 197–208.

Conway P J (2001). Chiropractic approach to running injuries. *Clin Podiatr Med Surg* 18: 351–362.

Dabbs V, Lauretti W J (1995). A risk assessment of cervical manipulation vs NSAIDs for the treatment of neck pain. *J Manipulative Physiol Ther* 18: 530–553.

de Schepper L (1994). *Musculoskeletal Diseases and Homeopathy*. Santa Fe, NM: Full of Life Publishing.

Drews T, Knieder R B, Drinkard B, *et al.* (1991). Effects of post event massage therapy on psychological profiles of exertion, feeling and mood during a four day ultraendurance cycling event. *Med Sci Sport Exerc* 23: 91.

EC Directive 65/65 EU Secretariat, Brussels.

Eltze Ch, Hildebrandt G, Johansson M (1982). Über die Wirsankeit der Vibrationsmassage beim Muskelkater. *Z Phys Med Baln Klim* 11: 366–376. (In Ernst E, Fialka V (1994). The clinical effectiveness of massage. *Forsch Komplementärmed* 1: 226–232.)

Ernst E (1998a). Spinal manipulation for low back pain. *Eur J Phys Med Rehabil* 8: 1–2.

Ernst E (1998b). Does post-exercise massage treatment reduce delayed onset muscle soreness? A systematic review. *Br J Sports Med* 32: 212–214.

Ernst E (2003). The benefits of arnica: 16 case reports. *Homeopathy* 92: 217–219.

Ernst E (2004). Should we use 'powerful placebos?' *Pharm J* 273: 795.

Ernst E, White A R (1998) Acupuncture for back pain: a meta analysis of randomized clinical trials. *Arch Intern Med* 223: 2235–2241.

Field T, Morrow C, Valdeon C, *et al.* (1992). Massage reduces anxiety in child and adolescent psychiatric patients. *J Am Acad Child Adolesc Psychiatry* 31: 125–131.

Freeman L W, Lawlis G F (2001). *Mosby's Complementary and Alternative Medicine: A Research-Based Approach*. St Louis, MI: Mosby, 297.

Godfrey C M, Morgan P P, Schatzker J (1984). A randomized trial of manipulation for low back pain in a medical setting. *Spine* 9: 301–304.

Heck A, Dewitt B A, Lukes A L (2000). Potential interactions between alternative therapies and warfarin. *Am J Health-Syst Pharm* 57: 1221–1227.

Hilbert J E, Sforzo G A, Swensen T (2003). The effects of massage on delayed onset muscle soreness. *Br J Sports Med* 37: 72–75.

Hill C L (1993). Barcelona Olympics – Chiropractic report. *N Z J Sports Med* 21: 8.

Hoehler F K, Tobis J S, Buerger A A (1981). Spinal manipulation for low back pain. *JAMA* 245: 1835–1838.

Halderman S, Rubinstein S M (1992). Cauda equina syndrome following lumbar spine manipulation. *Spine* 17: 1469–1473.

Hemmings B, Smith M, Graydon J, *et al.* (2000). Effects of massage on physiological restoration, perceived recovery, and repeated sports performance. *Br J Sports Med* 34: 109–114.

Jellin J M, ed. (2003). *Natural Medicines Comprehensive Database*. Stockton, CA: Therapeutic Research Facility.

Kaptchuk T, Eisenberg D M (1998). Chiropractic: origins, controversies and contributions. *Arch Intern Med* 158: 2215–2224. [Reprinted in: Fontanarosa P B, ed. (2000). *Alternative Medicine: An Objective Assessment*. Chicago: American Medical Association].

Kleinhenz J, Streitberger K, Windeler J, *et al.* (1999). Randomised clinical trial comparing the effects of acupuncture and a newly designed placebo needle in rotator cuff tendinitis. *Pain* 83: 235–241.

Kucera M, Barna M, Horacek O, *et al.* (2004). Efficacy and safety of topically applied Symphytum herb extract cream in the treatment of ankle distortion: results of a randomized controlled clinical double blind study. *Wien Med Wochenschr* 154: 498–507.

Leach M J (2004). A critical review of natural therapies in wound management. *Ostomy Wound Manage* 50: 36–40, 42, 44–46 passim.

Ledezma E, DeSousa L, Jorquera A, *et al.* (1996). Efficacy of ajoene, an organosulphur derived from garlic, in the short-term therapy of tinea pedis. *Mycoses* 39: 393–395.

Ledezma E, Marcano K, Jorquera A, *et al.* (2000). Efficacy of ajoene in the treatment of tinea pedis: A double-blind and comparative study with terbinafine. *J Am Acad Dermatol* 43: 829–832.

Lussignoli S, Bertani S, Metelmann H, *et al.* (1999). Effect of Traumeel S, a homeopathic formulation, on blood-induced inflammation in rats. *Complement Ther Med* 7: 225–230.

Marwick C (1997). Acceptance of some acupuncture applications. *JAMA* 278: 1725–1727.

Mitchell D R (2000). *Nature's Painkillers*. New York: Lyn Sonberg Book Associates.

Moreau C E, Moreau S R (2001). Chiropractic management of a professional hockey player with recurrent shoulder instability. *J Manipulative Physiol Ther* 24: 425–430.

Morrison L J, Gizis F, Shorter B (2004). Prevalent use of dietary supplements among people who exercise at a commercial gym. *Int J Sport Nutr Exerc Metab* 4: 481–492.

Murray M T, Pizzomo J E (1998). *Encyclopedia of Natural Medicine*, 2nd edn. Rocklin, CA: Prima Publishing.

Negi R S (1985). Homeopathy in sports medicine. *Hahnemanian Gleanings* 52: 244–248.

Pelham T W, Holt L E, Stalker R (2001). Acupuncture in human performance. *J Strength Cond Res* 2: 266–271.

Powell F C, Hanigan W C, Olivero W C (1993). A risk/benefit analysis of spinal manipulation for relief of lumbar or cervical pain. *Neurosurgery* 33: 73–78.

Preyde M (2000). Effectiveness of massage therapy for subacute low-back pain: a randomised controlled trial. *Can Med Assoc J* 162: 1815–1820.

Robertson A, Watt J M, Galloway S D (2004). Effects of leg massage on recovery from high intensity cycling exercise. *Br J Sports Med* 38: 173–176.

Ross J, White A, Ernst E (1999). Western minimal acupuncture for neck pain: a cohort study. *Acupunct Med* 17: 5–8.

Rutten L (2004). The benefits of arnica. *Homeopathy* 93: 63.

Shang A, Huwiler-Mütener K, Nartey L, *et al.* (2005). Are the clinical effects of homeopathy placebo effects? Comparative study of homeopathy and allopathy. *Lancet* 336: 726–732.

Shaw J (1987). Reflexology. *Health Visitor* 60: 367.

Solberg E E, Berglund K-A, Engen O, *et al.* (1996). The effect of meditation on shooting performance. *J Sports Med* 30: 342–346.

Stump J L, Redwood D (2002). The use and role of sport chiropractors in the national football league: a short report. *J Manipulative Physiol Ther* 25: E2.

Subotnick S (1991). *Sports and Exercise Injuries: Conventional, Homeopathic and Alternative Treatments*. Berkeley, CA: North Atlantic Press.

Terrett A G (1996). Misuse of the literature by medical authors in discussing spinal manipulative therapy injury. *J Manipulative Physiol Ther* 18: 203–210.

Tong M M, Altman P M, Barnetson R S (1992). Tea tree oil in the treatment of tinea pedis. *Aust J Dermatol* 33: 145–149.

Triano J, Schultz A B (1997). Loads transmitted during lumbosacral manipulative therapy. *Spine* 22: 1955–1964.

Tveiten D, Bruset S (2003). Effect of arnica D30 in marathon runners. Pooled results from two double-blind placebo controlled studies. *Homeopathy* 92: 187–189.

Vickers A J, Fisher P, Smith C, *et al.* (1998). Homeopathic arnica 30x is ineffective for muscle soreness after long-distance running: a randomized, double-blind, placebo-controlled trial. *Clin J Pain* 14: 227–231.

Weinberg R S, Comar W (1994). The effectiveness of psychological interventions in competitive sport. *Sports Med* 18; 306–318.

Wiktorsson-Moller M, Oberg B, Eksrand J, *et al.* (1983). Effects of warming up, massage and stretching on range of motion and muscle strength in the lower extremity. *Am J Sports Med.* 11: 249–252.

Wolfe F A (1999). *Reflexology*. New York: Alpha Books, 50.

Wood C (1993). Mood change and perceptions of vitality: a comparison of the effects of relaxation, visualization and yoga. *J R Soc Med* 86: 254–258.

Zollman C, Vickers A (2000). *ABC of Complementary Medicine. Massage Therapies*. London: BMJ Books, 32–35.

Further reading

Boon H, Smith M (1999). *The Botanical Pharmacy: The Pharmacology of 47 Common Herbs*. Kingston, Ont.: Quarry Press Inc.

Cash M (1996). *Sport and Remedial Massage Therapy*. London: Ebury Press.

Cash M, Ylinen J (1988). *Sports Massage*. London: Hutchinson.

Kayne S B (2002). *Complementary Therapies for Pharmacists*. London: Pharmaceutical Press.

Kayne S B (2005). *Homeopathic Pharmacy: Theory and Practice*, 2nd edn. Edinburgh: Churchill Livingstone.

Mootz R D, McCarthy K A (1999). *Sports Chiropractic* (Topics in Clinical Chiropractic Series). New York: Aspen Publishers.

Morgan L W (1990). *Treating Sports Injuries the Natural Way – Homeopathic Self-Treatment Handbook*. London: Harper Collins.

Thomas E (2000). *Homoeopathy for Sports, Exercise and Dance*. Beaconsfield: Beaconsfield Publishers.

Worwood V A (1990). *The Fragrant Pharmacy*. London: Macmillan.

Useful addresses

Aromatherapy

Aromatherapy Consortium
PO Box 6522
Desborough
Kettering
Northants NN14 2YX
Tel: +44 (0)870 7743477
http://www.aromatherapy-regulation.org.uk

Association of Medical Aromatherapists
11 Park Circus
Glasgow
Tel: +44 (0)141 332 4924

Chiropractic

British Chiropractic Association
Blagrave House
17 Blagrave Street
Reading
Berkshire RG1 1QB
Tel: +44 (0)118 950 5950
http://www.chiropractic-uk.co.uk

Herbalism

National Institute of Medical Herbalists
56 Longbrook Street
Exeter
Devon EX4 6AH
Tel: +44 (0)1392 426022
http://www.nimh.org.uk

Homeopathy

The Faculty of Homeopathy
Hahnemann House
29 Park Street West

Luton LU1 3BE
Tel: +44 (0)870 444 3950
http://www.trusthomeopathy.org

The Society of Homeopaths
11 Brookfield
Duncan Close
Moulton Park
Northampton NN3 6WL
Tel: +44 (0)845 450 6611
http://www.homeopathy-soh.com

Physiotherapy and complementary health (massage, reflexology and acupuncture)

Chartered Society of Physiotherapy
14 Bedford Row
London WC1R 4ED
Tel: +44 (0)20 7306 6666
http://www.csp.org.uk/physiotherapy/complementary

Other

Halliwick Association of Swimming Therapy in the UK
c/o ADKC Centre
Whitstable House
Silchester Road
London W10 6SB
http://www.halliwick.org.uk/
Halliwick is based on principles of hydrostatics, hydrodynamics and kinesiology. It promotes a holistic approach to swimming.

Part Three

Misuse of drugs in sport

7

History of doping in sport

Anthony C Moffat

Introduction

There have always been those who would try to gain an advantage over other competitors by taking substances they thought would improve their performance. This chapter looks at the history of doping in sport, with sections arranged in chronological order of when a particular form of doping was recognised. Each section then tracks that form of doping to the modern day, with the controls now in place and examples of some classic cases of doping and alleged doping in sport. Full details of current controls and dope testing procedures are covered in Chapter 8.

The word 'dope' probably comes from the Dutch word 'dop', meaning an alcoholic drink made of grape skins used by Zulu warriors to increase their abilities in battle. The word was used at the turn of the 20th century to describe the illegal drugging of racehorses (World Anti-Doping Agency, 2005), although in this case the doping was meant to reduce the racehorse's ability, whereas today doping means the deliberate act of improving performance.

Doping in sport used to be simply defined as:

- The use of an expedient (substance or method) that is potentially harmful to an athlete's health and is capable of enhancing their performance; or
- The presence in the athlete's body of a prohibited substance or evidence of the use thereof or evidence of the use of a prohibited method.

Today, doping is defined by the WADA (see p. 234 and Chapter 8) in the World Anti-Doping Guide as "the occurrence of one or more of the anti-doping rule violations set forth in Article 2.1 through Article 2.8 of the Code". The following constitute anti-doping rule violations (World Anti-Doping Agency, 2005):

1. The presence of a Prohibited Substance or its Metabolites or Markers in an Athlete's bodily specimen.
2. Use or Attempted Use of a Prohibited Substance or a Prohibited Method.
3. Refusing, or failing without compelling justification, to submit to Sample collection after notification as authorised in applicable anti-doping rules or otherwise evading Sample collection.
4. Violation of applicable requirements regarding Athlete availability for Out-of-Competition Testing including failure to provide required whereabouts information and missed tests which are declared based on reasonable rules.
5. Tampering, or attempting to tamper, with any part of Doping Control.
6. Possession of Prohibited Substances and Methods.
7. Trafficking in any Prohibited Substance or Prohibited Method.
8. Administration or Attempted administration of a Prohibited Substance or Prohibited Method to any Athlete, or assisting, encouraging, aiding, abetting, covering up or any other type of complicity involving an anti-doping rule violation or any Attempted violation.

How the Code grew to this extent is explained below. It should be noted that doping is a strict liability offence where the presence of a prohibited substance in an athlete's urine sample starts the disciplinary procedure.

Ancient history

Doping is certainly not new – the ancient Egyptians tried to improve their performance with a concoction of hooves of Abyssinian asses which were ground up, boiled in oil and flavoured with rose petals and rose hips (Hanley, 1983). Even at the ancient Olympic Games, athletes were reported to have taken stimulants of one form or another. For example, in the Olympic Games of 668 BC, Charmis, the winner of the 200-metre sprint, was said to have used a special diet of dried figs (Finley and Plecket, 1976). The ancient Greeks too were believed to have tried to enhance their performance by taking psychoactive mushrooms and fortifying drinks. It was Galen, in the 3rd century BC, who reported that Greek athletes used stimulants to enhance their performance (Verroken, 2003). Roman gladiators and medieval knights also used stimulants to continue fighting after sustaining injuries (Donohoe and Johnson, 1986).

The 19th century

Cycling has always been at the forefront of doping allegations and even as early as the 19th century cyclists often used strychnine, caffeine, cocaine and alcohol to increase their speed and endurance (World Anti-Doping Agency, 2005). The French especially were reported to use strong coffee as a source of caffeine to help them in endurance cycle races. This was later enhanced by the addition of cocaine and brandy during the races. One of the earliest suspected cycling deaths was that of Arthur Linton in 1886. His death was suspected of being caused by an overdose of dope given to him by his trainer during the Bordeaux to Paris race of that year, which he won. Although it appeared later that he died from typhoid fever, there was still a suspicion that strychnine was involved in his death (Donohoe and Johnson, 1986).

The swimmers in the Amsterdam canal races of 1865 were also suspected of taking some form of dope (Donohoe and Johnson, 1986).

Into the 20th century

By the turn of the century, doping was on the increase. In the 1904 Olympic Games in St Louis, the winner of the marathon, Thomas Hicks, was believed to have been aided by a cocktail of strychnine and brandy (Ackerman, 1991). In the next Olympic Games in 1908, Dorando Pietri was also suspected of taking strychnine in the marathon. He collapsed just in front of the finishing line and was helped over it by some spectators, which disqualified him from the event (Donohoe and Johnson, 1986). There were further instances of known or suspected doping during the next 20 years, including further deaths due to doping in cycling. In 1928 the International Amateur Athletic Federation took a major stand and became the first international sporting federation to ban the use of doping in their sport (World Anti-Doping Agency, 2005). Other sporting federations followed this example, but the bans were ineffective as there were no tests available to detect doping.

The problem continued to grow, and there was an outcry at the suspected doping at the 1952 Helsinki Winter Olympics in Oslo, when ampoules and syringes were found in changing rooms. Also at the 1956 Melbourne Olympics, one competitor showed the classic symptoms of strychnine overdose (Donohoe and Johnson, 1986). There were further fatalities, such as that of Danish cyclist Knud Jensen, who died in 1960 while competing in the 100-km team time-trial cycle race on the opening day of the 1960 Olympics in Rome after taking a combination of amfetamine and nicotinyl tartrate (Donohoe and Johnson, 1986; Ackerman, 1991).

It was suspected that the practice of power lifters and bodybuilders of taking anabolic steroids to increase their weight spread to athletes who competed in the power events in the 1950s and 1960s. By the early 1960s the pressure was building to do something effective about doping in sport.

The watershed of the 1960s

During the early 1960s, many sporting associations refused to acknowledge that doping took place in their sport because they thought it would bring their sport into disrepute. However in 1963, France introduced the first anti-doping law, followed by Belgium in 1965 (Donohoe and Johnson, 1986).

In the UK, there was vehement denial by many sporting authorities that doping was occurring in their sport. Professor Arnold Beckett was instrumental in setting up an anti-doping laboratory in 1965 at Chelsea College and convincing some sporting authorities to start testing procedures. That year the British Cycling Federation started the first testing in the Tour of Britain Milk Race. Over the next 3 years, three Spanish cyclists and one English cyclist were found to have amfetamine in their urine. This was followed in 1966 by testing at the World Cup Football Championship in London, under the auspices of the Federation Internationale de Football Association (FIFA), where nobody was found positive. The British Amateur Weightlifting Association wanted to show that their sport was free of doping and they started testing in 1967.

A number of conferences concerning doping in sport took place in the early 1960s, with the IOC taking a strong lead. The IOC subsequently introduced spot checks at the 1964 Olympic Games in Tokyo, although this was only in cycling. They set up the Medical Commission in 1967 to have responsibility for doping controls at Olympic Games and the IOC Medical Commission clearly stated that if a competitor was found guilty of doping, they would be disqualified from the event and any medal withdrawn.

The first mandatory drug testing was in 1968 at the Winter Olympics in Grenoble (86 tests) and in the same year at the Olympic Games in Mexico City (668) for all sports. The testing was mainly for stimulants and pain killers and no positives were found for these substances in either event. However, one competitor in the biathlon (Hans-Gunnar Liljenvall) was found to have a blood alcohol concentration above the permitted limit and lost the bronze medal as a result (Donohoe and Johnson, 1986).

Comprehensive testing began in 1972 at the Munich Olympic Games, when over 2000 urine tests were carried out. Nine positive results were found, with seven disqualifications. Stimulants were the only class of prohibited substances to be detected – one amfetamine, three ephedrine, two nikethamide and one phenmetrazine positive. Throughout the next 30 years the IOC, through its Medical Commission, was the world leader in promoting good sportsmanship, organising anti-doping procedures, certifying laboratories to conduct doping analyses and funding research into new analytical methods to detect doping.

Prohibited substances list

It was in 1967 that the IOC first published its list of prohibited substances. They defined doping based on the pharmacological action of drug classes. Rule 29A of the Olympic Charter states: "Doping is forbidden. The IOC Medical Commission shall prepare a list of prohibited classes of drugs and of banned procedures." There were five categories listing those substances believed at the time to be causing the greatest problem in doping in sport: psychomotor stimulants, sympathomimetic amines, CNS stimulants, narcotic analgesics and anabolic steroids. This was expanded to six classes in 1992 and over the years other classes of compounds have been identified as problems. Today there are nine classes of prohibited substances: stimulants, narcotics, cannabinoids, anabolic agents, peptide hormones, beta$_2$ agonists, agents with anti-oestrogenic activity, masking agents and glucocorticosteroids. The words "and other substances with similar chemical structure or similar pharmacological effect(s)" are part of the list to prohibit the use of other substances that have not yet been used in doping but could be.

In 1985 the classes of beta blockers and diuretics were added to the list of banned substances and in 1993 the beta blockers were moved to the class of "drugs subject to certain restrictions" as they were not widely used as doping agents.

Not all sporting authorities adopt the same classification and this can lead to problems in defining a suspected doping offence. For example, in the 1988 Tour de France, the Spanish cyclist Pedro Delgado tested positive for a substance that was banned by the IOC, but not by the International Cycling Union. He therefore did not receive any penalty.

Stimulants

By their very nature, stimulants must be taken very close in time to the event in order to have any effect and so the urine sample of the athlete will contain high concentrations of these drugs. Thus mandatory testing during the late 1960s and early 1970s was for mainly for stimulants, but it paved the way for the modern dope testing of today. During the 1960s it was widely reported that something like a third of professional cyclists and many of the top amateurs took stimulants. The death of the British cyclist Tommy Simpson in the Tour de France in 1967 brought the use of stimulants to the public's attention. He had taken metamfetamine and died on one of the mountainous stretches of the race due to heart failure and heat exhaustion. Amfetamines block the body's normal mechanism to stop exertion and so fatal consequences can ensue. His death was widely reported and the dangers of doping in events such as cycling were clearly identified and understood by the man in the street.

During the 1978 World Cup Football Championship in Argentina, Willie Johnson the Scottish footballer was found to have fencamfamin in his urine. He was sent home immediately, but fortunately the whole Scottish football team were not disqualified and continued to play.

There were hiccoughs along the way in enforcing anti-doping measures, such as in 1972 at the Summer Olympics in Munich when the American swimmer Rick DeMont was stripped of his gold medal because ephedrine was found in his urine. He suffered from asthma and used an anti-asthmatic medicine containing ephedrine to assist his breathing, which he had declared on his medical submission before the competition. Following the furore over that case, the IOC subsequently permitted the medical use of salbutamol, terbutaline and other bronchodilators at the 1976 Summer Olympics in Montreal (Ackerman, 1991).

The problem of strict liability is well illustrated by the case of Alain Baxter, which is fully described in Chapter 8. In 2002, he finished third in the men's slalom at the Salt Lake City Winter Olympics to win the first ever ski medal won by a Briton. However his urine sample, given after the race, tested positive for metamfetamine. He had bought a Vicks Inhaler in the USA, which contains the levo isomer of metamfetamine – the UK version does not contain this substance. Levo-metamfetamine does not have any performance-enhancing capabilities, unlike the dextro isomer which is a powerful stimulant (Figure 7.1).

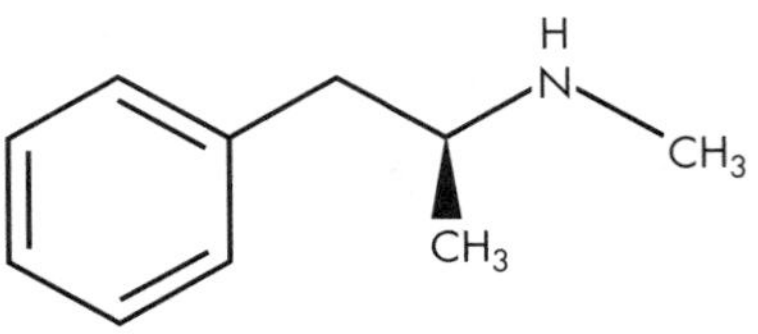

Figure 7.1 Metamfetamine (dextro-rotatory form).

Steroids

During the 1960s the use of anabolic steroids was increasing, in line with the increased size of athletes in the strength events such as shot-putting. Anabolic steroids are taken in the long term to increase muscle mass and strength and to assist recovery after heavy exercise and injury. They also increase aggression in the short term and may be used by athletes in explosive sports such as sprint events. Although their use became widely known, it was not until 1975 that the IOC included anabolic steroids in their list of banned substances. The first testing for steroids was at the Commonwealth Games in Christchurch in 1974. Professor Ray Brooks of St Thomas' Hospital, London, had developed a new radioimmunoassay for the detection of anabolic steroids in urine and this was used to test a number of competitors (Brooks *et al.*, 1979). Some of the urine samples tested positive, but the athletes were never named. In the 1976 Summer Olympics in Montreal, eight of the 275 samples tested were positive out of the over 2000 samples taken. This is in comparison with only three positive results for other banned substances out of 1786 samples tested (Barnes, 1980). This showed that the problem of anabolic steroids was real, but detectable. However, the problem grew as more and more athletes tested positive for anabolic steroids. In the preliminaries to the 1980 Moscow Olympics, the top three women's 1500-metre runners were banned from competition for life by the International Amateur Athletic Federation after being found guilty of taking anabolic steroids (Ackerman, 1991). One of the most notable cases was in 1988 at the Seoul Olympics when Ben Johnson won the 100 metres in a world record time and was later stripped of his gold medal because of the presence of anabolic steroids in his urine; he was also given a 2-year ban. In 1993 he was found positive again and given a life ban.

In 1993, the IOC changed the name of the prohibited class of anabolic steroids to anabolic agents and divided it in two, namely the androgenic anabolic steroids and the other anabolic agents (such as the beta-2 agonists, e.g. clenbuterol).

A major problem in detecting the use of steroids was that athletes could use them up to a week or so before an event, but then stop, so the steroid could not be detected in their urine when they were tested at the games. Out-of-competition testing was the only way to detect this type of doping (see below).

Testosterone

The main problem with detecting whether testosterone (Figure 7.2) was used as a doping agent was in interpreting the urine concentration because it appears naturally. However, a sister compound, epitestosterone (differing from testosterone only in the orientation of the hydroxyl group in the 17 position, Figure 7.3), is manufactured by the body at the same time as testosterone and excreted in the urine in approximately the same concentration.

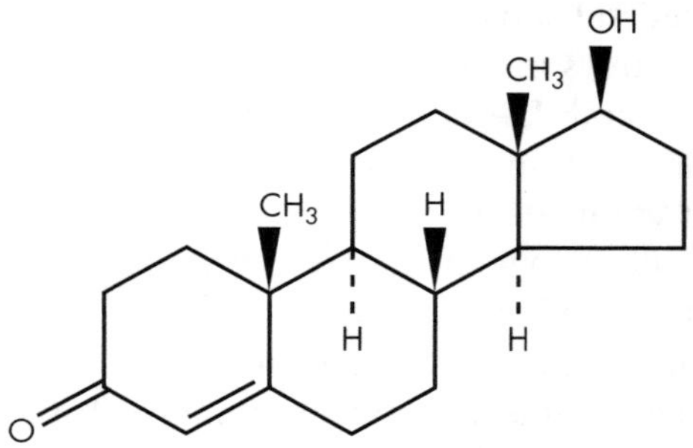

Figure 7.2 Testosterone.

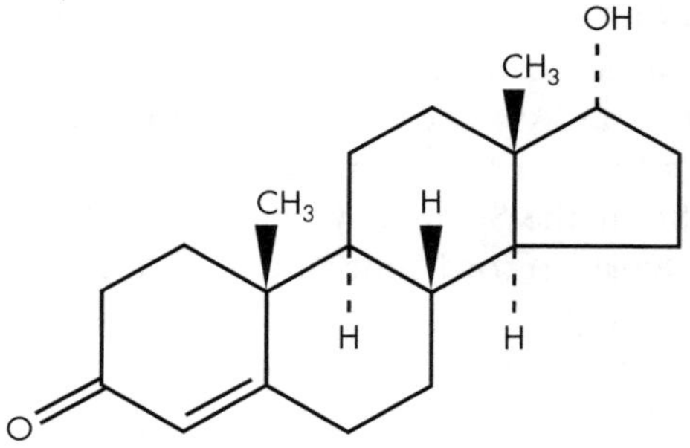

Figure 7.3 Epitestosterone.

The testosterone/epitestosterone (T/E) ratio is normally 1:2 in men and women, so the IOC set an upper limit for the ratio of 6:1 in 1983 and so included testosterone as a prohibited substance. This was the first time that a natural substance had been banned. This test was used for the first time from the 1982 Commonwealth Games in Brisbane and was used in the Olympics from 1984.

British athlete Diane Modahl tested positive for testosterone in Lisbon in 1992 and she was subsequently banned for 4 years. After lengthy appeals, this suspension was lifted with the Lisbon facility being declared inadequate. She resumed competing from 1996, winning a bronze medal in the 1998 Commonwealth Games. The British Athletics Federation, which had imposed the ban, spent so much money defending their decision that they went into administration.

Nandrolone

Nandrolone is a synthetic steroid that would not be expected to be found in normal urine samples. Chemically it is nortestosterone, i.e. testosterone without the methyl group in the 19 position (Figure 7.4). It has been among the three most commonly reported prohibited substances for many years (Table 7.1).

The use of the synthetic steroid nandrolone came to the public gaze in 1992 when it was detected in the urine of Dieter Bauman (Olympic 5000-metre champion). In 1999, the Olympic 100-metre champion Linford Christie tested positive after an athletics meeting in Germany and was subsequently given a 2-year ban, which was upheld by the International Amateur Athletics Federation. There have subsequently been a number of celebrated athletes also found positive, including Dougie Walker, Mark Richardson and Gary Cadogan.

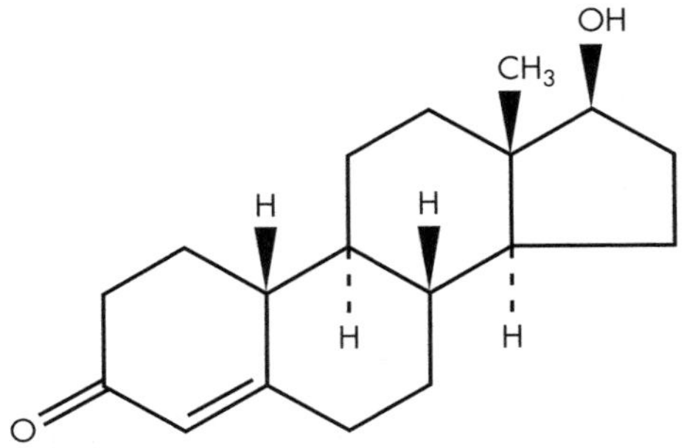

Figure 7.4 Nandrolone.

Table 7.1 Prohibited substances most commonly reported by IOC-accredited laboratories, in order of frequency.[a] Source: Cowan and Houghton, 2003 (numbers of reports in years shown)

Substance	1987	Substance	1990	Substance	1995	Substance	2000
Nandrolone	262	Nandrolone	192	Testosterone	293	Salbutamol	367
Pseudoephedrine	100	Testosterone	171	Cannabis	224	Nandrolone	325
Testosterone	83	Pseudoephedrine	123	Nandrolone	212	Testosterone	306
Ephedrine	58	Stanozolol	79	Methandienone	132	Cannabis	295
Phenylpropanolamine	57	Phenylpropanolamine	64	Salbutamol	132	Pseudoephedrine	136
Methenolone	42	Ephedrine	43	Pseudoephedrine	102	Ephedrine	129
Stanozolol	37	Codeine	32	Ephedrine	78	Stanozolol	116
Methandienone	27	Methenolone	25	Stanozolol	78	Terbutaline	110
Codeine	26	Amfetamine	24	Methenolone	39	Methandienone	75
Amfetamine	24	Methandienone	23	Clenbuterol	31	Lidocaine	64

[a] 1987 was first year of available data.

During 1999 there appeared to be an increase in the number of adverse findings concerning nandrolone – 17 British athletes tested positive for the steroid. As a result, UK Sport set up an Expert Committee under the Chairmanship of Professor Vivian James to investigate the current situation with regard to the testing of sports men and women for evidence of nandrolone abuse. The Committee reported in 2000, and made a number of recommendations. They recommended that the IOC should define the urine concentration of 19-norandrosterone (the metabolite of nandrolone detected in the urine) above which it considers that a doping offence may have been committed and that further studies should be carried out to investigate the factors influencing the endogenous production of nandrolone in human subjects. It was recognised that there was evidence that 19-norandrosterone is present naturally in low but detectable concentration in urine from some men and women and therefore concentration limits should be set at 2 ng/mL in men and 5 ng/mL in women. The Committee also noted that some dietary supplements contain nandrolone (or similar compounds), although they are not listed on the label (Expert Committee on Nandrolone, 2000). As suggested by the Committee, the IOC and the WADA changed the concentration limits in January 2003.

The Committee produced a further report in 2003, when they pointed out that there was further evidence that some dietary supplements contain banned steroids not included in the list of product ingredients. They went on to strongly advise competitors that using dietary supplements carries the potential risk of unknowingly ingesting a banned substance (Expert Committee on Nandrolone, 2003).

The possible contamination of supplements is well illustrated by Greg Rusedski's failed drugs test for nandrolone at a US tournament in July 2003. He insisted that he had never taken performance-enhancing drugs. At an independent tribunal in Montreal in March 2004 it was accepted that he was not to blame for his positive test and he had therefore not committed a doping offence. He had taken electrolyte tablets provided by his own governing body, the Association of Tennis Professionals (ATP), that were suspected of containing the nandrolone. He was the eighth tennis player in as many months to be exonerated in this way and the blame clearly rests with the ATP in not being vigilant in the supply of supplements to its players.

Tetrahydrogestrinone

Some scientists are constantly trying to invent new performance-enhancing drugs that are undetectable by current laboratory methodology. For example, early in 2003, the United States Anti-Doping Agency learned that athletes were using a new, and supposedly 'undetectable' steroid. Subsequently, Dr Don Catlin at the University of California at Los Angeles laboratory received a syringe purporting to contain this new steroid from a trainer of an athlete. Dr Catlin analysed the sample and identified it by analysis and then synthesis as tetrahydrogestrinone (THG) (Figure 7.5). He then went on to develop a method of testing for THG and this test has subsequently been used to analyse samples of urine from athletes in both race and out of race conditions.

The source of the THG was traced to the Bay Area Laboratory Co-operative (BALCO) of Burlingame, California, who specialised in nutritional mineral supplements for athletes. Britain's best sprinter, 26-year-old Dwain Chambers, was one of the first athletes to have THG detected in his urine. His nutritionist for the previous 2 years was none other than Victor Conte, BALCO's founder. In a high-profile test case, the UK Athletics disciplinary panel confirmed his 2-year ban for a doping offence. His defence, that THG was not specifically named as a prohibited substance, was not considered as sound. A link with gestrinone, a prohibited substance, had been proven and it produced the same effect in the body. Thus the use of designer drugs as doping agents was confirmed as an offence.

Urinary concentrations

It was recognised that there was a need to differentiate between the high concentration of a drug found in a urine sample from taking a large dose

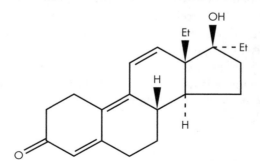

Figure 7.5 Tetrahydrogestrinone (THG).

of a drug for doping purposes and the lower concentrations from taking therapeutic doses or because they were metabolites of drugs taken for therapeutic purposes. For example, the Medical Commission of the IOC recognised that taking large doses of caffeine might improve performance and is harmful and therefore banned excess caffeine in the urine in time for testing in the Olympics in Sarajevo and Los Angeles of 1984. The level was originally set at 15 micrograms/mL, but this was reduced to 12 micrograms/mL in urine in 1988, which is the kind of concentration obtained by drinking ten cups of strong coffee. Other drug concentration limits have been set over the years and the list includes ephedrine, epitestosterone, methylephedrine, morphine, phenylpropanolamine and pseudoephedrine.

Out-of-competition testing

Athletes who take drugs just before a race may be exposed by the tests carried out on their urine samples taken the same day. However, if an athlete takes substances such as anabolic steroids to increase muscle mass and then stops a week or so before the event, there may be none in their urine to detect. To overcome this, out-of-competition testing was trialled in the 1970s and was first carried out in 1977 by Norway. It was formally brought into UK sport during the 1980s (Verroken and Mottram, 2003). The best procedure is random, unannounced testing while the athlete is training. In this way any prolonged use of steroids, or any other banned substance, can be detected.

By 1989, the IOC Medical Commission was supervising a programme of testing athletes at any time throughout the year involving 11 countries. Athletes were given up to 48 hours' notice to report to a testing laboratory in their own country and the procedure was observed by at least one representative from another country.

How it works in practice is amply demonstrated by Rio Ferdinand of Manchester United, who failed to turn up for a drugs test at the Manchester United training ground in September 2003 (see Chapter 8). Whether he was trying to evade detection or simply forgot because he was moving house that day is immaterial. He simply failed to comply with the requirement to provide a sample and was given an 8-month ban, which was upheld on appeal.

Deception

It became apparent in the 1980s that athletes were trying to avoid detection of taking banned substances by a variety of methods. Therefore the

IOC added pharmacological, chemical and physical manipulation to the list of prohibited methods in 1985. This deception included urinating at the end of a race, not providing a urine sample, someone else providing the sample, catheterisation to provide a different sample, and the use of diuretics (to dilute the urine). Probenecid and other masking agents were added in 1987.

Blood doping

Blood doping, or blood boosting, is the injection of blood cells into an athlete's body to increase its oxygen-carrying capability. Some athletes have been suspected of having some blood taken from their bodies and the separated blood cells put back later, before the race but when the body had recovered and replaced the blood that was taken. This is dangerous because it increases the viscosity of the blood and puts a much greater strain on the heart. There is an even greater risk if the blood injected is from another person, because there is a risk of a fatal haemolytic reaction.

Lasse Virren, the Finnish 3000-metre steeplechaser, broke the world record in the 1970s and was suspected of blood doping with his own blood taken a week or so earlier. In 1984 in Los Angeles, the American cyclist Pat McDonough admitted that he had used blood doping to increase his performance (Ackerman, 1991). In fact, one-third of the US cycling team received blood doping transfusions before the Los Angeles Olympic Games, where they went on to win a record nine medals. A report on Canadian television months later claimed evidence of doping.

Blood doping was banned by the IOC in 1985, although no detection method existed at that time. The first blood testing at the Olympic Games was at Lillehammer in 1994, where the test was for blood other than the athlete's (Verroken, 2003).

East Germany

It was long suspected that East German athletes had official support in using doping to improve their performance. For example, when Renate Vogel (1974 100-metre breaststroke world record holder) defected to the West in 1979 she told how steroids were handed round "along with the vitamin pills" (Donohoe and Johnson, 1986). In the early 1990s, a systematic doping plan was uncovered by German authorities in the Statsi files, the records of East Germany's secret police. The files showed that over 10 000 athletes received banned drugs as part of the government's policy to show that the new socialist government could produce impressive athletes, according to a report on Canadian television. Dr Werna Franke has produced evidence stating that the East German government files contained records of finance plans, treatment protocols, science meetings and correspondence relating to the programme. The documents also contained tables of the names of well-known athletes, the doses of steroids they had taken and the medals they had won. All the athletes in the lists were shown, by bar charts, to have been taking steroids at the same time, and to have stopped taking them at the same time, in order to compete in international events (Anon, 1994).

In 2000, two high-ranking East Germans were prosecuted for causing bodily harm to young athletes by doping them. Former East German sporting supremo Manfred Ewald was found guilty of doping more than 100 young athletes and given a suspended sentence of 22 months. Former East German sports medical officer Manfred Hoppner was given an 18-month suspended sentence at the same time.

Growth hormone

Growth hormone is a peptide hormone released from the anterior pituitary gland that promotes growth in youth. Athletes have used it in an attempt to increase protein synthesis and therefore the size of their muscles. It was originally prepared from human pituitaries but is now made by recombinant DNA technology. Tests to prove the administration of growth hormone are still being developed.

The peptide hormones and analogues, e.g. growth hormone (GH), corticotrophin (ACTH) and erythropoietin (EPO), were included in 1989 under the new class of peptide hormones.

Erythropoietin

Originally, natural erythropoietin (EPO) was used by athletes to increase their blood capacity. They moved to recombinant EPO when methods to detect its use were developed. However, methods are now available to differentiate the various forms of EPO used in doping (Lasne and Ceaurriz, 2000).

EPO abuse has been reported as being rife during the 1998 Tour de France and in the years following. The death of Marco Pantani, the 34-year-old Italian cycling champion, in 2004, has been attributed to a heart attack, as have the deaths of six other riders who also suffered heart attacks. The costs to human life of doping in this way are obvious.

The World Anti-Doping Agency

Following the scandal in the Tour de France in the summer of 1998, it was recognised that the fight against doping in sport was an international one that must involve not just sporting organisations but also governments. Thus, the IOC convened the World Conference on Doping in Sport in Lausanne in February 1999 to bring all the interested parties together – both sporting and government agencies. This conference produced the Lausanne Declaration on Doping in Sport, which advocated the setting up of an independent international anti-doping agency to be up and running by the Olympic Games in 2000 in Sydney. Subsequently, on 10 November 1999, the WADA was set up in Lausanne to consist of equal representatives from the Olympic movement and public authorities (see also Chapter 8). The Agency's headquarters were relocated to Montreal in 2001.

The WADA seeks "to foster a doping free culture in sport. It combines the resources of sport and government to enhance, supplement and coordinate existing efforts to educate athletes about the harms of doping, reinforce the ideal of fair play and sanction those who cheat themselves and their sport". Its key activities are (World Anti-Doping Agency, 2005):

- conducting unannounced out-of-competition doping control among elite athletes
- developing the World Anti-Doping Code
- funding scientific research to develop new detection methods
- observing the doping control and results management programmes of major events
- managing the Athlete's Passport Program
- providing anti-doping education to athletes, coaches and administrators
- fostering the development of National Anti-Doping Organisations.

The World Anti-Doping Code

Part of the major thrust of the WADA's activities is the formulation of the World Anti-Doping Code. Its intention is to harmonise the very different anti-doping policies, standards and laws of national governments.

The Code was approved at the World Conference on Doping in Sport in Copenhagen in March 2003 and by mid-2005, 170 governments had signed up to support it.

Pharmacy

Pharmacists have been instrumental in the fight against doping in sport, but probably none have done as much as Professor Arnold Beckett. He has been a tireless champion of using science to detect doping and in setting up competent systems to achieve this. In the 1960s he set up the Drug Control Centre at the Department of Pharmacy, Chelsea College, University of London, which now has a world-wide reputation for excellence and the dual roles of research into new methods for detecting doping and providing a service has continued under its present Director, Professor David Cowan, in its new home in the Department of Pharmacy, King's College, London. Professor Beckett was a member of the IOC's Medical Commission for many years, giving sound advice on the application of modern scientific methodology, as well as accurately predicting likely future trends that later became realities.

Pharmacists have a huge role to play in giving advice to sportspersons on which drugs to take and which not to take, as well as giving general advice about health and the treatment of sports injuries. A good example is the pharmacy that was set up for the XVII Commonwealth Games in Manchester in 2002, which was the largest sporting event ever held in the UK. Sixteen volunteer pharmacists were involved in providing advice on prohibited substances, monitoring athlete's medication, producing a formulary and dispensing medicines (see Chapter 9). Pharmacists also helped to interpret medication exemption requests from athletes. For example, gold medal-winning Kim Collins, the St Kitts and Nevis men's 100-metre sprinter, tested positive for salbutamol. He had failed to declare the medication before competing, which jeopardised his eligibility for the medal. The Commonwealth Games Federation Court decided that he should not be penalised after he underwent lung function tests that proved he was asthmatic (Anon, 2002a, b).

A first for pharmacy was when Dr Steven Kayne (the editor of this book) became the first pharmacist to gain an MSc in Sports Medicine in 2002.

It was in the 1980s that the Joint Formulary Committee for the *British National Formulary* (*BNF*) considered the possibility that the *BNF* could give advice to GPs on which medicines contained banned drugs. The problems of doing this were the huge numbers of OTC medicines on sale to the public (nationally and internationally) and the large amount of work necessary to keep the information up to date. However, in 1991, at the suggestion of Dr Michael Irani (Ashford Hospital), the topic was revisited and the Committee decided that the Sports Council's card 'Doping Control in Sport' should be included in the *BNF* as a service to prescribers and sportspersons. The card gave a list of the doping classes and methods as well as examples of permitted and prohibited substances. It was included in the *BNF* for the first time in September 1992 (No 24). Since then it has appeared in one form or another in the *BNF* and until recently appeared as UK Sport's 'Drug-Free Sport Advice Card', giving details of examples of permitted substances and classes of prohibited substances and methods (Mehta, 2005). It is now available from drug-free@uksport.gov.uk.

The future

Cheating athletes will always try to keep ahead of the Anti-Doping Code by trying performance-enhancing drugs that are not currently banned. It is for the WADA and other authorities to ensure that they write their regulations to include these substances as soon as they are discovered and to have a liberal interpretation of their rules so that cheats do not prosper.

Modern genetics has now moved to identifying genes that give good athletic performance and it is possible that gene doping will be seen in the future. There is the danger that scientists will isolate 'performance genes' and correct 'dysfunctional' ones or, worse still, create a genetic blueprint for a top athlete in their attempt to create better athletes. This would be gene doping defined as the non-therapeutic use of genes, genetic elements and/or cells that have the capacity to enhance athletic performance. It remains to be seen whether this becomes a reality.

References

Ackerman D L (1991). A history of drug testing. In: Coombs R H, West L J, eds. *Drug Testing: Issues and Options*. New York: Oxford University Press, 3–21.

Anon (1994). Out-of-competition testing needed. *Pharm J* 253: 413.

Anon (2002a). The XVII Commonwealth Games: (1) An insight into pharmacy preparations. *Pharm J* 269: 93.

Anon (2002b). The XVII Commonwealth Games: (2) A review of pharmacy operations. *Pharm J* 269: 211.

Barnes L (1980). Olympic drug testing: improvements without progress. *Physician Sports Med* 8: 21–24.

Brooks R V, Jeremiah G, Webb W A, *et al.* (1979). Detection of anabolic steroid administration to athletes. *J Steroid Biochem* 11: 913–917.

Donohoe T, Johnson N (1986). *Foul Play: Drug Abuse in Sport.* Oxford: Basil Blackwell.

Finley M I, Plecket H W (1976). *The Olympic Games: The First Hundred Years.* London: Chatto and Windus.

Hanley D F (1983). Drug and sex testing: regulations for international competition. *Clin Sports Med* 2: 13–17.

Lasne F, Ceaurriz J D (2000). Recombinant erythropoietin in urine. *Nature* 405: 635.

Mehta D K, ed. (2005). Drugs and Sport. *British National Formulary*, 49th edn. London: British Medical Association and Royal Pharmaceutical Society of Great Britain, 26.

UK Sport (2003). Nandrolone Progress Report to the UK Sports Council from the Expert Committee on Nandrolone. http://www.uksport.gov.uk/images/uploaded/Nandrolone_Progress_Report_Feb03.pdf (accessed 24 August 2005).

UK Sports Council (2000). Nandrolone Review: Report to the UK Sports Council from the Expert Committee. London: UK Sports Council.

Verroken M (2003). Drug use and abuse in sport. In: Mottram D R, ed. *Drugs in Sport*, 3rd edn. London: Routledge, 29–62.

Verroken M, Mottram D R (2003). Doping control in sport. In: Mottram D R, ed. *Drugs in Sport*, 3rd edn. London: Routledge, 307–356.

World Anti-Doping Agency (2005). http://www.wada-ama.org (accessed 24 August 2005).

Further reading

Coombs R H, West L J, eds (1991). *Drug Testing: Issues and Options.* New York: Oxford University Press.

Di Pasquale M G (1984). *Drug Use and Detection in Amateur Sports.* Warkworth: M G D Press.

Donohoe T, Johnson N (1986). *Foul Play: Drug Abuse in Sport.* Oxford: Basil Blackwell.

Lenehan P (2003). *Anabolic Steroids and Other Performance Enhancing Drugs.* London: Taylor & Francis.

Useful address

Drug-Free Sport
UK Sport
40 Bernard Street
London WC1N 1ST
http://www.uksport.gov.uk
drug-free@uksport.gov.uk

8

Drug use in sport and dope testing

David Mottram

Introduction

This chapter begins by describing the drugs and methods currently prohibited in sport, then looks at the procedures used in dope testing and finally presents four case studies involving British athletes.

The drugs and methods prohibited in sport

The World Anti-Doping Agency (WADA) List

Dope testing began in the 1960s and was controlled by the IOC (see Chapter 7). The classification and scope of the drugs included in the IOC's prohibited drug list changed over the years as trends in the use of doping substances and methods evolved and the methods for drug testing improved. In 2001 the World Anti-Doping Agency (WADA) was established as an independent organisation to oversee the control of drug misuse in sport, replacing the IOC in this role. The WADA launched its Anti-Doping Code in March 2003 and published a revised list of prohibited substances and methods at the beginning of January 2004. This list was revised in 2005 and is shown in Table 8.1.

The list in Table 8.1 applies to all sports and identifies those substances and methods that are prohibited within competition. For out-of-competition testing, the WADA identifies those substances and methods likely to be abused during training and limits its testing under these circumstances to anabolic agents, peptide hormones, beta-2 agonists, agents with anti-oestrogenic activity, masking agents and the prohibited methods M1–M3.

Changing trends in the misuse of drugs in sport has been reflected in the periodic revision of the list of doping classes and methods. The WADA has now introduced an annual review of the list and a 3-month notification is given before the revised list is implemented. Examples of

                ,s
                ,s
                ;s
              inoids
              lic agents
              ʌnabolic androgenic steroids (AAS)
          2. Other anabolic agents
S.5   Peptide hormones
        1. Erythropoietin (EPO)
        2. Growth hormone (hGH) and insulin-like growth factor (IGF-1)
        3. Chorionic gonadotrophin (hCG)
        4. Pituitary and synthetic gonadotrophins (LH)
        5. Insulin
        6. Corticotrophins
S.6   Beta-2 agonists
S.7   Agents with anti-oestrogenic activity
S.8   Masking agents
S.9   Glucocorticosteroids

Prohibited methods
M.1   Enhancement of oxygen transfer
        a. Blood doping
        b. The use of products that enhance the uptake, transport or delivery
            of oxygen
M.2   Pharmacological, chemical and physical manipulation
M.3   Gene doping

Substances prohibited in certain sports
P.1   Alcohol
P.2   Beta blockers
P.3   Diuretics

Source: http://www.wada-ama.org

drugs within each category are provided, but because new drugs regularly appear on the market and there is a growing trend towards 'designer' performance-enhancing drugs, the WADA has applied the term "and other substances with similar chemical structure or similar pharmacological effects" to its lists of examples, where appropriate.

The rationale for including substances and methods on the WADA list

The reasons for drugs being misused by athletes are many and various, however the justification for controlling the use of drugs was simply explained as "the use of doping agents in sport is both unhealthy and contrary to the ethics of sport".

If the motivation is performance enhancement, the type of drug used will depend on its pharmacological action and the sporting activity in which the athlete is involved. It is often difficult to understand why athletes use prohibited or restricted substances, because the potential benefits may be marginal and possibly inconsequential compared with the potential adverse effects. However, athletes generally exhibit a blinkered approach to drug taking and either choose to ignore side-effects or combine other substances in an attempt to counter side-effects.

A review of the pharmacology and potential performance-enhancing effects of the major groups of banned substances and methods is presented below (see also Chapter 7).

Prohibited substances

S.1 Stimulants

Stimulants have probably been misused in sport for the longest. Their main purpose has been to improve performance by the general action of CNS stimulation. Athletes may use stimulants to reduce tiredness and to increase alertness, competitiveness and aggression. They are considered to have a performance-enhancing effect within endurance or explosive power activities because they increase the athlete's capacity to exercise strenuously and reduce their sensitivity to pain. Stimulants are principally used on the day of a competition. There is, however, little scientific evidence available to suggest that stimulants do improve performance. The stimulant class includes psychomotor stimulants, sympathomimetics and miscellaneous CNS stimulants. Examples of this class include the amfetamines, ephedrine and cocaine.

Amfetamines are controlled under the UK Misuse of Drugs Act 1971. Athletes have probably used amfetamines to sharpen reflexes, reduce tiredness and increase euphoria. However they raise blood pressure which, with increased physical activity and peripheral vasoconstriction, makes it difficult for the body to cool down. If the body overheats and is unable to cool down, it dehydrates and blood circulation is compromised. This has led to a number of suspected amfetamine-related deaths in sport.

The sympathomimetic drug ephedrine is likely to be misused for its euphoric effect. Athletes who have tested positive for sympathomimetics have frequently protested their innocence, claiming inadvertent use as an OTC medication to treat cold or 'flu symptoms. Up until January 2004, the banned list included many examples of this class of drugs. However, the WADA removed drugs such as pseudoephedrine, phenylephrine and phenylpropanolamine from the January 2004 list. The rationale for this is based on evidence suggesting minimal benefits from these drugs and a likelihood that athletes would test positive for these drugs, despite a cut-off level having been specified (Chester *et al.*, 2003a, b). The WADA has nonetheless transferred these drugs to its 2004 Monitoring Programme in order to detect patterns of use in sport. The sympathomimetics that remain on the WADA's Prohibited List are subject to a urinary cut-off level and are only prohibited when the levels exceed 5 micrograms/mL for cathine and 10 micrograms/mL for ephedrine and methylephedrine.

Cocaine is likely to be used for performance enhancement for its euphoric effects and feeling of decreased fatigue. However, athletes are just as likely to test positive for cocaine through recreational use of the drug.

S.2 Narcotic analgesics

Narcotic analgesics act on the brain to reduce the amount of pain felt from injury or illness. In sports, the use of powerful pain-killing drugs might enable athletes to exert themselves beyond their normal pain threshold. There are considerable dangers associated with this – athletes may try to compete or train despite an existing serious injury, leading to further injury or to permanent damage.

Narcotic analgesics have strong addictive properties and as such are tightly controlled by legislation in most countries. The WADA regulations apply specifically to the more potent opiate analgesics including derivatives such as morphine, diamorphine (heroin) and pethidine. Less potent narcotic derivatives such as codeine, dextromethorphan, pholcodine and diphenoxylate are permitted.

S.3 Cannabinoids

The active constituent of marijuana is Δ^9-tetrahydrocannabinol (THC), whose central depressant effect decreases the motivation for physical effort and impairs motor coordination, short-term memory and perception (Reilly, 2003). The ban of this drug in all sports reflects the dangers to fellow competitors of competing under its influence of this drug as much as its questionable performance-enhancing properties. Athletes face the prospect of testing positive for cannabinoids through passive smoking in the period before competing.

S.4 Anabolic agents

In March 1993, the IOC changed its classification of anabolic steroids to anabolic agents and created two subgroups: (i) androgenic-anabolic steroids; and (ii) other anabolic agents, beta-2 agonists (e.g. clenbuterol). This reclassification followed reports of clenbuterol use by athletes as an anabolic agent as well as a stimulant. Clenbuterol has been shown in animal studies to increase skeletal muscle mass and reduce body fat (Matlin *et al.*, 1987).

The androgenic-anabolic steroids (AASs) are largely chemically-derived alternatives to naturally-occurring testosterone (George, 2003). Contrary to popular belief, oral administration of an AAS is more dangerous than injection. Oral forms have to be broken down in the liver first, leading to the risk of liver disease. Injectable forms are oil-based and fat-soluble, making their release into the body system slower, as fat stores are broken down. Orally active AASs are water-soluble and likely to have a shorter clearance time in the body, making them more popular among athletes. However clearance times are also likely to be dose-related and are difficult to calculate with any certainty.

The use of AASs by athletes is widespread, particularly in strength and power events, bodybuilding and stamina activities. The side-effects associated with these drugs are extremely serious, particularly the consequences of their long-term use (Tucker, 1997).

S.5 Peptide hormones and analogues

Peptide hormones are endogenous substances. It is therefore impossible to define a 'normal' level for these substances. These difficulties in detecting levels of abuse make them an attractive drug for athletes.

Human growth hormone (hGH) is used for its anabolic properties to increase size, strength or ultimate height, depending on the age of the user. It is a polypeptide hormone produced by the pituitary gland to maintain normal growth from birth to adulthood. It has a short (about 20 minutes) half-life, during which time it activates hepatic growth hormone receptors, mediating the production of insulin-like growth factor 1 (IGF-1). It is IGF-1 that is responsible for most of the anabolic action of hGH (Macintyre, 1987).

Erythropoietin (EPO) is a peptide hormone used by athletes for blood boosting (Armstrong and Reilly, 2003) that has become more readily available as a result of recombinant DNA technology. EPO is the major hormone regulator of red blood cell production, used in medicine in cases of kidney failure. The long-term effects of use in medicine or misuse in sport are unknown, however overload of the cardiovascular system is likely.

Other peptide hormones that are banned include human chorionic gonadotrophin (hCG), luteinising hormone (LH), corticotrophins including adrenocorticotrophic hormone (ACTH) and insulin. These peptide hormones are used to potentiate the endogenous levels of other hormones with ergogenic or other performance-enhancing properties. Endogenous levels of testosterone may be increased by the use of hCG and LH (Delbeke *et al.*, 1998). ACTH increases adrenal corticosteroid release. The powerful anti-inflammatory action of corticosteroids may be a useful aid to recovery from injury. Athletes might also seek the testicular stimulatory function of the gonadotrophins as a way to counter AAS effects. Insulin may increase muscle bulk through inhibition of muscle protein breakdown, in addition to its facilitation of glucose entry into cells (Sonksen, 2001).

S.6 Beta-2 agonists

Beta-2 agonists are first-line drugs in the treatment of asthma but also have potential performance-enhancing properties, particularly with respect to their bronchodilator activity. Clearly, it would be impossible to ban beta-2 agonists completely as this would prevent asthmatic athletes from competing in sport. The WADA therefore permits the use of formoterol, salbutamol, salmeterol and terbutaline.

However, these drugs are permitted by inhalation only, to prevent and/or treat asthma and exercise-induced bronchoconstriction. Medical notification for a TUE is also required (see also Chapter 10).

S.7 Agonists with anti-oestrogenic activity

This class of drugs is prohibited only in males, because of their testosterone-boosting activity; it includes aromatase inhibitors, clomifene, cyclofenil and tamoxifen.

S.8 Masking agents

Masking agents are products that have the potential to impair the excretion of prohibited substances, to conceal their presence in urine or to change haematological parameters. They include diuretics, epitestosterone, probenecid and plasma expanders (e.g. dextran, hydroxyethyl starch).

Athletes may use diuretics to modify the excretion rate of urine and to alter urinary concentrations of prohibited drugs. Epitestosterone may be taken with testosterone in order to maintain the ratio of these two substances in the urine, a criterion used in testing for testosterone misuse. Athletes have used probenecid in an attempt to mask the presence of drugs or their metabolites because of its ability to inhibit movement of molecules across kidney tissue.

S.9 Glucocorticosteroids

Glucocorticosteroids are potent anti-inflammatory substances. In their naturally-occurring form they are released by the adrenal gland during stress activity. The synthetically produced versions are used in medicine as analgesics and anti-inflammatories. In addition, corticosteroids are used in the treatment of asthma, a disease characterised by an inflammation of the respiratory tract. The use of glucocorticosteroids is prohibited when administered orally, rectally or by intravenous or intramuscular injection. Other routes of administration, such as topical use (aural, ophthalmological and dermatological), inhalation therapy (asthma, allergic rhinitis) and local or intra-articular injections are permitted but require a TUE (see p. 248).

Prohibited methods

M.1 Enhancement of oxygen transfer

Blood doping   Red blood cells or blood products containing red blood cells are administered intravenously in an attempt to gain unfair advantage in competition (Armstrong and Reilly, 2003). The intravenous administration of red blood cells (either from the same individual or from a different but blood type-matched person) would increase the oxygen-carrying capacity of the blood. Competitors in endurance activities such as marathon and long-distance running, cycling and skiing use this method. Similar effects are reported from training at altitude.

Blood doping carries considerable risk to the athlete. Injection of an additional volume of blood can overload the cardiovascular system and induce metabolic shock. Adverse effects can be compounded if blood from a second individual is used. A potentially fatal haemolytic reaction, with kidney failure or an allergic reaction, can result from mismatched blood. There is also an increasing risk of contracting infectious diseases such as AIDS or viral hepatitis.

The use of products that enhance the uptake, transport or delivery of oxygen An alternative method of enhancing the uptake, transport and delivery of oxygen is through the use of erythropoietin (EPO) or modified haemoglobin products such as microencapsulated haemoglobin and perfluorochemicals.

M.2 Pharmacological, chemical or physical manipulation

As the testing programmes to control the use of doping substances have increased in sophistication, one response from athletes has been to try to manipulate the test by using other substances to influence the quality of the urine. More often athletes have tried to provide a clean urine sample obtained from another person. Tightening of the collection procedures, particularly in relation to the time between notification and collection of the sample, have helped to control this practice.

Other methods of masking drug misuse include the inhibition of renal excretion, using drugs such as probenecid, or taking epitestosterone to ensure the testosterone/epitestosterone ratio remains within permitted limits.

M.3 Gene doping

Gene doping is defined as the non-therapeutic use of genes, genetic elements and/or cells in an attempt to enhance performance. There is no evidence that this procedure has yet been attempted but the procedure has been banned because of its potential.

Substances prohibited in certain sports

P.1 Alcohol

For most sports the use of alcohol would be detrimental to performance, so it is logical that it is only prohibited in certain sports, such as automobile sports, skiing and modern pentathlon. Many of these sports specify a threshold level for detection through breath and/or blood analysis. In low doses, alcohol has some sedative effects. Higher doses can cause poor co-ordination, reduced reaction time and mental confusion. As a potential doping substance to reduce anxiety, the dose would have to be carefully controlled. In sports such as archery, the use of alcohol may stabilise tremor but could adversely affect reaction time and increase the unsteadiness of the arm when aiming (Reilly, 2003).

P.2 Beta-blockers

Certain sports require an ability to control movements, such as gymnastics and wrestling. By moderating the cardiac output and muscle blood flow caused by the nervous system's response to stress and arousal, beta-blockers produce an anti-anxiety effect that is potentially useful in sports with high levels of anxiety, for example bobsleigh and skiing. One of the side-effects noted in the treatment of patients with beta-blockers was an ability to reduce muscle tremor. This would be of benefit in accuracy events and those where extraneous movement had to be kept under control, for example archery and shooting (Reilly, 2003).

P.3 Diuretics

In addition to their use as masking agents (Section S.8), diuretics may be taken to effect acute reduction of weight to meet weight class limits. In this respect they may offer a potential advantage in sports such as boxing, judo or weightlifting.

Specified substances

The WADA Code states: "The Prohibited List may identify specified substances which are particularly susceptible to unintentional anti-doping rule violations because of their general availability in medicinal products or which are less likely to be successfully abused as doping agents." A doping violation involving such substances may result in a reduced sanction provided the athlete can establish that the use of such a specified substance was not intended to enhance sport performance.

The specified substances in the January 2005 Prohibited List were:

- Stimulants: ephedrine, L-methamphetamine (lerometamfetamine), methylephedrine

- Cannabinoids
- Inhaled beta-2 agonists (except clenbuterol)
- All glucocorticosteroids
- Masking agents: probenecid
- All beta-blockers
- Alcohol

Therapeutic use exemption

The WADA Code permits athletes and their physicians to apply for a therapeutic use exemption (TUE). Through TUE they seek permission to use, for therapeutic purposes, substances or methods contained on the Prohibited List. A number of criteria must be met before TUE is granted:

- The athlete would experience a significant impairment to health if the substance or method were to be withheld.
- The use would produce no additional enhancement to performance other than a return to a state of normal health.
- There is no reasonable therapeutic alternative.

Clearly, the TUE Committee must face a considerable challenge in applying these criteria (see also Chapters 9 and 10).

Dope testing

The World Anti-Doping Agency

Responsibility for world-wide coordination of testing standards resides with the World Anti-Doping Agency (WADA). Until the Olympic Games of 2000 in Sydney there was no coordinated testing outside the Games, however the advent of the WADA has begun to have a significant impact on the way doping is controlled in sport. The WADA's Anti-Doping Code was adopted at the Copenhagen Declaration in March 2003 (http://www.wada-ama.org), which was attended by representatives from all major stakeholders in the fight against doping in sport.

Testing in and out of competition

Originally testing was scheduled within competition only. Athletes taking part in an event knew that they were likely to be selected for testing. To counter this, athletes started to reschedule their drug use to the training period and to calculate clearance times in the body. The extension of testing to the out-of-competition period was intended to address this trend.

Norway, in 1977, was the first country to conduct out-of-competition testing. It was introduced in the UK in the early 1980s. The key principle of out-of-competition testing is to give the athlete short or no notice of the test, to reduce any opportunity to manipulate the procedure.

While competition testing will involve the full range of substances, out-of-competition testing focuses on the anabolic agents, peptide hormones, beta-2 agonists, agents with anti-oestrogenic activity and masking agents. This focused analysis reduces laboratory costs. Out-of-competition testing programmes are also able to concentrate on athletes in representative teams and in the top ranking tables. In team sports, it is possible to organise testing at squad training sessions. For individual activities such as track and field athletics, swimming and weightlifting, testing may take place at any time, at the athlete's home, place of work or training venue. Out-of-competition testing is not appropriate for every sport.

Out-of-competition testing is not yet carried out world-wide. Establishment of the WADA represents a major step forward in the achievement of a world-wide programme of out-of-competition testing.

WADA accredited laboratories

On 1 January 2004 WADA took over the responsibility for accrediting testing laboratories. In 2005 there were a total of 33 accredited laboratories worldwide. They are listed in Table 8.2.

Accreditation of laboratories is dependent upon adequate facilities

Table 8.2 WADA accredited laboratories (January 2004)

Athens, Greece	Kreischa, Germany	Prague, Czech Republic
Bangkok, Thailand	Lausanne, Switzerland	Rio de Janeiro, Brazil
Barcelona, Spain	Lisbon, Portugal	Rome, Italy
Beijing, China	London, UK	Seibersdorf, Austria
Bloemfontein, South Africa	Los Angeles, USA	Seoul, Korea
Bogotá, Colombia	Madrid, Spain	Stockholm, Sweden
Cologne, Germany	Montreal, Canada	Sydney, Australia
Fordham, UK	Moscow, Russia	Tokyo, Japan
Ghent, Belgium	Oslo, Norway	Tunis, Tunisia
Havana, Cuba	Paris, France	Warsaw, Poland
Helsinki, Finland	Penang, Malaysia	

and expertise being available and the capacity of the laboratory for testing the numbers of samples required for a comprehensive control programme. For major sporting events the laboratories must be able to report on results within 24–48 hours of receiving the sample.

Where a country is hosting a major international sporting event and does not have a WADA accredited laboratory, that country may apply to have one temporarily installed in a non-accredited laboratory/facility for the duration of the event. The host city must provide the analytical facilities but the procedures are, partly, staffed and conducted by personnel from the WADA-accredited laboratory, with its director being responsible for all results.

The testing programmes

In the UK, the national organisation for doping control is UK Sport (http://www.uksport.gov.uk). Governing bodies are required to submit details of their competitive and training calendar, and of nationally ranked competitors, as a condition of recognition and funding. The service is also available to professional sports. A charge is made to these bodies.

In most countries, the responsibility for organising testing has moved from sport and the governing bodies of individual sports to a government-funded organisation. An independent, accountable national body has the potential to deliver testing on behalf of national and international federations and to work in conjunction with WADA.

Procedures for drug testing

However a competitor is selected, as a winner, randomly or as part of a programme of out-of-competition testing, the sample collection procedure should follow the same principles. If such principles and policies are not sound and adhered to they become the target of lawsuits (Uzych, 1991).

The general procedure for drug testing is show in Figure 8.1 (Verroken and Mottram, 2003).

Selection of competitors

For testing within competition, the selection normally includes those competitors who are placed in the first three or four of an event, additional randomly selected competitors, all team members or a combination of these. For out-of-competition testing, selection may be from

Selection and notification of the athlete

↓

Attending the doping control station

↓

Completion of documentation

↓

Supervised provision of urine sample

↓

Sample divided into A and B bottles

↓

Transfer to the laboratory

↓

Testing of the A sample

POSITIVE   NEGATIVE

Finding reported   No further action and B
                                          sample destroyed
↓

Hearing by governing body
(B sample analysed if required)

↓

Sanction if doping offence confirmed

Figure 8.1 Flow chart for doping procedures.

a register of eligible competitors or from a targeted group within the register.

Notification

The competitor is notified, in writing, that they have been selected for testing. The sampling official must accompany the competitor to the doping control station. Where there is delay because of award cere-monies, press conferences, treatment for injury, etc., competitors must be chaperoned to prevent pharmacological, chemical or physical manipulation or substitution of urine. A coach or other team official may accompany the competitor to the doping control station.

Documentation

The competitor's identity and time of arrival at the doping control station are recorded. The competitor is invited to declare any medica-tions or other substances taken in the previous week, including prepa-rations that may have been obtained from a pharmacy, health food shop or other source.

Providing the sample

The competitor is provided with sealed, non-alcoholic and caffeine-free drinks, to prevent allegations of spiking of drinks. The competitor selects an individually sealed collection vessel. Collection of the urine takes place under the direct observation of a sampling officer. The competitor should produce a sample of at least 75 mL.

The competitor then selects two pre-sealed glass bottles labelled A and B. Normally two-thirds of the sample is placed in bottle A and one-third in bottle B. Both bottles are closed and sealed with numbered seals (Figure 8.2).

Once the samples have been sealed, the documentation is com-pleted and checked by the sampling officer and the competitor, who receives a copy of the form. Another copy, excluding the name of the competitor but recording their gender, the volume of urine, the bottle and seal numbers and any medications declared is enclosed with the samples sent to the laboratory.

Transfer to the laboratory

The samples and accompanying documentation are transported in sealed transit bags to a WADA laboratory, along with a chain of custody document. On arrival at the laboratory the seal numbers are checked and recorded (Figure 8.3). The A sample is prepared for analysis while the B sample is stored at low temperatures (normally 4°C) pending the result of the analysis of the A sample.

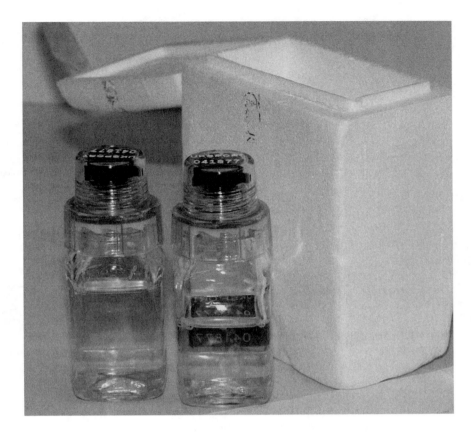

Figure 8.2 Samples of urine A and B.

Laboratory testing procedures

In general, drug-testing procedures are divided into two categories: screening and confirmatory. Screening procedures ascertain whether the sample contains any of the prohibited substances. Confirmatory tests are used to specifically identify the nature and the quantity of the prohibited substance(s) present.

The essential equipment and methods that WADA accredited laboratories must employ are:

- gas chromatography (GC)
- high pressure liquid chromatography (HPLC)
- mass spectrometry (MS) in combination with gas chromatography (Figure 8.4)

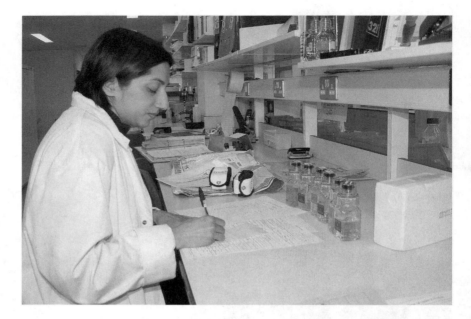

Figure 8.3 Recording samples in the laboratory at the Drug Control Centre, King's College, London.

- high resolution MS or tandem MS
- immunoassay equipment
- additional or alternative equipment recommended by WADA according to new scientific developments.

Reporting test results

If the test result is negative, the governing body should advise the competitor of the result and the laboratory will destroy the B sample.

In the case of a positive result, reports are released by the analysing laboratory to the relevant governing body and the competitor notified. The competitor may be invited to explain the finding and if they dispute the A sample finding, will be invited to attend and/or be represented at the analysis of the B sample, together with a representative of the governing body. The B sample analysis looks specifically for the substance(s) reported in the A sample. The analytical data is reported to the governing body as before.

Where a positive result is confirmed, the athlete may be suspended and invited to appear and/or be represented before a disciplinary

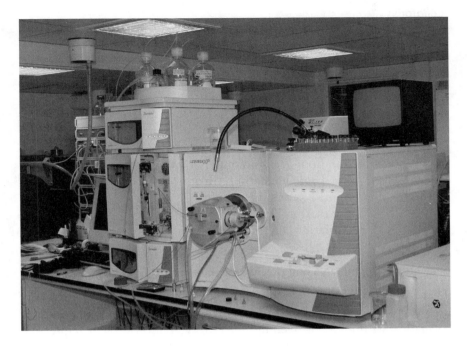

Figure 8.4 Mass spectroscopy and gas chromatography used in the analysis of samples at Doping Control Centre, King's College, London.

hearing. Following the hearing, decisions are made about the disciplinary action and the penalties that will apply. The competitor has the right to appeal.

Refusal or failure to provide a sample follows the same investigation and disciplinary procedures as for a positive result.

Sanctions

According to WADA regulations, athletes who test positive may be subject to two forms of sanction, disqualification and/or ineligibility.

Disqualification

If an anti-doping rule violation occurs during or in connection with a sports event, the ruling body may disqualify the athlete of all her/his individual results obtained at that event. This includes forfeiture of all medals, points and prizes.

Ineligibility

For all prohibited substances and methods, except those listed as specified substances:

- First violation: 2 years ineligibility
- Second violation: lifetime ineligibility
- For specified substances where an athlete can establish that the use of such a specified substance was not intended to enhance sport performance, the period of ineligibility is:
    — First violation: at a minimum, a warning and reprimand and no period of ineligibility from future events and at a maximum, 1 year's ineligibility
    — Second violation: 2 years ineligibility
    — Third violation: lifetime ineligibility

Nutritional supplements and positive dope tests

There is a well-established culture of substance taking in sport. Many athletes have used nutritional supplements in an attempt to enhance performance without contravening WADA regulations (see Chapter 3). Unlike drugs, nutritional supplements are not required to have scientific and clinical evidence that they are effective before marketing (Clarkson, 1996). There may be no legal requirement for manufacturers to list the content of nutritional supplements, and so they frequently make unsubstantiated claims that their products have ergogenic properties (Beltz and Doering, 1993), making it difficult for an athlete to determine whether taking such a preparation would contravene the doping regulations (Herbert, 1999). There are many preparations that may contain banned drugs (Ayotte, 1999) (see also Chapter 9).

Some products are likely to do more harm than good. Indeed, studies in which diet was manipulated to induce metabolic acidosis by reducing carbohydrate intake or increasing fat and protein intake have resulted in impaired performance (MacLaren, 1997).

Creatine has been the subject of many studies (see Chapters 1 and 3), but whether it is capable of producing ergogenic effects is equivocal (Clarkson, 1996; Balsom, 1997; MacLaren, 2003). Williams (1994) suggested that cut-off limits could be applied to nutrients that are shown to be ergogenic, however this could pose an impossible task for dope testers.

In recent years, the sport nutritional industry has offered a number of natural and, they claim, legal steroids. These include precursors for testosterone such as dehydroepiandrosterone, androstenedione, androstenediol, 19-androstenedione and 19-androstenediol (Ayotte, 1999). These substances may lead to metabolites in the urine, resulting in a positive test or altering the testosterone/epitestosterone ratio that again may trigger a positive result. These steroidal supplements are available through the Internet. A study in 2002 indicated that, from analysis of 634 'non-hormonal' nutritional supplements, 14.8% contained prohormones, mainly of testosterone and/or nandrolone, which would produce urinary metabolites sufficient to trigger a positive test result (Shanzer, 2002).

In recent years, there have been a significant number of high-profile cases involving athletes who tested positive for nandrolone and who subsequently claimed that the drug must have been present in nutritional supplements (Ferstle, 1999a, b, c).

Clearly, athletes take a considerable gamble when using nutritional supplements, because WADA adopt the rule of zero tolerance or strict liability, whereby athletes must take responsibility for what is present in their body, from whatever source.

Case studies

In this section, a number of recent high-profile cases are reviewed in order to illustrate some of the important issues relating to drug use in sport and dope testing.

Alain Baxter – alpine skier

The background

- Alain Baxter won a bronze medal in the men's slalom skiing event at the Winter Olympic Games in Salt Lake City in February 2002 (Figure 8.5). However, he then tested positive for metamfetamine. The IOC stripped Baxter of his bronze medal.
- Baxter had used an American product (Vicks Vapor Inhaler) as a nasal decongestant to treat a cold. This product contains lev-metamfetamine, the levo-isomer of metamfetamine, a relatively inactive isomer compared with the dextro form. It was previously known as L-desoxyephedrine. Baxter claimed that he was unaware the product contained a banned substance. The product looked similar to a product that Baxter had used in the UK, which does not contain the banned drug.

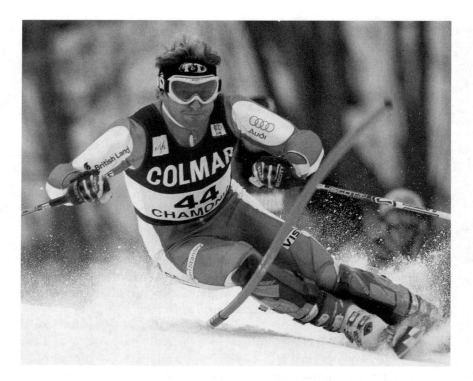

Figure 8.5 Scottish alpine skier Alain Baxter competes for Great Britain. (Courtesy of Olivier Morin/AFP/Getty Images.)

- In June 2002, the International Ski Federation (ISF) accepted that Baxter had taken the drug inadvertently but imposed a ban from all competitions of 3 months.
- In August 2002, the Court of Arbitration in Sport upheld Baxter's appeal and lifted his 3-month ban.
- Alain Baxter also appealed to the IOC with regard to regaining his bronze medal. The IOC's Court of Arbitration accepted that Baxter "did not intend to obtain a competitive advantage" by using the inhaler but refused to overturn the medal disqualification.
- The British Olympic Association ruled in March 2003 that Alain Baxter will be eligible for selection in future Olympic Games.

The issues

- Unlike some other OTC sympathomimetics such as ephedrine and phenylpropanolamine that were also on the banned list at that time, there was no urinary cut-off level for metamfetamine. The cut-off levels allow athletes to avoid sanctions if the drug levels in the urine are below the prescribed level.

- The Prohibited List made no mention of isomers of banned substances.
- The IOC and WADA have a policy of strict liability (it is the athlete's responsibility to ensure that no banned substance appears in the test results, regardless of the reason).
- Athletes should always get any medicines (prescription or OTC) checked for prohibited substances by their team doctor or other healthcare professional before taking them.

The consequences

- WADA now stipulate in their list of prohibited substances, under the section on stimulants, "including both their optical (D- and L-) isomers where relevant".
- The WADA Code, which came into operation in January 2004, included a new section on sanctions relating to 'specified substances', which include "substances which are particularly susceptible to unintentional anti-doping rules violations because of their general availability in medicinal products", including L-metamfetamine. The burden of proof is on the athlete to provide evidence that the taking of the drug was inadvertent.

Dwain Chambers – sprinter

The background

- The 'undetectable designer steroid' tetrahydrogestrinone (THG) was discovered in June 2003 when Don Catlin developed a test for it at the WADA/IOC accredited laboratory in Los Angeles, after he had been sent a syringe containing the substance.
- Dwain Chambers provided an out-of-competition urine sample for the International Association of Athletics Federation (IAAF) on 1 August 2003 at a training camp in Saarbrucken, Germany. It was claimed that Chambers was targeted for testing following a tip-off by an American anti-doping official. The sample contained THG.
- Chambers claimed that he had ingested the THG unwittingly in a supplement given to him by Victor Conte, the owner of the Bay Area Laboratory Co-operative (Balco) in San Francisco.

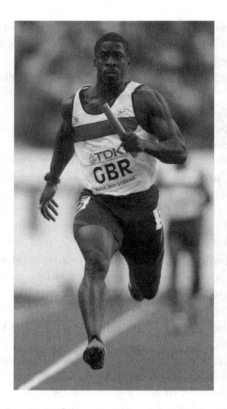

Figure 8.6 Dwain Chambers of Great Britain in action during the men's 4 × 400 m relay. (Courtesy of Phil Cole/Getty Images Sport/Getty Images.)

- The B urine sample was tested, in Los Angeles, on 7 November 2003 and confirmed the presence of THG.
- On 24 February 2004, Dwain Chambers' case was heard by UK Athletics. Chambers' legal team argued that the THG was not specifically listed on the WADA/IOC Prohibited List. Chambers was given a 2-year ban by UK Athletics and under British Olympic Association rules would be banned from all subsequent Olympic Games.

The issues

- The 'strict liability' rule was adhered to in this case.
- To what extent are 'back-street' laboratories working on 'undetectable' performance-enhancing drugs?

- Athletes are clearly prepared to take drugs that have not undergone any safety checks, let alone controlled clinical trials, thereby exposing themselves to additional health risks.
- Drugs do not have to be specifically named on the Prohibited List in order to be covered by WADA or Sports Federation rules.

The consequences

- Retrospective testing of B samples was conducted by the IOC on samples from as long ago as the 2002 Winter Olympic Games in Salt Lake City. This suggests that B samples are retained by testing laboratories for longer periods than might have been expected.
- WADA have revised the wording within their Prohibited List. They considered the use of the word 'analogue' to describe any new drugs within a doping class to be restrictive as it implied an analogue to have both a similar chemical structure *and* similar pharmacological effect. Because 'designer steroids' have been administered to athletes, despite the lack of studies on their pharmacological effects, WADA has replaced the words 'analogues' and 'mimetics' in Sections S4 and S5 with the wording ". . . and other substances with similar chemical structure *or* similar pharmacological effect(s)".
- On 29 April 2004 Britain was stripped, by the IAAF, of its silver medals for the 4×100 metres relay at the 2003 World Championships in Paris, as Chambers had competed in this race after having provided his positive urine sample. Darren Campbell, Christian Malcolm and Marlon Devonish therefore also paid a penalty for Dwain Chambers' doping offence.

Greg Rusedski – tennis player

The background

- Greg Rusedski tested positive for nandrolone in July 2003. He claims it was a result of taking 'contaminated' electrolyte supplement pills that the Association of Tennis Professionals (ATP) had been giving out to tennis players through its trainers.
- The ATP withdrew these pills in May 2003 after the emergence of a large number of nandrolone positive results from tennis players between September 2002 and May 2003. Many of these players were below the cut-off level and were therefore not sanctioned, another six were above it but were exonerated by the ATP.

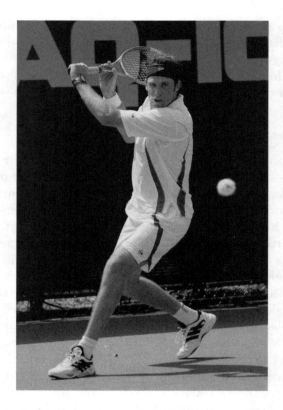

Figure 8.7 Greg Rusedski competing in the NASDAQ 100 Open. (Courtesy of Clive Brunskill/Getty Images Sport/Getty Images.)

- The ATP issued a general warning to players about the 'contaminated' pills but did not see fit to warn each player individually that they may test positive by using these pills.
- The ATP Anti-Doping Tribunal exonerated Greg Rusedski on 9 March 2004 on the basis that it could not prosecute this case when it had created the situation itself by the action of its trainers distributing these 'contaminated' supplements.

The issues

- It was not possible to establish whether the positive test results of Greg Rusedski and other tennis players were directly as a result of taking the 'contaminated' electrolyte supplement pills as the ATP claimed. The ATP commissioned an anti-doping expert, Richard

Young, to investigate the source of the nandrolone. He found no trace of nandrolone in around 500 pills tested. His conclusion was ambiguous: "While the circumstantial evidence points to nandrolone-related contamination of the electrolyte-replacement products as the source . . . there is insufficient evidence to prove that the electrolytes were the cause of the test results. Similarly there is not sufficient evidence to prove they were not the cause."

- Is ATP's treatment of their athletes consistent with the treatment of athletes in other sports? Should 'strict liability' rules have been applied?
- This is another example illustrating the culture of substance taking in sport and the dangers to athletes of testing positive through taking unregulated and inconsistently labelled supplements.
- In July 2004 WADA issued a review of Young's report, concluding that the facts did not support the legal reasoning behind the ATP tribunal decision. The full text may be viewed at http://www.atptennis.com/en/media/reports/WADA_review.pdf

The consequences

- The ATP and other sports organisations need to tighten their rules with regard to the supply of supplements to their players and advice given on their use.
- The ATP needs to harmonise its rules in line with the WADA Code.

Rio Ferdinand – professional footballer

The background

- Rio Ferdinand failed to turn up to a routine out-of-competition drug test on 23 September 2003. This was conducted by UK Sport on behalf of the Football Association (FA). Ferdinand claimed that he forgot about the test.
- On 19 December 2003, Ferdinand was given an 8-month ban, to begin on 12 January 2004 and was fined £50 000 by an FA disciplinary committee.
- An appeal by Rio Ferdinand was heard on 18 March 2004, when the player claimed he had undergone a retrospective drug test 36 hours after the missed test, and that this test had proved negative. The appeal committee upheld the original sanction.

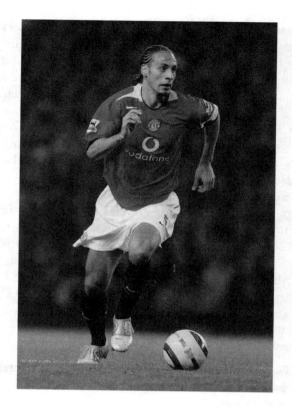

Figure 8.8 Rio Ferdinand of Manchester United. (Courtesy of Matthew Peters/ Manchester United/Getty Images.)

The issues

- According to WADA rules, Rio Ferdinand should have received a 2-year ban. However, the English FA (as a national body within FIFA) had not signed up to the WADA Code, at that time.
- FIFA had declined to sign up to the WADA Code at the Copenhagen Declaration in March 2003, principally on the grounds that it considered WADA's sanctions to be too severe. Despite having not signed up to the WADA Code, FIFA warned the FA not to make Ferdinand's sanction too lenient.
- Rio Ferdinand's claim that he was 'clean' at the time of the missed test was irrelevant as a missed test is treated as a positive result, regardless of whether the player had banned substances in his system.

The consequences

- The Rio Ferdinand case further strained relationships between the FA and UK Sport. Subsequent to the Ferdinand case, UK Sport has suggested that it may make its reporting systems more transparent. Consequently, the FA is considering breaking free from UK Sport and conducting its own drug-testing programme. Such a move would further antagonise relationships between the FA and WADA.

References

Armstrong D J, Reilly T (2003). Blood boosting and sport. In: Mottram D R, ed. *Drugs in Sport*, 3rd edn. London: Routledge, 205–225.

Ayotte C (1999). Nutritional supplements and doping controls. *New Studies in Athletics* 14: 37–42.

Balsom P D (1997). Creatine supplementation in humans. In: Reilly T, Orme M, eds. *Esteve Foundation Symposium. Vol. 7: The Clinical Pharmacology of Sport and Exercise*. Amsterdam: Excerpta Medica, 167–177.

Beltz S D, Doering P L (1993). Efficacy of nutritional supplements used by athletes. *Clin Pharm* 12: 900–908.

Chester N, Reilly T, Mottram D R (2003a). Physiological, subjective and performance effects of pseudoephedrine and phenylpropanolamine during endurance running exercise. *Int J Sports Med* 24: 3–8.

Chester N, Mottram D R, Reilly T, Powell M (2003b). Elimination of ephedrines in urine following multiple dosing: the consequences for athletes, in relation to doping control. *Br J Clin Pharmacol* 57: 62–67.

Clarkson P (1996). Nutrition for improved sports performance. Current issues on ergogenic aids. *Sports Med* 21: 393–401.

Delbeke F T, Van Eenoo P, DeBackere P (1998). Detection of human chorionic gonadotrophin misuse in sport. *Int J Sports Med* 19: 287–290.

Ferstle J (1999a). Explaining nandrolone. *Athletics Weekly* 15 September, 16.

Ferstle J (1999b). Nandrolone, part II. *Athletics Weekly* 22 September, 26–27.

Ferstle J (1999c). Nandrolone, part III. *Athletics Weekly* 29 September, 14–15.

George A J (2003). Androgenic anabolic steroids. In: Mottram D R, ed. *Drugs in Sport*, 3rd edn. London: Routledge, 138–188.

Herbert D L (1999). Recommending or selling nutritional supplements enhances potential legal liability for sports medicine practitioners. *Sports Med Alert* 5: 91–92.

Macintyre J G (1987). Growth hormone and athletes. *Sports Med* 4: 129–142.

MacLaren D P M (1997). Alkalinizers: influence of blood acid-base status on performance. In: Reilly T, Orme M, eds. *Esteve Foundation Symposium. Vol. 7: The Clinical Pharmacology of Sport and Exercise*. Amsterdam: Excerpta Medica, 157–165.

Maclaren D P M (2003). Creatine. In: Mottram D R, ed. *Drugs in Sport*, 3rd edn. London: Routledge, 286–306.

Matlin C, Delday M, Hay S, *et al.* (1987). The effect of the anabolic agent, clenbuterol, on the overloaded rat skeletal muscle. *Biosci Rep* 7: 143–148.

Reilly T R (2003). Alcohol, anti-anxiety drugs and sport. In: Mottram D R, ed. *Drugs in Sport*, 3rd edn. London: Routledge, 256–285.

Schanzer, W. (2002). *Analysis of Non-Hormonal Nutrititional Supplements for Anabolic-Androgenic Steroids – An International Study*. Cologne: Institute of Biochemistry, German Sport University Cologne (available from http: //multimedia.olympic.org/pdf/en_report_324.pdf).

Sonksen P H (2001). Hormones and sport. Insulin, growth hormone and sport. *J Endocrin* 170: 13–25.

Tucker R (1997). Abuse of androgenic anabolic steroids by athletes and body builders: a review. *Pharm J* 259: 171–179.

Uzych L (1991). Drug testing of athletes. *Br J Addict* 86: 25–31.

Verroken M, Mottram D R (2003). Doping control in sport. In: Mottram D R, ed. *Drugs in Sport*, 3rd edn. London: Routledge, 307–356.

Williams M H (1994). The use of nutritional ergogenic aids in sport: is it an ethical issue? *Int J Sports Nutr* 4: 120–131.

Further reading

Mottram D R, ed. (2003). *Drugs in Sport*, 3rd edn. London: Routledge.

Part Four

The application of sports pharmacy
in practice

9

Pharmacy for elite athletes at international games

Mark C Stuart

Introduction

Most community pharmacists will only have a modest involvement in sport and exercise and their clients will not reach the heights of double gold medal winner Kelly Holmes (Figure 9.1). However, opportunities for a far more visible contribution do exist in elite competition and in this chapter some of the factors involved in this specialised practice are outlined.

Major competitive environments

Each of the competition and training venues at international games has separate medical facilities, under the management of a venue medical

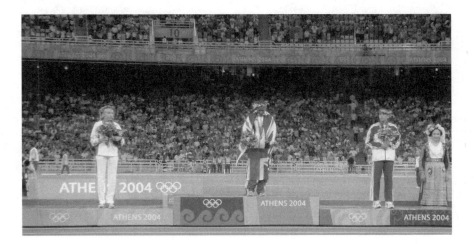

Figure 9.1 Britain's double gold medallist Kelly Holmes (centre) at the medal ceremony in Athens in 2004.

manager. Medical staff are constantly present on the playing field to attend to injured athletes and can include doctors, nurses, physiotherapists, massage therapists and ambulance personnel. Separate medical teams consisting of doctors, nurses and staff trained in first aid are responsible for the medical care of spectators. The provision and distribution of medicines for use at all competition venues presents a huge logistical task that the pharmacy services are responsible for.

Every 4 years the world's fittest and fastest sports stars come together to compete at the summer Olympic and Paralympic Games, which are quite rightly considered to be the 'greatest show on earth' (Figure 9.2).

Two years after each summer Olympic Games, the Winter Olympics and the Commonwealth Games are staged (Figure 9.3). These are massive events on a human and technological scale, and are watched by billions of people around the globe, providing an opportunity for proud host countries to showcase their nation to the world.

In the couple of weeks before the Games, thousands of athletes arrive at the athletes' village, which will be their home for the next

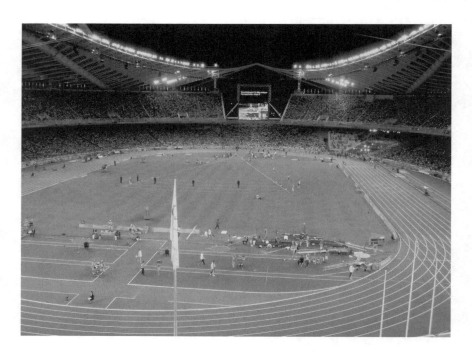

Figure 9.2 The Olympic Stadium, Athens 2004.

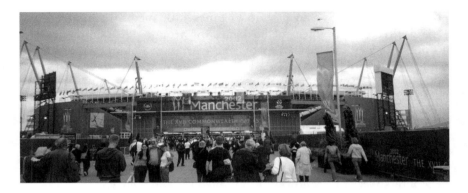

Figure 9.3 City of Manchester Stadium, Commonwealth Games 2002.

3 weeks or so. Each team, which can range in size from just one or two athletes to hundreds, is individually welcomed to the Olympic Village with an official ceremony from the host city. The national anthems of the host and visiting country are sung and their flags are raised. The athletes' village quickly comes to life with exotic accents and thousands of athletes parading proudly in bright and colourful tracksuits in national colours; the atmosphere is electric with anticipation in the days before competition.

The athletes' village is the hub of athlete life at international games. It is built as a complete self-contained city and is designed to make the athletes' stay as welcoming and comfortable as possible. Along with comprehensive medical services, facilities also usually include a bank, florist, hair salon, Internet cafe, religious services, gym, library, cinema, photo-developing and tourist information, as well as many bars, dance clubs and live entertainment venues. Roving street performers entertain the athletes and team officials as they walk around the mini-city. Massive dining halls serve food from all around the world, catering to all religious and cultural dietary requirements with unlimited food available 24 hours a day to athletes in order to fit around their hectic training schedules. Medical staff who are on duty also eat free alongside the athletes.

The provision of medical services

Providing medical services and catering to the pharmacy requirements of the thousands of athletes and millions of visiting spectators at these events is a unique challenge, on a scale unrivalled by any other public event. At the 2000 Sydney Olympic Games 4500 medical volunteers and 8 paid directors provided medical care for around 12 000 athletes and 13 000 officials at 35 Olympic venues around Sydney. At the 1996 Games in Atlanta, 4000 medical volunteers provided care to 11 000 athletes from 197 countries. It was estimated that 2.2 million visitors converged on Atlanta for these Games.

For the Athens 2004 Games, around 3000 medical staff were required to run the medical programme. This included 400 specialist doctors, 400 nurses, 400 physical therapists, 200 masseurs, 40 dentists, 30 opticians and 20 podiatrists. In addition, 170 ambulances and three helicopters were on stand-by for any medical emergency.

Athletes' medical services

Purpose-built medical centres are the core of medical services at Olympic and Commonwealth Games (Figure 9.4). Termed the 'Polyclinic', this complex is usually located within the athletes' village or in very close proximity to it and is open for a couple of weeks before, during, and a week after the Games finish. The Polyclinic is the main medical facility for athletes and team officials, and acts as the central control and co-ordination point for the many other medical facilities. In addition to the Polyclinic within the athletes' village, medical services are also provided at each competition venue for the athletes.

The full spectrum of medical services and specialities are represented in the Polyclinic and it is staffed by healthcare professionals with experience and expertise in sports medicine. Along with the world's best athletes, many of the healthcare professionals here are the world's leading experts in sports medicine. It is a unique environment that showcases both sporting and medical excellence.

The Polyclinic provides the ideal medical situation, in which an injured athlete has immediate access to a closely-knit medical team with the best diagnostic and treatment equipment available at their fingertips. Within the space of an hour, an athlete may have a consultation with a doctor specialising in sports medicine, an ultrasound or MRI scan interpreted by a radiographer, a session of physiotherapy or nursing intervention, and leave with free prescribed medicine after being counselled by a pharmacist. This perfect situation is often far removed from the reality of medical treatment available outside this environment, where such a comprehensive, efficient and instant service is rare.

Medical services in a Games Polyclinic include emergency medical services, sports medicine, general practice, medical imaging (X-ray,

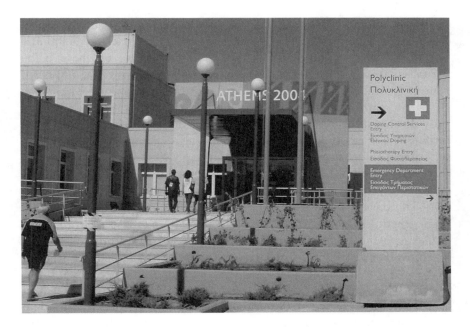

Figure 9.4 Polyclinic, Athens Olympics 2004.

ultrasound, CT scanning, MRI), dentistry, eye services (ophthalmologists, opticians, optometrists), physiotherapy, massage therapy, hydrotherapy, podiatry, pathology, medical records, interpreter services, doping control, gender verification, and pharmacy. All of these medical services are provided free to the athletes and team officials for the duration of the Games.

At the 2000 Olympic Games in Sydney, around 20 000 visits were made to the Polyclinic in the athletes' village over a period of a month. There were 3619 doctor consultations, 2884 physiotherapy treatments and 5622 visits to the pharmacy, making the pharmacy one of the busiest medical services at the Games. At the 1996 Olympic Games in Atlanta, 2474 athletes and Olympic staff were assessed in the Olympic Village Polyclinic.

Traditionally, dental and eye services are always in high demand and are kept very busy throughout the Games. It enables athletes from areas where such treatment may be limited, such as developing countries, to access routine dental and optical treatment. At the 1996 Olympic Games in Atlanta there were 910 dental appointments resulting in 400 free dental fillings to athletes and team officials. A total of 620 pairs of spectacles and 50 sets of contact lenses were also prescribed and issued. At the Sydney Games, there were around 1800 visits each to dental and optometry services in the Polyclinic, figures similar to these being common at other Games. The provision of these services, often for routine treatment, is considered an unofficial obligation of the host city.

The main focus of medical treatment at international games is to provide care for newly acquired injuries or disease rather than treating or diagnosing existing complaints. This is also reflected in the demands on other medical staff present, such as the physiotherapists or massage therapists who are usually kept extremely busy tending to newly acquired injuries.

The busiest times for the Polyclinic correspond with training and event schedules. During the Games, there are often two sessions of a particular sport each day, with training sessions most popular in the morning. The Polyclinic is most frequently visited by athletes either very early in the morning, before competition and training, or late in the evening when they return after the day's events. The hours of the medical centre and the pharmacy reflect these schedules; opening early at 6:30am and closing at 11pm with an on-call pharmacist available throughout the night.

Medical facilities for athletes are not just confined to the Polyclinic. Each competition venue will have an independent medical facility for the athletes close to the field-of-play or poolside. For open water events such as sailing, boats carrying medical supplies and personnel are deployed. For road sports such as cycling (Figure 9.5) and marathons, mobile medical facilities are necessary to provide medical cover for the event.

The Polyclinic will also have the support of a network of designated local hospitals that can accept patients requiring medical care that it cannot provide. The medical services at the Athens Games worked closely with the Greek Ministry of Health and Welfare to ensure that the resources of local hospitals could be utilised if required.

Daily clinics for VIPs and officials

Mobile clinics are provided for VIP guests and officials during Olympic and Commonwealth Games. In Manchester, a GP ran a clinic for 2 hours every morning and afternoon at both the Technical Officials Village (TOV) and also at the hotel designated for VIP visitors. A doctors bag containing a small number of drugs such as analgesics and antihistamines, and a variety of first-aid materials, was maintained daily by pharmacists in the Polyclinic. After the clinic, the doctor would present any

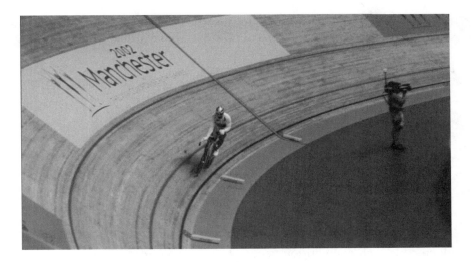

Figure 9.5 Cycling velodrome, Commonwealth Games, Manchester 2002.

prescriptions to the Polyclinic pharmacy for dispensing. A courier service would then deliver the medicines to the patients.

A similar service was provided in Sydney at the hotel where Olympic officials were staying. The clinic was staffed by a doctor and a nurse with an ambulance available onsite, and able to visit other hotels around Sydney if required.

Spectator medical care

At the Atlanta and Sydney Olympic Games and the Commonwealth Games in Manchester, separate medical services were provided for athletes and spectators. In Manchester, the St John Ambulance Service provided medical care for spectators at the various stadiums and other venues. In Atlanta, Red Cross volunteers trained in first aid were stationed throughout the crowds. Teams of paramedics were also available at each venue to provide emergency treatment if required. Medical care for spectators at these games mostly consisted of issuing simple analgesic drugs and minor dressings; however cardiac defibrillators were available in the event of a cardiac emergency.

In Atlanta, a total of 30 000 people (including athletes) were treated at first-aid stations and clinics over the period of the Games, with 10 723 patients being examined by doctors. With extreme summer temperatures experienced in Atlanta, many people required medical care for heat-related illness and this accounted for around 10% of medical encounters. However, injury accounted for about a third of all medical cases.

The Polyclinic pharmacy

The planning process

In the year and a half before the Commonwealth Games in Manchester, a pharmacy working group, consisting of pharmacist representatives from NHS hospitals in the Greater Manchester area and other experts in sport medicine, met regularly. As well as establishing the pharmacy procedures and operations for the Games, they were responsible for compiling the list of emergency drugs that would be made available to doctors at each competition venue. The list contained a comprehensive assortment of life-saving drugs for use in an acute emergency (Table 9.1).

Before the Games, the drugs, along with needles and syringes, were systematically packed into portable medical bags by the pharmacists for immediate use by the duty doctors if necessary (Figure 9.6). Fortunately, drugs from the emergency packs were hardly used, with the exception of paracetamol, which was frequently replenished. However, in one

Table 9.1 Drugs contained in the emergency drug pack for use by doctors at competition venues of the XVII Commonwealth Games, Manchester 2002

Product	Quantity
Adenosine 6 mg in 2 ml amps	6
Adrenaline 1 in 10 000, 1 mg in 10 ml prefilled syringe	1
Atropine sulphate 3 mg/10 ml prefilled syringe	1
Benzylpenicillin 600 mg powder for reconstitution	1
Diazepam 5 mg rectal tube	2
Adrenaline Epi-Pen Auto Injector Adult 0.3 mg in 0.3 ml	1
Glucose 50%, 50 ml prefilled syringe Mini-Jet	1
Glyceryl trinitrate sublingual spray 400 micrograms/dose	1
Hydrocortisone 100 mg powder for reconstitution	2
Ketamine injection 100 mg/ml vial	1
Ketorolactrometamol 30 mg/ml vial	1
Metoclopramide 10 mg/2 ml injection	1
Midazolam 10 mg/2 ml injection	1
Naloxone 2 mg in 2 ml prefilled syringe	1
Paracetamol 500 mg tablets	16
Salbutamol 500 micrograms/ml injection	1
Water for injection 5 ml	2

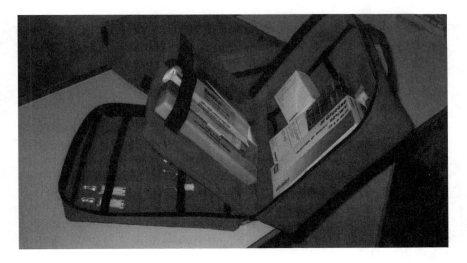

Figure 9.6 Emergency drug pack, Commonwealth Games, Manchester 2002.

instance, a volunteer staff member was promptly administered adrenaline (epinephrine) after developing an anaphylactic reaction to a bee sting. He was then taken to the Polyclinic ward for additional treatment and monitoring.

The provision of controlled drugs of addiction was a consideration for the Manchester pharmacy team. It was considered necessary for a strong opioid analgesic to be available for use by doctors at the venues in the event of an emergency; however safe storage conforming to legal requirements was not available at the competition venues. This problem was overcome by issuing the drugs to individual doctors. Kits containing two prefilled syringes of morphine were issued at the beginning of the doctor's shift and signed back into the pharmacy at the end of the doctor's period of duty. At the Polyclinic pharmacy the legal requirements for safe storage were met by installing a safe in the pharmacy bolted into a specially poured concrete slab beneath the floor.

In addition to the drugs used for emergency situations, general first aid requirements for the athlete medical facilities were managed by the Polyclinic pharmacy. Each venue medical manager was responsible for the secure storage and replenishment of used drugs from the Polyclinic pharmacy when needed using an official requisition form.

Many of the smaller venues had only one main medical room, however the City of Manchester Stadium, with a capacity of 38 000 spectators, had two main medical rooms for the athletes and separate

Table 9.2 Medicines available for use by doctors at each medical facility at the competition venues of the XVII Commonwealth Games, Manchester 2002

Pharmacy stock list for competition venue medical rooms

Sodium chloride 0.9% sachets 25 ml (pack of 25)
Sterile water for irrigation 150 ml (6)
Sodium chloride 0.9% for injection, 500 ml bags (5)
Glucose 5% for injection, 500 ml bags (5)
Paracetamol tablets 500 mg (2 × 100)
Paracetamol syrup for children 120 mg/5 ml, 100 ml (2)
Ibuprofen syrup for children 100 mg/5 ml, 100 ml (2)
Loratadine tablets 10 mg (1 box of 21 tabs)
Co-codamol 30/500 tablets (24)
Ibuprofen 400 mg tablets (2 × 24)
Salbutamol 100 micrograms inhaler (3)
Volumatic device for use with salbutamol inhaler (1)
Eye wash kit (3)
Multistix GP test strips (1 box of 25 strips)
Chlorphenamine syrup 4 mg/10 ml, 100 ml (1)
Medicine spoons (1 bag)
Medicines formulary (1)
Pharmacy requisition form (to request replenishment of stock if required) (5)

spectator medical facilities situated on each level of the stadium. A standard list of medicines was issued to each competition venue medical facility for use by the doctors on duty (Table 9.2).

For the 2002 Commonwealth Games, the shooting events were held at the National Shooting Centre in Surrey. This venue was a few hours from Manchester, so to overcome delays in providing medicines from the Polyclinic pharmacy to the athletes and officials living there, doctors at the venue were issued a supply of formulary drugs to dispense. Daily deliveries from the Manchester Polyclinic would replenish stock and take prescription records back to the Polyclinic.

Unusual swarms of biting insects and seasonal allergies caused the greatest problem for competitors at the shooting venue in Surrey – large numbers of tubes of hydrocortisone and sting-relief cream and dozens of antihistamine prescriptions were prescribed.

Facilities provided

The Polyclinic pharmacy is mainly geared to the specific pharmacological requirements of sports medicine and is stocked to be able to provide immediate and necessary care for the 'games family' members. The 'games family' is defined as athletes, team officials, and accompanying members of each country's team and inevitably includes people of varying health.

The Polyclinic pharmacy is run by volunteer pharmacists who work in 8-hour shifts for an average of about 5 days each. Around 40 pharmacists covered the Olympic and Paralympic Games in Sydney, and 14 pharmacists were responsible for running the Polyclinic pharmacy at the Manchester Commonwealth Games. In Athens, the Polyclinic pharmacy was staffed by 12 Greek pharmacists and 10 pharmacy students from Athens University.

Most athletes who are taking long-term medicine for pre-existing conditions will generally be prepared for the few weeks of living away from home. There is less emphasis placed on providing a comprehensive drug selection for long-term or chronic conditions, or those associated with geriatric or paediatric medicine. A limited supply of the most common but necessary medicines used by the general population, such as antihypertensive drugs, are kept, but are usually only used for the purpose of assisting a patient who has left their regular drugs at home.

The pharmacy is responsible for providing the drug and therapeutic substance requirements for all of the medical disciplines present in the Polyclinic. Items dispensed may include dental prescriptions for antibiotics and analgesia, and various eye drops prescribed by the optometrists and ophthalmologists. In Manchester, the Polyclinic pharmacy was also involved with the supply of diagnostic agents for eye services and specific drugs for use in dental procedures. For all prescriptions, only a 1-week supply of drugs or a full course of antibiotics are issued to patients.

The Polyclinic pharmacy may also cater to the unique supply requirements of physiotherapy, podiatry and massage therapy. At the Manchester Games, isopropyl alcohol (rubbing alcohol), enormous volumes of massage oil, ultrasound gel and bandage removal solvents were among products accessed through the pharmacy suppliers, to be used by the physiotherapy and massage services. Chemical agents used for podiatry procedures, such as liquid phenol, were also supplied by the pharmacy. This close interaction between pharmacists and allied healthcare professionals is a situation often unique to the Games environment. Encounters with such preparations are unusual in community pharmacy, but are an interesting facet of sports pharmacy at such events.

At Olympic Games, pharmacy staff have access to interpreter services. Often the athletes do not speak the language of the host country and an interpreter may be required to provide adequate counselling to the patient. It is particularly important for an athlete to understand the medication they are taking, especially when restricted drugs that require notification before competition are dispensed. At the Sydney Olympic Games, 6227 occasions of interpreter service were provided to the medical staff by 23 interpreters.

The Games formulary

For each Commonwealth Games and Olympic Games a list of drugs for use throughout the event is drawn up beforehand, using similar criteria to a hospital or Primary Care Trust formulary. However, there is greater emphasis on providing a comprehensive range of the types of drugs used by athletes compared to a standard hospital formulary. The formulary also lists the permitted, prohibited or restricted status of all the drugs it contains.

A copy of the Games formulary is sent to each team of the participating country in the months before Olympic or Commonwealth Games to inform the accompanying medical personnel of the drugs that will be available. The formulary also contains advice to team doctors about the procedures for prescribing at the Games.

As anti-inflammatory medication is the most frequent class of drugs prescribed for sports injury, their use during the Games is an important consideration for the formulary. Where a hospital formulary may have a concise range of anti-inflammatory medication, a Games dispensary would stock almost the complete range of drugs in this class.

The international availability of certain drugs in the participating countries, and the familiarity of visiting doctors with drugs available locally, is another important issue to be taken into account. The range of medicines stocked in the pharmacy needs to reflect those known and used by the global medical community as well as those frequently used in the host country.

Altering an athlete's regular treatment, such as anti-inflammatory medication, very close to competition brings with it the risk that it may not be as effective therapeutically as familiar treatment and may present different side-effects. A change in medication at this point means the athlete must quickly adjust to the new therapy. This may add to the psychological stress of the finely-tuned athlete unfamiliar with the new treatment. Although of little concern in most patients, for an elite athlete whose winning performance depends on absolutely perfect physical and psychological conditions, these situations are often avoided where possible. A broad range of drugs commonly used in sports medicine, such as anti-inflammatory analgesics, allows the team doctors to prescribe their drug of choice to the athlete.

The licensed indications and the use of drugs for therapeutic use can differ between countries, which may restrict the suitability of some drugs to be included on the formulary. This was the case in Manchester, where drugs that selectively inhibit cyclo-oxygenase-2 including rofecoxib and celecoxib were not included on the formulary, even though some visiting foreign athletes were familiar with their use for soft tissue injury. In the UK they were licensed for pain and inflammation in osteoarthritis; the initiation of treatment for such a disease would not be expected in such an environment.

Pharmacy dispensing systems

For recent Games, the pharmacy dispensing system has become an important tool in eliminating the chances of unknowingly dispensing a prohibited drug. At both the Atlanta and Sydney Games, all prohibited and restricted drugs were flagged in the pharmacy computer and would alert the dispensing pharmacist at the time of processing a prescription for such drugs.

A sophisticated system was developed for the Manchester Games, which was linked to the main Games accreditation database. This enabled details of the patient, doctor and pharmacist to be retrieved using the unique accreditation numbers assigned to all athletes, officials and staff, allowing fast, accurate and safe dispensing.

Drug distribution

The medical services, in particular the pharmacy, rely on daily deliveries from local wholesalers to maintain the supply of drugs at international games. This high level of security creates an interesting logistical challenge to maintain regular pharmacy deliveries.

In Manchester, vehicles with pharmacy deliveries were thoroughly searched by a team of bomb experts before being permitted on site, or X-rayed if deliveries were carried in. Drivers required special passes, time-slots and pharmacist escort while in the athletes' village. Similar security was in place for the Sydney Games, posing similar issues for drug delivery.

To deliver pharmacy supplies to the competition venues around the main Sport City site in Manchester, golf buggies proved a practical mode of transport for pharmacists, something that would probably only be seen at such events.

Regular drug distribution to the rest of the host city also needs careful consideration and planning in light of the fact that millions of visitors are expected during the Games. For the Athens Games, the Olympic Organising Committee and pharmacists representing the pharmaceutical industry and local businesses came to an agreement on the operation of local pharmacies and the restocking of essential medicines around Athens. The number of pharmacies open at the weekends and overnight was increased, especially around Olympic venues, downtown Athens and the port of Piraeus. Local pharmacies were also restocked during evening hours.

Prescribing procedures

The issuing of prescriptions

Prescribing and dispensing drugs for elite athletes is undertaken very cautiously, given the many regulations that apply to drug use in sport. Unique prescription forms are used for all medication in the Polyclinic and require signatures from the doctor, pharmacist, athlete, and sometimes team officials before a drug is handed over.

At Commonwealth and Olympic Games, all drugs are issued using a prescription written by a doctor, regardless of whether the drug is available over-the-counter or not. This practice effectively eliminates the potential for an athlete to inadvertently take a prohibited substance, as some can be found in OTC preparations. It also enables comprehensive medication records to be kept for individual athletes.

If a restricted or prohibited drug is considered necessary for an athlete, the athlete is informed about the substance and the consequences of taking it. The athlete must then sign the prescription to acknowledge acceptance of the treatment. The dispensing pharmacist, prescribing doctor, and sometimes the head of athlete medical services are also required to sign the prescription following the issue of a drug whose use is restricted in sport. Restricted drugs may require notification to the Games medical commission, using a TUE form, before the athlete competes (see below).

As an additional precaution, all restricted and prohibited drugs are labelled as such at the time of dispensing. They are often also stored separately to drugs that are permitted, further minimising the risk of dispensing them inappropriately.

A total of 1017 prescriptions were dispensed from the Manchester Commonwealth Games Polyclinic for 5000 athletes. At the Sydney Olympics, with around 12 000 athletes, 4244 prescriptions were dispensed and 3600 were dispensed at the Atlanta Games, where close to 11 000 athletes competed. In Athens, the Polyclinic pharmacy processed around 100–150 prescriptions daily and catered for the pharmaceutical requirements of over 17 000 athletes and team officials.

Prescribing by visiting doctors

Each team present at international games usually has at least one doctor accompanying the athletes, sometimes more. The laws of the host country will often govern the rights that visiting doctors have in relation to prescribing and supply of drugs to the athletes they are looking after.

For the Sydney Olympics, 1109 visiting team doctors were given prescribing rights for the period of the Games. Similar rights were granted to visiting team doctors in Athens. This enabled them to prescribe drugs from the Games formulary for members of their own team only.

In Manchester, such prescribing rights were not possible by UK law, so all prescriptions had to be written by doctors registered in the UK. To acknowledge the input of a foreign team doctor into the medical decisions made for an athlete, the prescription had a separate section for them to sign. However, the UK-registered doctor was ultimately responsibile for the prescription issued to the patient.

Similarly, at the 1996 Commonwealth Games in Kuala Lumpur, only prescriptions written by doctors registered with the Malaysian Medical Council were honoured. Team physicians were advised to procure temporary registration for the period of the Games with the Malaysian Medical Council.

Drug exemptions for therapeutic reasons

Athletes are required to submit a TUE form before competition if they are using a restricted drug such as a beta-2 agonist or corticosteroid injection (see also Chapters 8 and 10). They are usually completed by the team doctor and provide the Medical Commission with details of the diagnosis, drug, dose, frequency and reasons for use. Results of lung function tests may be provided by a pulmonary specialist to support the use of beta-2 agonists in asthma.

Failing to submit a TUE form declaring the therapeutic use of a restricted drug would result in a doping violation should the athlete test positive for these substances. During the Manchester Games, gold medal winner Kim Collins, a sprinter from St Kitts and Nevis, failed a drug test after testing positive for salbutamol, but failing to submit a TUE form. His case went before the Commonwealth Games Federation Court, where the offence was dropped because he could prove retrospectively that the inhaler was used for asthma.

Misinformed athletes are sometimes under the impression that they can take any therapeutically used drug they like, as long as they declare it on a TUE form. This is certainly not the case, as some drugs such as diuretics and oral corticosteroids are prohibited regardless of the health status of the athlete.

One unknowing athlete competing in a clay-pigeon shooting event declared his regular medicine on a TUE form, which was identified by a pharmacist as being a combination product containing atenolol. Beta-blockers are specifically prohibited in shooting because of their ability to minimise tremor, so improving accuracy. The athlete was taking the drug to treat ventricular arrhythmia and it was deemed highly inappropriate to change from atenolol to an alternative such as amiodarone, which would require close monitoring at the initiation of therapy.

The athlete was to compete in a clay-pigeon shooting event, where, compared to stationary target shooting, having a steady hand was of uncertain advantage. The sport relies greatly on reaction and speed, and it is possible that beta-blockers may even slow down the reaction time for the athlete. Given his genuine medical circumstances and the nature of this particular shooting event he was given a rare medical exemption and allowed to compete.

Interestingly, in contrast to the last case, a number of shooters submitted TUE forms for salbutamol, where one of the common side-effects of this drug is shaking hands.

The Games pharmacy in Manchester was responsible for the collection of TUE forms for athletes taking restricted drugs for legitimate medical use. Pharmacists were responsible for identifying the drugs declared on the forms, before they were to be considered case by case by the Commonwealth Games Medical Commission. Many of the preparations requiring pharmacist identification were those with proprietary names not available the UK.

From observation, it would seem that the level of awareness of the list of prohibited substances, doping issues in sport, and notification requirements of different drugs, is different across the various athlete groups. It seems apparent with the types of pharmacy enquiries at the Manchester Games that sports with a lower public profile, such as lawn bowls or shooting, are less aware of some of these issues and are more vulnerable to the inadvertent use of banned drugs. Similarly, athletes from developing countries also appear to be less educated with respect to prohibited substances. Athletes competing in high public profile events such as athletics, swimming and rugby seem to have a good knowledge of doping control issues.

Patterns of drug use

Athletes at international games are in peak physical condition, often in the prime of their youth, eating a near-perfect diet and would qualify as some of the healthiest individuals on the planet. The pattern of drug use and the types of drugs used at international sporting events is therefore understandably far removed from the prescribing patterns seen in an average community pharmacy.

The medical services quickly gain momentum in the days before the Games. The athletes are most focused in the time leading up to what might be their once-in-a-lifetime event. For most, this will be the culmination of many years of intense training, a lifetime of ambitious dreams, and the highlight of their sporting career. It is no wonder that the slightest sign of ill health at this stage can be extremely traumatic for the athlete. This anxiety and obsession about a perfect physical state is reflected in the initial demands on medical services.

In Atlanta, Barcelona and Seoul, medical operations began 13 days before the opening ceremonies and continued until 3 days after the closing ceremony. Patterns of demand were similar for all three Games, with medical services slow in the first week, allowing time to test procedures and equipment and for staff to familiarise themselves with the facilities. The demands on medical services peaked just before the opening ceremony and continued until the end of the first week of competition. After this time there was typically a gradual decline until the closing ceremony, then a dramatic drop. However, the demand for MRI and ultrasound imaging increased steadily throughout the whole period.

Similarly, at the Manchester Commonwealth Games, the pharmacy was busiest at the start of the Games. Antibiotic prescriptions accounted for the majority of the prescriptions dispensed before the competition, followed closely by NSAIDs. After the opening ceremony, the daily number of antibiotic prescriptions dropped considerably but the daily number of anti-inflammatory drugs remained relatively consistent.

Contracting a cold or respiratory tract infection before competition could be potentially detrimental to an athlete's performance, particularly for athletes competing in aerobic sports. In Manchester, the number of antibiotics dispensed for respiratory conditions peaked dramatically on the day before the opening ceremony. One theory is that this peak indicates that athletes were more likely to seek medical attention for symptoms of infection before their event than afterwards, when they were perhaps less concerned with contracting a respiratory illness because they had already competed.

This trend also reflects the anxiety intensity of the athletes before competition and illustrates the immediate nature of sports medicine at this level. Some would see the main aim as enabling the athlete to be at optimum health for their event. There is pressure on prescribers from athletes and coaches to act on the most minor of symptoms of infectious disease when competing at this level where the stakes are so high. Understandably, athletes can get extremely paranoid if they experience the slightest sniffle a couple of days before their one chance of a gold medal.

Even in the week preceding the Games, most athletes are still engaged in strict training schedules and, although less frequent before competition, the medical team can expect to treat a number of musculoskeletal injuries. After competition starts, anti-inflammatory drugs become the most frequently dispensed drugs, and their use escalates as the Games progress. This pattern would be expected, as athletes are at a greater risk of injury when they exert to their extreme limits during the event.

Based on figures from recent international Games, anti-inflammatory drugs are by far the most widely used class of drugs, accounting for around 20% of all prescriptions dispensed during the course of such Games. Diclofenac is the single most prescribed drug, accounting for about half of all the prescriptions for anti-inflammatory drugs.

In Atlanta, over 3600 prescriptions were dispensed, with 219 processed on one day. The most commonly dispensed drugs were ibuprofen, amoxicillin, naproxen, paracetamol, cimetidine, clotrimazole, diazepam, terfenadine, cough suppressants and throat lozenges.

The use of injectable local anaesthetics and corticosteroids is not uncommon for sporting injuries, particularly those affecting the joints. A number of prescriptions for drugs such as lidocaine and methylprednisolone are usually dispensed during the course of the Games for severe injuries, where they are injected intra-articularly (into the joint) for treatment of acute pain and inflammation. These drugs can be subject to abuse because they can enable an otherwise injury-free athlete to exert themselves past natural pain limits. Such use contravenes sporting ethics and can put the athlete at risk of more serious injury.

It is necessary to notify the Games medical commission of the use of injectable corticosteroids. The notification forms require a diagnosis from the treating doctor and an explanation justifying their use. These forms must be presented before competition, or at the earliest opportunity after treatment. The pharmacy at the Manchester Commonwealth Games was responsible for the collection and collation of these forms for the Games Medical Commission.

It is not surprising that fungal infections are relatively common in athletes competing at this level and the demand for antifungal preparations supports this fact. Such preparations account for around 5% of all dispensed medication in a Games medical centre. Hours of intense, sweaty training creates the warm and moist conditions perfect for opportunistic fungal infections. The use of public training facilities with shared showers and changing rooms can add to the risk of acquiring a fungal infection. As with the general population, the incidence of fungal infections varies with the seasons and Games held in warmer, tropical climates would typically see a higher demand for antifungal drugs. There were a greater percentage of antifungal drugs prescribed at the Sydney Games than there were for those in Manchester.

The athlete's home country is often on the opposite side of the globe to the host city. Extreme seasonal variations contribute to the considerable incidence of allergy and hay fever among athletes at international Games. The 2000 Olympics were staged during springtime in Australia, and allergy medications were some of the most frequently dispensed medicines from the Polyclinic pharmacy.

At the time of the Sydney Olympics, there were two considerations to be taken into account when prescribing drugs for seasonal allergies. Firstly, many of the decongestants such as phenylephrine, phenylpropanolamine and pseudoephedrine, were considered to be performance-enhancing and were prohibited in sport at the time (phenylephrine, phenylpropanolamine and pseudoephedrine have since been removed from the Prohibited List). Secondly, many of the antihistamines cause drowsiness; a side-effect that may impair performance in some athletes.

The effect of local environmental conditions and climate on prescribing trends was also evident in Athens. Loratadine was commonly dispensed for allergies, and simple lubricating eye drops were also in high demand for irritated eyes as a result of the dry and dusty atmosphere.

The benefit of treatment for the athlete and the risk of performance impairment can influence the drugs chosen. This risk/benefit ratio requires careful consideration by the prescriber in consultation with the athlete. For example loratadine, with a small risk of drowsiness, might be prescribed for a long-distance runner with severe hay fever, whose performance may be more impaired from the symptoms of the hay fever than any side-effect caused by the drug. Decisions based on similar logic are commonplace within the setting of elite sport, where a millisecond lost can be the difference between gold and silver.

Jetlag is common in athletes arriving at the athletes' village in the days before the Games and must be carefully managed to ensure minimum disruption to the athlete's strict training and rest schedule. Some teams have the benefit of spending time in the host country for the weeks before the Games to allow acclimatisation to local conditions such as temperature and altitude. However, many arrive within a few days of their event, perhaps due to the cost of athlete accommodation. The athletes usually adjust using non-pharmacological approaches, due to the obvious performance-inhibiting effects of sedative drugs that could persist the following day, although some coaches and officials request short courses of medication such as temazepam or sedating anti-histamines to help with jetlag.

Drugs for dental use

Before 2004, the use of local anaesthetic drugs was permitted only by the local or intra-articular injection route, but it was also necessary to notify the Games Medical Commission if they were used. This regulation had implications for the use of local anaesthetics for dental procedures. Although local injection was permitted, dentists at the Manchester Games routinely completed notification forms for every patient who required local anaesthetics to be administered. Regulations have since changed and local anaesthetics (with the exception of cocaine) are no longer restricted in sport.

Winter Games considerations

Planning for a pharmacy at a Winter Olympic Games must take into account the unique environmental factors that freezing temperatures and altitude conditions present. The formulary for such an event would reflect the pharmacological requirements of health problems associated with these conditions.

At the 2002 Salt Lake City Winter Olympics there were around 11 000 people – including spectators – treated at 35 medical stations located throughout the venues. Around 2000 athletes and team officials were treated in the Polyclinic. The majority of cases were 'flu and respiratory infections, but 43 cases of altitude sickness and 16 cases of frostbite were treated.

Public health issues

Infectious disease outbreaks

With the high density of athletes living in the Olympic Village and sharing training facilities, dining areas and leisure amenities, a mass outbreak of an infectious disease is a real possibility during international Games, where infection could spread quickly among residents. Athletes may sleep in rooms accommodating more than one athlete, further adding to the risk of transmission of any infection. Establishment of prevention and infection control measures is extremely important.

The possibility of an infectious disease surfacing is an important consideration for the pharmacy services, where an effective array of antibiotic drugs must be available in the case of such occurrences. The selection of such drugs to be kept by the pharmacy must take into account possible differences in antibiotic resistance between visitors from foreign countries. There may be visitors from close to 200 countries living in the environment of the athletes' village, and there is the possibility of intercontinental disease transmission.

At the 1996 Atlanta Games, eight cases of malaria were reported and one case of an athlete with malaria with thrombocytopenia requiring hospitalisation for 5 days. There were also three cases of hepatitis, and one case of filariasis. Several athletes requested HIV tests, with no positive results. At the Manchester Games, a purpose-built observation ward in the Polyclinic was used for overnight observation of an athlete with malaria, with the pharmacy promptly obtaining the appropriate anti-malarial treatment. This four-bed ward in the Polyclinic would be used to quarantine the athlete from the rest of the team should an infectious disease be diagnosed. Fortunately it was not necessary to use it for this purpose.

Rigorous reporting systems are implemented to notify suspected medical conditions that may pose a threat to public health. In Atlanta these were reported to the state Division of Public Health, so immediate public health interventions could be initiated.

Disaster planning

It is a disturbing fact that international Games can be the target for terrorist attack. The bombing at Centennial Olympic Park in Atlanta during the 1996 Games resulted in two deaths and 111 people injured. Eleven Israeli athletes were killed in Munich during a terrorist attack in the athletes' village at the 1972 Olympic Games. In 1997, four Australian athletes were killed when a bridge collapsed at the Maccabiah Games in Israel. The possibility of such horrific events must be taken seriously when preparing for international games.

In Atlanta, the possibility of a terrorist attack was recognised and reflected by the stocking of some drugs in the pharmacy. Pralidoxime chloride and atropine was available for the treatment of nerve gas poisoning and decontamination facilities were available in the event of gas or radioactive contamination.

In Manchester, no special agents specifically used for treatment of biological or chemical attack were stocked by the Polyclinic pharmacy. However, tight links with local public health services meant that in the event of a disaster on a mass public scale, medical services would be taken over by the National Health Service and patients would be redirected to local hospitals, who maintained detailed contingency plans.

Nutritional supplement monitoring

Because the pharmacy is the medicines information point for athletes at international games, pharmacists are often presented with bottles of vitamins or other nutritional supplements and asked if they are permitted in sport (see also Chapter 8). Such products are often recommended by coaches or team-mates, and most athletes take one or more supplements to optimise their health and performance.

The advice that must be given to athletes by pharmacists is one of caution, as recent studies have revealed prohibited substances in many commonly available nutritional supplements. The number of athletes claiming they are absolutely certain that their product is contaminant-free is alarming, given the fact that many contaminated products have been found.

Pharmacists at the Manchester Games were responsible for ensuring that there were no products in the dining room or available from shops in the athletes' village that could lead to an inadvertent positive drug test. Of particular concern was the availability of herbal and other nutritional supplements within the athletes' village, as such products have been linked to positive drug tests.

Pharmacists met with catering officials to identify any herbal products intended for use during the Games. Teabags containing various herbs including ginseng were found and promptly removed from the athletes' dining hall. It was imperative that the village complied with international warnings to athletes about the risks of taking herbal preparations that could not be guaranteed contaminant-free.

All food shops within the village were examined by the pharmacists for similar products. One small food shop was asked to remove an energy drink containing high amounts of caffeine and amino acids from sale because at the time, an athlete could test positive for caffeine after excessive consumption. The high caffeine in the drink could potentially have led to an athlete unfamiliar with the ingredients to test positive for caffeine. Sensibly, caffeine has since been removed from the list of prohibited substances.

Dilemmas for pharmacists

Many of the duties and patient encounters experienced in a Polyclinic pharmacy are far from removed from the routine work of a community or hospital pharmacist. The medical situations that arise are often unique and unexpected, and can provide an extremely stimulating, but also perplexing, environment to work in. In the days before competition, pharmacists at the Manchester Games faced an interesting dilemma.

The Games pharmacists were involved in sourcing information and advising an athlete who was to compete in a shooting event. The athlete had just taken up residence in the athletes' village and had been given the news that he had tested positive for a prohibited drug in an out-of-competition test conducted by the doping authorities in his home country before the Games.

The athlete, distressed by the test results and the possibility of being sent home without competing, presented to one of the Games doctors. He claimed the only medication he was taking was blood pressure tablets, which he declared to the doping control authorities at the time of testing. The athlete was enormously upset by the fact that his lifelong dream of competing at this level may be shattered.

The tablets he was taking were presented to the pharmacy for identification. They were found to be a formulation containing a combination of enalapril and the diuretic, hydrochlorothiazide, which is a prohibited drug in all sports. It was now clear that hydrochlorothiazide was the drug that resulted in the positive doping offence. His doctor decided to immediately change the athlete to a tablet containing just enalapril and monitor his blood pressure closely.

His event was not for another week, so he would not have any further tests until then, however there was also no definite guarantee that the diuretic would be undetectable a week after stopping it. Pharmacists attempted to estimate the elimination time of hydrochlorothiazide in order to advise him appropriately. For diuretics, there is no minimum level that constitutes an offence, so *any* trace of the drug would constitute another doping offence.

The distraught athlete had another problem. Even if his system was completely free of the diuretic by the time he was to compete, it would still not protect him from the risk of a doping offence at the Games, as a number of random out-of-competition tests were being independently conducted by WADA in the week before the Games.

The consequences of a positive test at the Games could be a 2-year ban from competition and public international embarrassment, because positive test results are made public.

There were two choices for his country's team officials. Either send the athlete home, or allow him to compete the following week in the hope that the drug would be completely eliminated. There was also always a risk of him being selected for a random out-of-competition test in the meantime.

The athlete did compete the following week, but did not win a medal, nor was he ever selected for a drug test. This case illustrates how pharmacists can be key facilitators in complex ethical, legal and medical issues for athletes at international games. In this situation, they were involved in foreign drug identification, clinical guidance on suitable drug alternatives, and monitoring when the therapy was changed. Additionally, they used pharmacokinetic data to estimate drug elimination for the athlete, and were also involved in counselling the athlete on anti-doping regulations.

Unique medical encounters

Unusual requests for treatment and prescribed drugs by elite athletes are common at international games. A minor condition can be exaggerated to 'medical emergency' status in the context of elite sport. The urgency of treatment is often governed by the athlete's competition schedule and can be far removed from the usual priority given to these conditions outside the Games environment.

During the Manchester Games, a concerned boxer presented a prescription at the pharmacy for a course of aciclovir tablets and cream, to be used for a suspected cold-sore, with typical initial tingling symptoms. The athlete had genuine reason for concern because with a cold-sore he could not compete because of the risk of infection to his opponent. It seemed extreme treatment for a problem that is not usually a huge concern for most people, but given that the athlete's chance of a gold medal and even his career, could be jeopardised because of it, one can sympathise with the aggressive treatment.

Another unusual request was for chloramphenicol eye drops for a shooter who had developed conjuntivitis. The condition became a matter of urgency for the athlete, as the infection was causing blurred vision in the eye that he used to aim the gun. Left untreated, the infection may have impaired his performance considerably.

Also during these Games, a hysterical coach was prescribed a few diazepam tablets for an anxiety attack. Her condition was triggered when she received news that the athlete she was coaching was withdrawn from competition when it was revealed she was a different nationality to the one she was representing.

Imported drugs for team use

Many teams, especially the larger ones, often bring all the medication they might need and may only access the Polyclinic pharmacy for drugs that they did not bring with them. Around 80% of teams at the Sydney Games brought their own health teams with them.

The host country's laws on the importation of drugs for therapeutic use must be adhered to when a participating team imports drugs for their athletes. Often import permits must be obtained by teams who wish to bring their own supply of medicines, as was the case for the Sydney Olympics.

At these Games, National Olympic Committees were required to submit to the government a list of medications, herbal preparations and traditional medicines that they intended to import. Some substances need supporting documentation by a doctor, some require temporary registration before importation, and some were prohibited from being imported into Australia without a permit or import licence. These included narcotics, psychotropics, growth hormones, anabolic androgenic steroids and erythropoietin.

In Athens, each national Olympic committee was requested to declare all medicines it planned to bring into Greece eight months before the Games, to ensure that there could be no inadvertent breach of customs and importation laws.

A freely available drug in one country may be considered a narcotic in another, with legal implications for importation requiring consideration. For example, codeine phosphate is considered a controlled drug in Greece and Australia, but is not so tightly regulated in the UK. This is another factor for consideration for teams bringing their own medicine supplies.

Safe sex

The pharmacy at Olympic and Commonwealth Games is traditionally the centre of safe sex campaigns for the athletes' village, which guarantees to always attract media attention. In Atlanta, posters and pamphlets in 17 languages were used to promote safe sex and 50 000 condoms in Olympic colours were distributed at the Polyclinic. In Sydney, 70 000 condoms were distributed, compared with 12 000 in Salt Lake City, and 130 000 in Athens. A record 150 000 condoms were available for distribution in Manchester to 5000 athletes, equating to 30 allocated for each athlete. 'Will they have enough energy left to actually compete?' was the *Mail on Sunday* headline during these Games. Athletes use the free issue to stock up and take them home with them.

In Manchester, information was available from the pharmacy about local community services such as family planning, sexual health and counselling services. The morning-after pill was on the pharmacy formulary but was rarely prescribed.

Pharmacist education

For the pharmacists and other healthcare professionals volunteering for Olympic and Commonwealth Games, it will often be their first experience of managing the treatment of elite athletes in such an environment. A number of training sessions are provided in the months before the Games to enable the volunteers to confidently assume this unique role.

In the Games environment, athletes rely heavily on the knowledge and advice of pharmacists in relation to drugs banned in sport. Pharmacists must be familiar with the list of prohibited substances, and the regulations for the provision of drugs that may have a restricted status. Pharmacists must also be aware of drugs that require notification to the Medical Commission before competition, such as beta-2 agonists and corticosteroids, in order to advise athletes appropriately. Training on the use of specialised computer dispensing programmes that are unique to the Polyclinic pharmacy is also necessary.

It is not only the pharmacists working in the athletes' village that are approached by athletes during the Games for information on treatment and doping issues. The athletes are free to explore the host city and may present to any local pharmacy or hospital outside the village. In

Manchester, an education programme was implemented for pharmacies outside the village likely to encounter athletes during the Games. An education pack containing the list of prohibited substances and information on abuse of drugs in sport was distributed to pharmacies in close proximity to the village, at the airport, and local hospitals.

Confidentiality and the media

The eyes of the world are focused on the athletes for the 2 weeks of an Olympic or Commonwealth Games and a medical or doping scandal can quickly make international headlines. Reporters may approach medical staff if there is news of a top athlete being injured. In sports medicine, as with all other branches of medicine, patient confidentiality must be observed. The right to privacy relating to medical advice or treatment received by an athlete must be respected.

The issue of patient confidentiality can present the healthcare professional with some difficult ethical decisions when dealing with elite athletes. For example, if a pharmacist knows that an athlete is taking a performance-enhancing drug for non-medical reasons, should they inform the sporting authorities?

Pharmacists have a duty of care to the athlete as an individual patient and must have the intention to protect or improve the athlete's health. Confidential medical information should never be disclosed unless there is a risk of death or serious harm to another person. However, pharmacists have the right to refuse treatment that may be harmful, or carry risks for the athlete. Patient confidentiality is an important factor in establishing the patient's trust, creating a situation where the pharmacist can offer counselling and advice on the safe and ethical use of drugs, in the best interests of the athlete's health.

In the Games environment, a pharmacist could be asked in confidence about a performance-enhancing drug an athlete is using, or they may recognise that an athlete's medication is prohibited. In this situation, patient confidentiality must be maintained and the pharmacist must provide the best duty of care to that individual. This may involve counselling the patient on the risks associated with drug abuse, advising on safe practices, or referring the athlete to appropriate help.

A unique opportunity

Being a pharmacist at international games provides a unique opportunity to be part of a medical team for the world's best athletes. This environment provides exposure to a wide range of sport-related conditions, encompassing both minor and acute conditions. It enables the pharmacist to work closely with a team of other international specialists to treat disease and injury.

Medical decisions in the environment of elite sport can be influenced by many factors, some of which are subject to difficult ethical issues uncommon in normal medicine. Sports medicine can provide challenges to treatment, particularly with respect to the tight regulations and restrictions on drug use in sport.

Further reading

Brennan R J, Keim M E, Sharp T W, *et al.* (1997). Medical and public health services at the 1996 Atlanta Olympic Games: an overview. *Med J Aust* 167: 595–598.

Clements A (2003). Medical support for the greatest show on earth. *Brit Travel Health Assoc J* 5: 52–54.

Eaton S B, Woodfin B A, Askew J L, *et al.* (1997). The Polyclinic at the 1996 Atlanta Olympic Village. *Med J Aust* 167: 599–602.

KSL Television & Radio Coverage (2002). Thousands treated for medical needs. http://2002.ksl.com/news-6801i.php?p=1 (accessed 25 July 2005).

New South Wales Health Department (2000) *NSW Health Services for the Sydney 2000 Olympic and Paralympic Games*. Sydney: NSW Health Department.

Stiel D, Trethowan P, Vance N (1997). Medical planning for the Sydney 2000 Olympic and Paralympic Games. *Med J Aust* 167: 593–594.

Stuart M, Skouroliakou M (2004). Pharmacy at the 2004 Olympic Games. *Pharm J* 273: 319.

Sydney Organising Committee for the Olympic Games, Olympic Co-ordinating Authority (2001). *Official Report of the XXVII Olympiad*. Sydney: SOCOG.

UK Sport (2002). *The XVII Commonwealth Games, Manchester, 2002. A Summary Report of Anti-Doping Operations*. London: UK Sport.

World Anti-doping Agency (2005a). *2005 List of Prohibited Substances*. http://www.wada-ama.org/rtecontent/document/list_2005.pdf (accessed 1 August 2005).

World Anti-doping Agency (2005b). *The 2005 Monitoring Program*. http://www.wada-ama.org/rtecontent/document/Monitoring_Program_2005.pdf (accessed 1 August 2005).

10

The role of the pharmacist in sport and exercise care

Steven B Kayne

Introduction

This chapter seeks to build on the knowledge gained by reading the rest of this book and to provide practical information to allow pharmacists to exploit the opportunities that exist in sport and exercise medicine. It is also meant to offer a summary of what has gone before. Inevitably some material will be repeated briefly for convenience but original chapter references are given.

The disciplines involved in sport and exercise pharmacy are essentially extensions of a pharmacist's current activities as providers of health care, including:

- a public health role in promoting and maintaining good health
- offering a proactive medicines management service
- provision of first aid to treat a range of minor injuries
- provision of treatment and advice on minor ailments
- giving advice on specialised health matters
- providing items for sale.

Reason for sporting activity

Considering the reason for individuals taking part in sports activities can often help with an assessment of the likely severity of the condition and the urgency with which an individual will seek treatment.

Competitive sport

George Orwell is reputed to have said:

> Serious sport has nothing to do with fair play. It is bound up with hatred, jealousy, boastfulness, disregard of all rules and sadistic pleasures in witnessing violence; in other words, it is war minus the shooting.

Individuals whose sole aim is to improve their overall fitness should be advised to approach competitive sport with extreme caution! The additional psychological pressures of competition can significantly alter one's attitude. Most problems in this sector are dealt with by club medical staff or sports injury clinics. There may be a number of ethical considerations associated with providing assistance to elite athletes (see Chapter 5).

Health

Appropriate regular exercise will help an individual enjoy enhanced well-being and encourage recovery from a medical condition. A specially designed 'exercise prescription' will emphasise the necessary elements of activity. Accidents caused by over-exuberance will usually be referred to a GP but clients may present in the pharmacy with simple sprains and strains or allergies (see Chapter 2).

Recreational sport

This is the enjoyment of sport for social aspects or for some gentle exercise to fill leisure time. People in this group are most likely to consult their local pharmacist for advice on injuries and illnesses.

The enthusiastic spectator

Here there is no intentional involvement in sport – other than enthusiastic support for other participants. Injuries due to over-exuberant behaviour or the effects of drinking alcohol to excess may lead to a consultation with a pharmacist.

Promoting and maintaining a healthy lifestyle through exercise

Physical activity is sometimes called 'habitual sports activity' (HSA), particularly when it forms an important part of people's leisure activities. Sport and exercise, both structured activities, are often considered as two subcategories of HSA, and are ideal for those who are otherwise unable to achieve the desired levels of activity in their working life. Department of Employment surveys have shown that the average annual holiday entitlement for most full-time employees has doubled over the last 25 years, from 2 to 4 or more weeks, and the average number of hours in a basic working week has dropped from 43 to around 35 hours. There is therefore more leisure time available for a greater number of people than ever before. More campaigns are required to bring to the attention of individuals the need to devote some of this time to regular physical activity.

Despite the considerable health benefits from activity that were discussed in Chapter 2, for many people participation in sport or exercise is a daunting prospect, even if they have already been convinced that it will be beneficial to their health. They may fear that exercising will be uncomfortable or painful, or they may worry about potential injuries. Many of those who have not played any sport since school are likely to be extremely lacking in confidence or too embarrassed to learn or 'relearn' a new skill. Lack of time is an important factor in many people's lifestyles, and it may be necessary to reorganise other activities.

The pharmacist can, where necessary, emphasise that it is not necessary to run marathons to become fit, and explain the overload principle of training (i.e. it is only necessary to regularly increase physical activity above usual levels for a minimum of 20 minutes three times a week). The pharmacist can also suggest, for those who wish to learn a sport, that perhaps the best way is to join a beginner's class, so that everyone will be at a similar level of playing skill, and possibly fitness. The social advantages of participating in a sport, particularly if it involves membership of a sports club, could also be stressed. People's goals and capabilities vary enormously, and the pharmacist's initial function is to assess what these are.

There are many different ways of exercising and the pharmacist could find out what local facilities are available through the local council offices, adult education centres or private clubs, and pass the information on to those interested.

Not everyone has the time or the inclination to take up a sport, and some people may prefer solitary exercise rather than group exercising. One of the most popular, convenient and least obtrusive ways of exercising is walking (see Chapter 2).

As long as the pace is brisk and faster than normal walking pace, and forms a regular part of an individual's normal routine, there will be a training effect. The most enjoyable way is to specifically 'go for a walk', particularly in areas of interesting scenery. For those truly pressed for time, there are ample opportunities throughout the course of a normal day's work to 'walk rather than ride'. Stair-climbing instead of using a lift or walking short distances instead of taking a car, bus or train is of great benefit; the extra time taken is probably negligible compared to the time wasted in rush-hour traffic or waiting for public transport.

There is the additional benefit of boosting the body's levels of vitamin D by carrying out physical activities outdoors. Activities such as bowling offer gentle exercise and a social environment for older people.

Medicines management

Prescribing prohibited substances

It is necessary for athletes to be aware that a banned substance remains banned even when prescribed by a physician for a justifiable medical purpose, unless a TUE has been granted (see also Chapters 8 and 9). There may be instances where a patient has not told a prescriber that he or she intends to participate in a registered sporting event, and turns instead for advice to the pharmacist dispensing the prescription.

A TUE may be either abbreviated or standard. An abbreviated TUE applies to the following prohibited substances and permitted routes of administration only and is usually granted by the sport's governing body, on receipt of a form signed by the athlete's physician:

- Beta-2 agonists (formoterol, salbutamol, salmeterol and terbutaline) administered by inhaler only to prevent and/or treat asthma and exercise-induced asthma/bronchoconstriction.
- Glucocorticosteroids administered by non-systemic routes such as local and intra-articular injections, topical (other than dermatological preparations), anal, aural, ophthalmic and inhalation.

A standard TUE requires comprehensive supporting documentation to support the use of any other prohibited substance. This would include a medical history, examinations, laboratory investigations, imaging studies, and copies of original reports and/or letters. The application may be considered by a panel of physicians.

Because sports organisations have varying policies, athletes must consult the current list of banned substances and make sure a banned drug is not prescribed. In addition there may be further restrictions imposed by other national or international organisations, and some sport-specific restrictions. For example, beta-blockers are prohibited in competition in bridge, chess and curling and both in and out of competition in archery and shooting. Permitted levels of alcohol in the blood vary from zero (motorcycling) to 0.2 g/L (billiards).

The problems that can occur when an athlete does not follow the appropriate procedures for obtaining a TUE are outlined in Chapter 9. Further information on the TUE scheme may be found at http://www.wada-ama.org/rtecontent/document/TUE_ENG_QA.pdf

Care must be exercised when prescribing antihistamines if they are contained in multi-ingredient preparations, because they may be combined with stimulants such as ephedrine. Propecia, a product used to combat hair loss, contains finasteride, a substance that is banned as a masking agent.

Adverse effects

It may be necessary to advise on the effects of any medication on performance or ability to partake in sports or strenuous exercise programmes. Some drugs (e.g. morphine) depress the rate of respiration, which ultimately slows down the rate of gaseous exchange between the alveoli and the blood. Alterations in fluid and electrolyte balance affect the plasma concentrations of some drugs (e.g. lithium), and toxic effects may arise if the patient becomes dehydrated during intense exercise. Studies have shown increased absorption of medication from transdermal delivery systems (e.g. glyceryl trinitrate patches) during hard physical activity, which may be related to an increase in cutaneous blood flow and increased skin temperature. The so-called muscle-building herbs (e.g. yohimbine) can raise blood pressure, bowel evacuation, sweating and coughing.

Potential interactions between herbal supplements and prescribed and OTC medication should be considered (see also Chapter 6).

Treating a range of sport- and exercise-related injuries in the pharmacy

Advice to participants on reducing the risk of injury

Attention to many of these factors may reduce the risk of injuries to a large extent (see also Chapters 2 and 4). Injuries may result from intrinsic or extrinsic risks, which are summarised in Table 10.1. Judicious questioning may identify risks that can be minimised to prevent similar injuries occurring again.

Common injuries sustained during sport and exercise

The most common injuries arising during sports or exercise for which clients may seek assistance include those listed in Table 10.2, all of which have been covered in detail in Chapters 4 and 5.

The type of injury occurring during sport and exercise generally

Table 10.1 Examples of risk factors for sports and exercise injuries

Intrinsic or personal risks

Age	Affects ability to pursue exercise to varying intensity.
Anatomy	Body shape and size. Misalignment of feet and/or legs or other parts of the body.
Disabilities	Presence of debilitating disease – diabetes. Handicap.
Fitness	Insufficient aerobic capacity, strength and flexibility.
Existing weaknesses	Insufficient rehabilitation from previous injury (sprains and strains); arthritis, old fracture etc.

Extrinsic or environmental risks

Climatic conditions	Temperature and altitude.
Equipment	Inappropriate for surface (grass, synthetic, wood, etc.); ill fitting, poor quality, or poorly maintained.
Training programme	Inappropriate duration, frequency and intensity.
Training surface	Hard, irregular contours, sloping, etc.

Table 10.2 Common injuries arising from sports and exercise

Trauma
Abrasions and lacerations
Bruises
Dislocation
Fractures
Ligament injuries (sprains)
Muscle injuries (strains)
Tendon injuries

Over-use syndromes
Bursae injuries
Inflammation of muscles
Inflammation of tendon and attachments
Joint problems
Stress fractures

Miscellaneous
Blisters
Burns – friction
Cramp
Delayed onset muscle soreness (DOMS)

varies with the type of activity being undertaken. Trauma is more likely to occur during combat or contact sports (e.g. boxing, judo or rugby), whereas over-use injuries are more commonly a feature of sports involving repetitive movements (e.g. golf or tennis).

Providing advice to people with existing medical conditions involved in sport and exercise

Patients suffering from anaemia, chronic disorders of the cardiovascular, renal or respiratory systems, metabolic disorders or thyroid disorders should be advised to consult their GP for a full examination before undertaking any exercise programme. It is generally considered that exercise is contraindicated in such disorders until the condition has been brought under control. Medical assessment is also advised for patients recovering from acute conditions, and in those with hypertension or musculoskeletal disorders.

Asthma

Asthma attacks occur in almost 90% of people who have chronic asthma and in 40% of individuals who have allergic rhinitis or atopic dermatitis (Feinstein *et al.*, 1996). Breathlessness and wheezing characteristically occur after exercise, or may arise a few minutes into continuous exercise. Known precipitating factors should be avoided, and prophylactic therapy administered. Treatment options for asthma include non-pharmacological measures that address the exercise environment and warm-up routines, as well as drugs. Four beta-2 agonists are permitted by inhalation only to prevent and/or treat asthma and exercise-induced asthma/bronchoconstriction (see above) with an abbreviated TUE.

Sodium cromoglicate and nedocromil are also allowed for the treatment of asthma but isoprenaline is banned.

Cardiac defects

Sport and exercise may uncover cardiac defects or disease (see Chapter 2). Cardiac disorders (e.g. ischaemic heart disease, myocardial disease and valvular heart disease) reduce the cardiac reserve of the heart. Faulty valves (either as a result of incompetence or stenosis) increase the workload of the heart muscle under normal conditions, and exercising causes further increases. A person with valvular heart disease is therefore unable to cope with the same level of physical activity as someone with a normal heart. Chronic myocarditis may lead to cardiomyopathy and possibly cause sudden death during exercise. However, a controlled and supervised exercise programme may be of benefit in preventing further cardiac damage following myocardial infarction.

Diabetes

Exercise may precipitate hypoglycaemia in type I diabetes mellitus, and it can occur up to several hours after physical activity unless preventive measures are taken. A patient should be medically assessed before undertaking a programme of sport or exercise. It may be necessary to reduce the insulin dose before anticipated exercise and to inject at a site not being exercised (to minimise the increase in absorption that occurs from exercising muscles, presumably as a result of increased blood flow). Doses should not be administered less than 1 hour before exercise. Some diabetics, especially those with low body weight, may need to ingest carbohydrate before exercising and during prolonged sessions, and a meal should always be taken within 3 hours of completing the activity. It may be helpful for those who wish to regularly undertake vigorous exercise to monitor their blood-glucose concentrations before, during and after exercise, in order to assess their personal response to physical activity and to allow reasonably accurate predictions of future requirements to be made.

All insulin-dependent diabetics involved in competitive sport are required to apply for a standard TUE.

Type II diabetics on diet therapy alone do not generally experience problems related to altered blood-glucose concentrations, and need only observe the same precautions related to taking up exercise as the general population. However, those on oral antidiabetic agents may experience hypoglycaemia during prolonged physical activity, and should first seek medical advice.

With proliferative retinopathy, a common complication of the disease, exercise may result in retinal or vitreous haemorrhage (Horton, 1991). Strenuous exercise can lead to soft tissue or joint injuries in persons with peripheral neuropathy (Bell, 1992). Unnoticed injuries from ill-fitting footwear may also cause concern in diabetic patients.

Exercise has, however, been shown to be beneficial in both types of diabetes mellitus and should be encouraged. Vertigo during exercise may simply be related to stress or it may be indicative of a serious disorder (e.g. iron-deficiency anaemia or cardiac disease), particularly if it occurs on changes in posture. Exercise is contraindicated until medical investigations have been carried out.

Diabetes UK provides a number of information leaflets on physical activity (see end of chapter for web address).

Epilepsy

In the past patients suffering from epilepsy were advised against certain forms of exercise. Depending on the frequency and severity of seizures and with sensible precautions (e.g. making a lifeguard aware of the possibility of a seizure before swimming), it is now acknowledged that stable individuals can exercise effectively and become involved in sport.

There are a number of epilepsy triggers that can precipitate a seizure minutes or hours after exercise if the body is unnecessarily strained. Exercise-related risk factors could include:

- extreme fatigue
- lack of sleep
- dehydration
- electrolyte loss (because of severe dehydration)
- hyperthermia (elevated body temperature)
- hypoglycaemia (low blood sugar levels).

Advice that may be given to avoid exercise-related epilepsy triggers include:

- Drink plenty of water before, during and after exercise.
- Don't push yourself to the point of physical exhaustion.
- If you are feeling very hot and tired, slow down or stop.
- Make sure you have at least two rest days every week.
- Make sure your diet is nutritionally adequate.
- Get plenty of rest and good-quality sleep.
- Take all steps to avoid head injuries.
- Don't abuse alcohol.
- Make sure you take your medication according to your doctor's directions.

Infection

Exercising is also contraindicated during infections, particularly viral infections, because there is often an associated risk of myocarditis. The extra workload placed on the inflamed heart results in reduced exercise tolerance, characterised by breathlessness and fatigue, and can be responsible for sudden death during exercise. Exercise may also prolong convalescence and increase the incidence of post-viral depression (e.g. after 'flu or Epstein–Barr virus infection). Patients should not resume exercising until fully recovered.

Ostomy patients

Sympathetic community pharmacists may be approached by ostomy patients for help or advice on sports participation. To facilitate swimming it may be necessary for the prescriber to change the dimensions of appliances and/or supply seals with enhanced waterproof characteristics. Appropriate swimwear may be purchased from several sources.

Some contact sports are also possible with the help of a belt to secure the bag firmly. However, contact sports can be dangerous and having extra concerns about whether the stoma may be damaged or the ostomy bag ripped off or punctured, does not help the sportsman's peace of mind. Advice to watch for the effects of dehydration would be appropriate and any OTC medicines required should be supplied in liquid or crushable tablet form. Hollister produce an excellent leaflet on sport and fitness for ostomy patients.

Respiratory conditions

Exercise tolerance is reduced in those with respiratory problems, e.g. obstructive airways disease, because more work is required to force air through constricted passages. Also, any disorder that increases the dead space of the lungs reduces the efficiency of respiration. Fluid accumulates in the air spaces of the lungs in pulmonary infections, reducing the efficiency of gaseous exchange. Emphysema results in reduced elasticity of the alveoli, which lowers the amount of air expelled. Some diseases (e.g. bronchitis and emphysema) influence the distribution of blood to different parts of the lungs, which reduces exercise tolerance because alveolar gaseous exchange is dependent on adequate perfusion. Similarly, exchange can only take place across healthy alveolar walls, and any disease that affects the lining (e.g. emphysema, pulmonary fibrosis or viral infections) reduces the efficiency of respiration. Carbon dioxide diffuses into the alveoli faster than oxygen diffuses into the blood, so the primary effect of impaired gaseous exchange is reduced oxygenation of the blood rather than an increase in the blood-carbon dioxide concentration. Exercises may, however, be beneficial in the management of obstructive airways disease but full medical supervision is necessary.

Treating a range of sport- and exercise-related ailments

A pharmacist presented with a request for advice by an athlete for the treatment of a minor ailment should check the relevant list of banned substances issued by the WADA before counter-prescribing (see Chapter 8). As with prescription medication, competitors have a responsibility to make themselves fully aware of all regulations governing a specific event and present the information to the pharmacist before purchasing medicines or having a prescription dispensed.

The following brief review of common conditions presented by sports persons will give an indication as to the items that should be stocked in a sports section in the pharmacy (see below).

Allergic rhinitis or hay fever

This may be caused by contact with grasses or pollens in spring or early summer and may lead to allergic conjunctivitis. Antihistamines that cause little or no drowsiness are preferable, so that athletic performance is preserved as far as possible. OTC products to treat hay fever may contain corticosteroids and a TUE certificate is necessary before they can be used.

- **Allowed** – antihistamines, nasal sprays containing a corticosteroid (see above) or xylometazoline, eye drops containing sodium cromoglicate.
- **Banned** – products containing ephedrine or pseudoephedrine.

Exercise-induced asthma

Exercise-induced asthma (EIA) is one of the most common conditions among active children, adolescents and young adults (Kaplan, 1995). EIA can impede physical activity; common symptoms are fatigue and poorer performance than training would predict. The condition usually peaks about 5–10 minutes after exercise and abates after 30–60 minutes. The severity of the attack is related to the intensity of exercise, but further exercise 2–4 hours later (the refractory period) fails to elicit the same intensity of response. This property is made use of by some asthmatic athletes, who induce asthma some time before an event. EIA does not necessarily occur every time a susceptible individual exercises, but may be precipitated by specific factors. Cold, dry conditions are more likely to induce an attack than a warm, moist atmosphere, and it is noteworthy that swimming is less likely to induce asthma than running. EIA may also be related to stress or the presence of certain allergens (e.g. pollens) in the air.

- **Allowed** – formoterol, salbutamol, salmeterol and terbutaline inhalers (subject to abbreviated TUE; see above).

- **Banned** – products containing sympathomimetics (e.g. ephedrine, fenoterol, isoprenaline).

Vitamin C has also been studied in the context of EIA (Cohen *et al.*, 1997). Despite using very large doses, studies showed variable protection; a minority of patients were partially protected.

Coughs and colds

The important issue here is that coughs and colds cannot be treated with any product containing sympathomimetics.

- **Allowed** – all antibiotics, steam and menthol inhalers, cough mixtures containing antihistamines, codeine, pholcodine, guaifenesin, dextromethorphan.
- **Banned** – products containing sympathomimetics (e.g. ephedrine).

Diarrhoea

The strict routine observed in training schedules may be upset by bouts of diarrhoea caused by sudden changes in eating habits. Diarrhoea can also be brought on by anxiety and stress, in which case CAM might offer a remedy (see Chapter 6). Oral rehydration therapy with a suitable antidiarrhoeal should cure the problem. Hyoscine may be used as a gastrointestinal antispasmodic and as an antiemetic.

- **Allowed** – diphenoxylate, loperamide, products containing electrolytes (e.g. Dioralyte or Rehidrat).
- **Banned** – products containing opioids (e.g. morphine).

Skin conditions

Topical corticosteroids are permitted for the treatment of skin conditions but there are partial restrictions imposed on the use of other corticosteroid formulations (see Chapter 8).

Common fungal infections include athlete's foot (*Tinea pedis*), ringworm of the body (*Tinea corporis*) and ringworm of the groin (*Tinea cruris*). The latter, popularly known as 'jock itch', starts on one side of the groin and may spread to the other side, then to the buttocks, thighs and abdomen.

For patients with a dry rash a broad-spectrum antifungal cream will help, while if the skin is moist and painful a powder might be better.

Sprays and paints are also available. Patients should be given clear instructions on how to manage the condition.

Head lice (*Pediculosis capitis*) can be a problem; they are spread by direct contact with hair and in the sports environment possibly by combs, brushes and by sharing protective headgear.

Verrucae are caused by a virus that penetrates moist skin and are most commonly found on the soles of the feet. They are caught from others by walking barefoot across changing rooms or showers. A range of OTC products is available.

Soft tissue injuries and pain

Occasional tension headaches resulting from stress may be treated with analgesics but it is important to obtain a full history before counter-prescribing to exclude the possibility of a more serious condition.

- **Allowed** – aspirin, codeine, dihydrocodeine, ibuprofen, paracetamol, all NSAIDs (see chapter 5).
- **Banned** – products containing opioids (e.g. dextropropoxyphene) (see Chapter 8).

Vomiting

Vomiting may be treated with domperidone and metoclopramide.

Advice on contracting disease

Two conditions on which advice is sought are HIV-AIDS and hepatitis.

HIV-AIDS and sport

According to the World Health Organization consensus statement on AIDS and sport, no evidence exists for a risk of transmission of HIV virus when any affected persons do not have bleeding wounds or other skin lesions, and there is no documentary evidence of HIV being acquired through participation in sport. However, if a lesion is observed or a bleeding wound occurs in any participant, it is prudent for attention to be given immediately. The area should be cleansed with disinfectant and securely covered. HIV is not believed to be transmitted through sweat, urine, respiratory droplets, swimming bath water or toilets. The possibility of injecting steroid abusers acquiring HIV through injecting practices has given cause for concern. This has implications for pharmacists through needle exchange schemes.

Hepatitis

Many sporting authorities strongly recommend that all sports participants playing under adult rules in high-level competition and personnel working in team areas be vaccinated against hepatitis B and that any blood spills be swabbed with suitable antiseptics.

Advice during pregnancy

Exercise during pregnancy may pose some risks for the mother or foetus, although if carried out sensibly and in moderation, has been shown to be of benefit (see Chapter 2). A pregnant woman should seek medical advice to assess whether or not it is safe for her to exercise. Absolute contraindications include any factors that predispose to prematurity (e.g. incompetent cervix, more than one fetus, or a history of premature labour), or any factors that cause decreased oxygenation of the uterus or placenta (e.g. pregnancy-induced hypertension or smoking). Relative contraindications should be assessed on an individual basis, taking into account all other factors present, and include anaemia, arrhythmias, diabetes mellitus, essential hypertension, thyroid disorders or extremes of weight. Vigorous exercise by pregnant women has been seen to produce fetal bradycardia and should therefore be avoided. Hyperthermia may have an adverse effect on the fetus and pregnant women should avoid exercising to such a level or in conditions that significantly raise the core temperature. For the same reason, post-exercise saunas or hot baths are not recommended.

Advice to the elderly

The decline in physical fitness with aging was once considered to be resistant to change. Hollman stated that commencement of exercise in a person unaccustomed to sport caused slight effects of adaptation after age 40 but practically no change after 60 (Hollman, 1995). However opinion now favours the view that at least 50% of such observations may be due to disuse atrophy (Smith, 1995). The potential of exercise as an intervention for maintaining functional capacity in the elderly has now been established.

Disadvantages of exercise in the elderly include symptoms caused by over-exertion or inappropriate types of exercise (e.g. loadbearing, non-loadbearing, aerobic or anaerobic). Existing medical conditions such as those outlined above may be exacerbated by over-enthusiastic activity.

Advice on doping

The opportunity to impress on youngsters proactively the dangers and futility of attempting to improve performance by taking drugs should not be missed.

The status in sport of any UK-licensed medication may be checked by logging on to UK Sport's Drug Information Database (DID) at http://www.uksport.gov.uk/did or by e-mailing drug-free@uksport.gov.uk. By entering the substance name, the athlete will be informed whether a substance is permitted or prohibited in or out of competition. This should be done well before competition so alternative therapeutic strategies may be chosen before the event.

The DID is the most comprehensive and up-to-date drug information service available to athletes anywhere in the world. In the UK enquiries may also be made by phone (+44 (0)800 528 0004; responses given within 24 hours Monday to Friday). A card giving advice on drug-free sport may be accessed at http://www.uksport.gov.uk/images/uploaded/AdviceCardJano5.pdf – the information included on the card is frequently updated and is also included in the *BNF*.

Advice on needle exchange schemes

Needle exchange schemes were set up primarily for opiate abusers, but now include all drug misusers. Sports injectors generally use short narrow-gauge needles.

Advice on where to get further specialist help

For those who may have difficulties coping with sport and exercise (e.g. the elderly, or physically or mentally handicapped), specialist help is available from various organisations. The pharmacist can help by passing such information on and by displaying some of the many leaflets available from such organisations.

Sale of sports equipment

There is an extensive range of items that may be requested within a sports and exercise context. Obviously it is impractical for the average community pharmacist to keep anything more than a selection of items. The following will help in deciding what stock to assemble.

Bandages

Types of product available

There are two main groups of bandages: the non-extensible and the extensible:

- **Non-extensible bandages:** These are the traditional 'fixed' or unyielding bandages formerly manufactured from materials like linen, flannel and calico. The latter still exist as triangular bandages used for arm slings. The most widely used dressing of this type is the white open weave (or WOW) bandage, made from loosely woven cotton, or cotton and viscose. Although largely superseded by extensible bandages, they do still have a wide range of applications, including covering superficial skin abrasions.
- **Extensible bandages:** This group contains by far the greater number of the two types of bandages. It includes compression bandages, retention bandages and support bandages.

Compression bandages (Table 10.3) are an important element of the Rest-ice-compression-elevation (RICE) regime for soft tissue injuries (see Chapter 4). In the treatment of oedema, it is possible to limit the loss of fluid from the capillaries to the surrounding tissue by the application of

Table 10.3 Examples of high compression bandages

Trade name	Manufacturer	Compression	Material
Blue line Elastic web	Various	Very high	Heavy cotton, rubber, rayon
Red line Elastic web	Various	Very high	Heavy cotton, rubber
Elastoweb	S&N	Very high	Heavy cotton, rubber
Setopress	Seton	High	Polyamide, elastane, cotton
Tensopress	S&N	High	Viscose, elastane, cotton
Varico	Seton	Very high	Elastic web with foot loop

a surface pressure of 15–20 mmHg without increasing vascular resistance and reducing blood flow. The consequences of inappropriate or excessive pressure can be severe, involving skin necrosis and, in extreme circumstances, even amputation (Callum *et al.*, 1987).

The effects of different levels of compression have been studied widely and has resulted in a range of hosiery to accommodate different requirements. For many years the compression bandages available in the UK Drug Tariff were limited to a small number of heavy products such as Blue line and Red line webbing. Although these bandages can maintain high levels of pressure they are difficult to apply correctly and uncomfortable to wear. Bandages such as Setopress (Seton) and Tensopress (S&N) overcome these problems.

Retention (or securing) bandages are used to keep other dressings in the correct position but with the advantage over WOW in that they are lightweight and have the ability to conform to the injured area. The first bandages to be introduced were cotton conforming bandages BP, made from simple woven fabrics that were crimped mechanically or chemically to give a degree of extensibility. A range of new highly extensible bandages made by incorporating lightweight elastomeric yarns into the warp have recently been introduced to the market. There are also retention bandages of a stockinette type (e.g. Seton's highly conformable Tubifast, indicated for retaining and securing dressings), as well as the adhesive bandages that are mainly used for strapping purposes. Most of the retention bandages shown in Table 10.4 can also be used to give light support in the treatment of superficial sprains and strains.

Support bandages are designed to maintain retention and control of the tissue without compression. They are usually applied to an injured limb to contain swelling or the development of some deformity. The fabric needs to be rather firmer than the retention bandages described above and have a more limited extensibility. Non-extensible bandages can also be used for this purpose, but extensible bandages are easier to apply and more comfortable for the patient. For greater efficiency of support some bandages are coated with an adhesive to hold them in place. It is advisable to suggest to customers that if adhesive bandages are to be applied to hirsute ('hairy') limbs, the area should first be shaved to ensure less painful removal.

This group, examples of which are included in Table 10.5, contains bandages for both light support (sprains and strains) and for firm support (fractures). Most of the support bandages listed in Table 10.5 can also act as *light* compression bandages.

Table 10.4 Examples of Type 1 retention bandages and tubular bandages

Trade name	Manufacturer	Material
Bandages		
Crinx	S&N	Cotton conforming bandage
Easifix	S&N	Polyamide and cellulose contour bandage
K-Band	Parema	Knitted polyamide and cellulose contour bandage
Kling	J&J	Cotton conforming bandage
Slinky	Seton	Polyamide and cellulose contour bandage
Stayform	Robinson	Polyamide and cellulose contour bandage
Tubular		
Netelast	Seton	Elastic net tubular stockinette bandage
Tubifast	Seton	Lightweight tubular bandage
Tubiton	Seton	Viscose rayon and unbleached cotton tubular bandage
Tubegauze	Seton	Bleached cotton yarn tubular bandage
Vulkan Professional Pro	Vulcan	Grip stockinette

Table 10.5 Examples of support bandages

Trade name	Manufacturer	Material
Light support (sprains)		
Crepe bandages	Various	Cotton, wool
Elastocrepe	S&N	Cotton crepe bandage
Elastoplast	S&N	Elastic adhesive bandage
Flexocrepe	Robinson	Cotton crepe bandage
Flexoplast Bandage	Robinson	Elastic adhesive bandage
Lestreflex	Seton	Elastic, ventilated diachylon
Rediform	Salts	Elasticated tubular stockinette
Tensogrip	S&N	Elasticated tubular stockinette
Tubigrip	Seton	Elasticated tubular stockinette
Firm support (fractures)		
Gypsona	S&N	Plaster of Paris bandage
Varico	Seton	Elastic web bandage

Some examples of tubular bandages ('stockinettes') with support functions have also been included. Cotton heavyweight stockinette bandages are also used as a base for plaster of Paris and some other types of bandages. Suspensory bandages also perform a supporting function and are widely used by men in contact sports.

Support bandages are often used as retention bandages when a much cheaper alternative would be more appropriate. Examples of these products are shown in Figure 10.1.

Application of bandages

Training in the application of bandaging is vital if the correct amount of compression is to be achieved, especially with the more modern

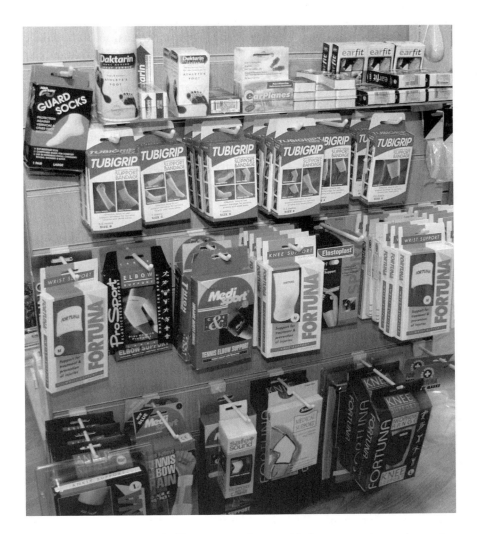

Figure 10.1 Display stand of footcare products and light compression and retention bandages.

bandages that will maintain pressure levels for extended periods. Companies like SSL International (Seton Healthcare 0161 652 2222) can provide educational material and videos to help with this. Bandages should be applied in the form of a spiral with a 50% overlap between turns, effectively producing a double layer of bandage at any point on the limb. The amount of pressure exerted depends very much on the operator's technique and can vary widely. Crepe support bandages are often used as light compression bandages, an application for which they were not designed. The degree of compression achieved is determined initially by the radius of curvature of the leg and the tension in the fabric during application. This means that initially a crepe bandage will provide the proper amount of compression if used correctly. However, the bandage does not have sufficient elasticity to accommodate all the changes in leg dimension during normal muscular activity. The pressure applied by the bandage will rise quickly, falling to zero when activity ceases and the muscles relax. This cyclical process will be repeated, and although the resulting 'pulses' of pressure may facilitate blood flow in the active individual, the bandages will be much less effective in inactive individuals. There is also a tendency for crepe bandages to work loose (Thomas, 1993).

As bandages have developed over the years they have become more specific and now often perform much more than just a passive function. Pharmacists can play an important part in advising on what is available and, just as importantly, how to use the products effectively.

Sports drinks

Chapter 3 covers the use of sports drinks as a source of energy; this chapter discusses formulation issues. The sport and energy drinks market is huge – approaching £1 bn annually in the UK. Advice on sports and energy drinks is frequently requested, particularly by athletes in non-elite and recreational groups who are confused by the range of products available.

The first energy drink launched in the UK in 1920 was Glucozade (later renamed Lucozade), a product designed to give supplementary glucose to sick children. A similar Scottish product known as Ferguzade disappeared from the market in the late 1970s.

Energy drinks now use caffeine, taurine, and in some cases, glucuronolactone to achieve a quick energy fix. All three of these exist naturally in foods but are present in much higher concentrations in energising drinks. The amount of caffeine in these drinks has been reviewed by the European Commission's Scientific Committee on Food (SCF) and declared safe for general consumption. However, the SCF found that children who consume two cans daily of such a drink may become irritable and anxious. An initial rush of carbohydrate may cause a subsequent fall in blood concentration below the original levels. The drinks are not recommended for pregnant women as the effect of caffeine on the fetus is still unknown. Examples include Lucozade Energy, Red Bull, Pure Power and Rhino's.

There are also ranges of energy bars in various flavours (e.g. Power Bar and High Five) and one-shot gel sachets (e.g. Clif Shot and Power Gel).

The first sports drink to be commercially available in the 1970s was Quaker's Gatorade. Much research has been conducted to determine the benefits of consuming fluid replacement beverages during exercise. The major components that can be manipulated to alter its functional properties are type and concentration of carbohydrate, electrolyte composition and concentration, palatability, osmolarity and other additives. Examples include Lucozade Sport (12 variants including powder and concentrate), isostar, High Five, and Boots Isotonic. PowerAde and Gatorade are used widely by elite athletes.

For exercise of less than 60 minutes, plain water is fine. For more prolonged efforts, sports drinks are claimed to be superior to water in replacing fluid losses (Gatorade website) especially as ingestion of plain water tends to diminish the desire to continue drinking. Athletes are likely to drink far more of a specially formulated palatable product that has additional beneficial functions than simply replacing fluid loss.

Fluid ingestion during exercise has two main functions:

- Supplying fluid to replace losses incurred by sweating and replacing the electrolytes lost in sweat.
- Providing a source of carbohydrate fuel to supplement the body's limited stores.

Choice of drink

The choice of drink formulation depends on five factors.

Type and concentration of carbohydrate The type of carbohydrate present in the drink does not appear to be critical; glucose, sucrose and oligosaccharides have all been used successfully. There may be some advantage to be gained from using glucose polymers (Sole and Noakes,

1989), for this should allow an increase in concentration without an accompanying increase in osmolarity, but there is some doubt as to whether this theoretical consideration occurs in practice (Hargreaves and Briggs, 1988). Fructose also appears to have theoretical advantages, providing a readily available source of substrate without stimulating insulin release and consequent inhibition of fatty acid mobilisation. In fact insulin production is suppressed during exercise, negating this argument. Comparisons between glucose and fructose ingested by fed subjects during exercise show that the rate of oxidation of fructose is less than that of glucose. Mixtures of sugars have also been suggested (e.g. glucose, sucrose and maltodextrin) as being effective in maximising absorption (Shi et al., 1995).

The substrate requirement will depend on the intensity and duration of exercise. While running low on substrate is likely to affect performance but is not usually life-threatening, fluid imbalance is potentially much more serious. Increasing carbohydrate content to make more fuel substrate available will tend to increase osmolarity (see below) and decrease the rate at which water can be made available to deal with dehydration. High sugar content may also cause gastrointestinal disturbances (Davis et al., 1988) and above a threshold limit it will not increase available substrate and reduce fatigue (Wagenmakers et al., 1993). Another disadvantage of high sugar content (and also low pH caused by citrus flavouring agents) is the risk of increased dental caries (Milosevic, 1997). Carbonated drinks contain 100–120 g/L sugar and are often associated with abdominal cramps and diarrhoea (Lamb and Brodowicz, 1986).

Maughan (1991) claims that even dilute glucose solution in the range of 40 g/L will slow the rate of gastric emptying; the highest rates of oral water replacement are said to be achieved with dilute solutions of glucose and sodium salts. Researchers suggest variations in the total hourly minimum dosage of carbohydrate capable of improving performance that range from 37 to 150 g.

In general, research has suggested that the correct concentration of carbohydrate in a drink is about 5–7%. Most commercial sports drinks fall within this range.

The American College of Sports Medicine recommend drinking 100–200 mL of fluids containing around 6% carbohydrate every 15–20 minutes during exercise.

Drinking larger amounts of fluid has been shown not to be beneficial in a South African study designed to replicate a 2-hour running race (Haley et al., 2000).

Presence of electrolytes   Sweat contains proportionally more water and less sodium than blood plasma. Exercise and heat exposure may cause an imbalance of electrolytes in the plasma, leading to a range of symptoms including lethargy, fatigue, headaches and nausea.

The ingestion of small amounts of sodium during exercise may help maintain and restore plasma volume during exercise and recovery and also helps to retain water in the extracellular space without causing thirst. Carbohydrate-electrolyte drinks are often referred to as being 'isotonic'.

Palatability   Beverage characteristics such as taste, aroma, tartness, mouthfeel and sweetness can all influence palatability and voluntary fluid consumption (see above). The addition of electrolytes (e.g. sodium compounds) may adversely affect taste but this can be mollified by replacing chlorides with other anions. Cool, pleasantly flavoured sweetened drinks are generally preferred (Hubbard *et al.*, 1984).

Osmolarity   The osmolarity of ingested drinks is important because it can affect gastric emptying and the passage of intestinal water, factors that affect the process of rehydration. Increased osmolarity of the gastric contents (by increasing carbohydrate or electrolyte content in a sports drink) will tend to delay emptying.

Other ingredients   Many commercially available sports drinks contain minerals and vitamins to increase the functionality of the product, but these are not thought to be necessary providing the athlete has a balanced diet. Some ergogenic materials (e.g. caffeine, glutamine) and herbs (ginkgo biloba, ginseng and kola nut) may also be present. The inclusion of glycerol together with water may lead to an increased total body water content.

Custom formulation

It is possible to obtain custom-made sports drinks if nothing on the market satisfies a client's requirements (see http://www.custom-sportsdrinks.com/index.html). Suitable formulae for making one's own drink are:

- **Isotonic** – 200 mL of orange squash (concentrated orange), 1 litre of water and a pinch of salt (1 g). Mix all the ingredients together and keep chilled.
- **Hypotonic** – 100 mL of orange squash (concentrated orange), 1 litre of water and a pinch of salt (1 g). Mix all the ingredients together and keep chilled.

- **Hypertonic** – 400 mL of orange squash (concentrated orange), 1 litre of water and a pinch of salt (1 g). Mix all the ingredients together and keep chilled.

First aid kits

Chapter 9 describes the contents of a professional medical kit used in international competition. Many low-key events will not have professional medical help available, and it will be the responsibility of the coach to administer first aid, followed by medical referral where necessary. A community pharmacist may be asked by local clubs for advice about items necessary to stock a first aid bag to facilitate the provision of on-site treatment at a sporting event.

Table 10.6 suggests items that may be included in a sports medical bag to cover the basic requirements of sports injury first aid.

Hot and cold packs

Hot and cold packs (see Figure 10. 2 for examples) are frequently used in soft tissue injuries and are components of a typical first aid kit.

Strapping and taping products

The type of taping technique and the choice of material used should depend on the treatment aim, the anatomical site to be strapped, the nature of the injury, and the size of the patient (see Chapter 4). This decision may often be based largely on custom, superstition and comfort (both physical and mental).

Athletic tape is manufactured in various sizes and textures and can be elastic or non-elastic. Elastic wraps and tape are available in varying widths, and wraps come in lengths to accommodate large body areas such as the hip and trunk. Some elastic bandages are self-adhesive. Non-stretch tape (i.e. Leukotape or Vulcan Meditape) is produced in varying tensile strengths. Where skin sensitivity or allergies to the tape are likely, underwrap is used for comfort and protection. A hypoallergenic tape (i.e. Strappal Zinc Oxide) is an alternative. Sprays and dressings can be used to help fix the strapping in place.

The following are examples of products associated with taping and strapping procedures (see also Chapter 4):

- **Adhesive spray** – used to firmly secure a tape job.
- **Chiropody felt** – this can be used to protect sensitive areas, or as a 'horseshoe' in a compression support for the ankle.

Table 10.6 Suggestions of items to include in a medical sports bag to administer basic first aid in the event of sports injury. Source: Kayne (2001)

Item	Purpose	Examples	Comments
Wound cleansing			
Disinfectants and cleansers	to cleanse and disinfect skin and wounds	Cetrimide Chlorhexidine Povidone-iodine Sodium chloride 0.9% (sterile solutions may also be used for eye irrigation)	Chlorinated solutions (e.g. dilute sodium hypochlorite solution) are no longer recommended for wound cleansing as they are considered too irritant
Swabs	to apply the disinfectants and cleansers	Gauze Swab BP Absorbent Cotton BP Absorbent Cotton Gauze BP	Absorbent cotton hospital quality should not be used for wound cleansing
Wound dressing			
Absorbents	to absorb wound exudate and provide protection	Absorbent Cotton BP Absorbent Lint BPC Calcium Alginate Dressings (Drug Tariff) Gauze and Cotton Tissue BP Perforated Film Absorbent Dressing BP	
Haemostatic dressings	to stop bleeding	Calcium Alginate Dressings (Drug Tariff)	
Tulle dressings	to apply to abrasions, burns and other skin injuries, usually beneath an absorbent dressing	Paraffin Gauze Dressing BP Chlorhexidine Gauze Dressing BP	

(Continued)

Table 10.6 (Continued)

Item	Purpose	Examples	Comments
Retention bandages	to hold dressings in place and to aid in the application of pressure to stop bleeding	Cotton Conforming Bandage BP Elastic Net Surgical Tubular Stockinette (Drug Tariff) Elasticated Tubular Bandage BP Open-wove Bandage BP	
Standard dressings	comprises an absorbent pad and retention bandage in one complete sterile dressing, used for wounds that are bleeding severely	Triangular Calico Bandage BP	May also be used as a sling A selection of sizes is recommended, including an eye pad
Adhesive dressings ('plasters')	an absorbent pad (which may be medicated) surrounded partly or completely by a piece of extension plaster, used to cover minor wounds	Elastic Adhesive Dressing BP Semipermeable Waterproof Plastic Wound Dressing BP	
Surgical adhesive tape	to secure dressings	Elastic Surgical Adhesive Tape BP Permeable Non-woven Surgical Synthetic Adhesive Tape BP Zinc Oxide Surgical Adhesive Tape BP	May also be used as a skin closure for for small incision wounds May also be used to immobilise small areas

Table 10.6 (Continued)

Item	Purpose	Examples	Comments
Management of soft-tissue injurie			
Cooling aids	to reduce the blood-flow in soft-tissue injuries and minimise further damage and swelling	Ice Ice-packs Cooling sachets	
Compression bandages	to provide pressure to reduce the flow of blood and inflammatory exudate	Cotton Crepe Bandage BP Crepe Bandage BP Elastic Adhesive Bandage BP	
Support bandages	to provide support for an injured area during active movement	Cotton Crepe Bandage BP Crepe Bandage BP Elasticated Tubular Bandage BP Open-wove Bandage BP	Provides light support only
Miscellaneous			
Wide-necked thermos flask or insulated bag	to carry ice or ice-packs		
Bucket, sponge and towel	for general cleaning purposes		
Scissors, safety pins and forceps	to cut up dressings and for general surgical use		

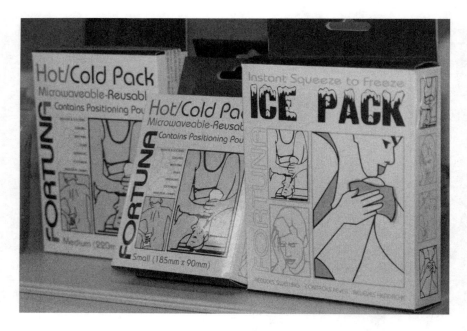

Figure 10.2 Examples of hot and cold packs.

- **Cohesive strapping** – as the name suggests, this strapping sticks to itself, which is practical because no underwrap (see below) is required.
- **Elastic adhesive bandages** – adhere to body contours and their elastic properties mean that they can 'give' a little with tissue changes.
- **Underwrap** – a thin foam material applied before the tape on sensitive areas.
- **Zinc oxide tape** – this material doesn't 'give' and is therefore ideal to provide restraint and reinforcement.

Examples of strapping products are given in Table 10.7. Items such as adhesive remover, bandage scissors and tape cutters are appropriate additions to the above list.

Nutritional supplements

A complete list of nutritional supplements was provided in Chapter 3. The following list summarises some OTC products that are particularly popular with bodybuilders and may not be familiar to pharmacists. It

Table 10.7 Products associated with strapping

Product	Manufacturers (range of product widths)
Elastic adhesive bandage	Smith & Nephew Elastoplast Henry Schein Vulkan Cohesive (washable)
Non-stretch tape: high tensile strength, ideal for immobilising joints	Strappal Zinc Oxide: hypoallergenic (1.25–5 cm) Leukoplast Zinc Oxide: water repellent (1.25–5 cm) Leukotape (2–5 cm) Vulkan Meditape Pro Zinc Oxide Leukotape P: flesh coloured Vulkan Professional P Tape: flesh coloured
Lightweight tapes	Vulkan Meditape Zinc Oxide (1.25–5 cm) Vulkan Medilastic E.A.B. (2.5–7.5 cm) Vulkan Professional Fixation tape Vulkan Medilite E.A.B. (2.5–7.5 cm)
Air and water permeable tapes	Leukopor – hypoallergenic BSN Hypafix (2.5–10 cm)
Associated products	Underwrap (comfort) Smith & Nephew Tensospray (adhesion) Leukotape Removal

should be noted that this market is not confined solely to athletes; security officers, club 'bouncers' and young men wishing to enhance their image also supplement their diet. There are many other products available, as a search on the Internet will reveal. Figure 10.3 shows a gondola in a Scottish pharmacy displaying nutritional supplements and sports drinks.

Amino acid tablets

Amino acids are the building blocks that make up protein. It was suggested that taking amino acids directly would be more efficient than digesting protein. Amino acid tablets are less popular today than when they first appeared, but are still widely available.

Carbohydrate supplements

There are numerous carbohydrate supplements available on the market. They are usually taken with milk or water (see Chapter 3).

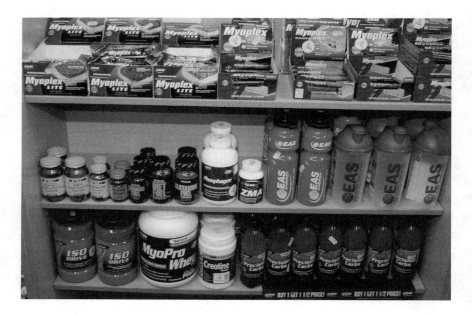

Figure 10.3 Display of food and drink supplements in a pharmacy.

Creatine

Creatine monohydrate, the supplement form of creatine, is one of the most talked-about sports supplements of the last few years. It is a white, flavourless and odourless powder and is a combination of three amino acids – arginine, glycine and methionine. It can also be found in high quantities in some foods (tuna, herring and beef), although not high enough to be considered a method of supplementation (see also Chapters 1 and 3).

Essential fatty acids (EFAs)

Omega 6 and Omega 3 are two essential fatty acids that are needed for many bodily functions and processes and are considered to be an important element of the diet because they are not produced in the body. Major sources of Omega 6 EFAs are food oils such as sunflower and corn oil, and sources of Omega 3 EFAs are fish oils and flax seed oil.

The latter is popular amongst athletes as a supplement as it is thought to shorten recovery time for fatigued muscles after exertion and increase the body's production of energy. The dietary essential fatty acids common to flax seed oil are converted by the body to prostaglandins which are important for regulating steroid production and hormone synthesis.

Fat loss 'stacks'

Especially popular around summer time, fat loss supplements are designed to accelerate fat loss when dieting and work by increasing metabolism. They are usually in capsule form, taken 3–4 times a day. Many of these fat loss supplements are based around ephedrine, caffeine, asprin or their herbal equivalents. People with existing heart problems should be careful of such supplements. Some of the latest stacks raise your metabolism but not via your heart, thereby making them a safer alternative.

HMB (beta-hydroxy beta-methylbutyrate)

HMB is a metabolite of the branched chain amino acid leucine. It is not a steroid or a drug and can be found in many foods (vegetables and meat). It is also manufactured by the body. HMB appears to increase the body's ability to build muscle and burn fat and is claimed to have a positive effect on protein metabolism.

L-Glutamine

Glutamine is a non-essential amino acid with a unique structure and is taken for several reasons including an ability to increase protein synthesis, which in basic terms means the ability to build muscle. It spares muscle tissue.

Meal replacement powders (MRPs)

Very similar to weight-gaining powders, but have greater nutritional value via additional vitamins and minerals. A number of companies have started supplying MRPs in sachets or small packets. While these offer convenience over larger tubs, they are often more expensive, and so choice depends on an individual's priorities.

Multivitamin and mineral tablets

Athletes who restrict their dietary intake may be at risk of an inadequate supply of vitamins or minerals (see Chapter 3). This may occur in sports requiring weight loss or strict weight maintenance. It may also occur if eating patterns are disrupted for example during extended travel or a busy competition schedule. Although there is no evidence that supplementation of an existing health diet enhances performance the perception is often that it does and many athletes take vitamins and minerals regularly.

Prohormones

Prohormones are precursors to testosterone. In simple terms, they are the closest legal sports supplement to anabolic steroids and large gains can be obtained from them. There are many different types of prohormones, but they are not recommended as supplements for beginners.

Protein powders

One of the most popular products taken to build muscle mass is protein powder, usually mixed with milk or water. The drink has a high protein content and is relatively low in fat and carbohydrate. Protein drinks are often used for convenience – some people find it easier and less filling to drink it rather than eat it. Various types of protein powder are available including egg protein, soy protein, milk protein and whey protein. Whey protein is claimed to be one of the best sources of quality protein. Protein drinks are usually available in a variety of flavours.

Protein bars have become popular over the last couple of years. These are snack bars (often coated lightly in chocolate) that are high in protein. Most protein bars also have quite a high sugar/carbohydrate content but a variety of low-carb bars have slowly begun to appear on the market.

Ribose

Ribose is a carbohydrate used by the body to produce energy. Still relatively new, ribose has yet to prove itself as a valuable supplement in the long term.

Vitamin C (ascorbic acid)

Taking vitamin C in doses of 1000 mg per day may reduce the secretion of cortisol, allowing muscles to grow and keeping testosterone levels high, helping the body keep up that level of performance.

Vitamin C is not stored appreciably in the body and excess amounts are eliminated rapidly through the urine. It is therefore usually suggested that athletes take either a timed-release vitamin C tablet, or spread the intake throughout the day. Vitamin C works best in conjunction with bioflavonoids, calcium and magnesium and OTC variants often contain one or more of these.

Weight gainers

Weight gainers are high-calorie shakes/drinks used to aid or supplement calorific intake to ensure it is sufficient for growth. Early weight gainers were loaded with sugar, but as technology has improved, so has the quality of the supplements. The majority of today's weight gainers use complex carbohydrates. Many people like to manufacture their own weight gainers by mixing a protein powder and a complex carbohydrate supplement together in a single drink.

All-in-one supplements

All-in-one supplements are becoming very fashionable. They are essentially a variety of different supplements mixed together for convenience. It is often worth comparing the price of the individual supplements against the price of the all-in-one alternative.

Getting started

In its simplest form, creating a sports section in the pharmacy requires gathering together a number of suitable OTC medicines (see above) and first aid products on a shelf and erecting a sign.

At the other end of the scale there would be a substantial stock holding accompanied by merchandising and widespread advertising campaigns through local sports clubs and newspapers.

There is evidence that the public – and indeed athletes – do not think of pharmacies as a potential port of call for advice on sport- and exercise-related problems despite the fact that in many cases these closely resemble the very things pharmacists are dealing with on a day-to-day basis as a result of domestic mishaps (Kayne and Reeves, 1994). For example, soft tissue injuries and abrasions account for the majority of injuries sustained by non-elite athletes, yet in a sample of 148 sports people only 2% of rugby players, 6% of ice skaters and no football players admitted to making the pharmacy their first point of contact

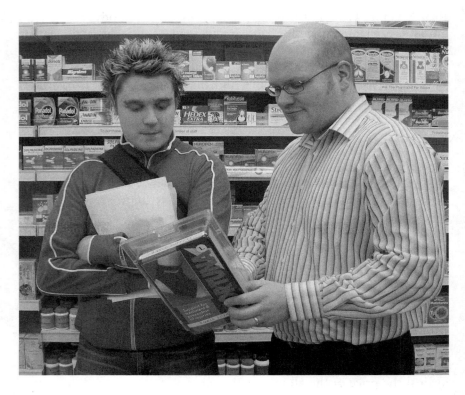

Figure 10.4 Giving advice in the pharmacy.

following a sports injury. The reason given for this was "not believing the pharmacist had sufficient knowledge". Amongst those people who did consult a pharmacist, 88% were satisfied with the quality of assistance.

Although merchandising in-store is going to be of obvious benefit, it is the ability of pharmacists to respond to sport- and exercise-based queries that must be given the highest priority to ensure a customer base can be built up (Figure 10.4). Making local clubs aware of a new interest would be appropriate.

Learning more

The Centre for Pharmacy Postgraduate Education (CPPE) in England offers a distance learning package available for self-study (see below).

References

Bell D S (1992). Exercise for patients with diabetes, benefits, risks, precautions. *Postgrad Med* 92: 183–184, 187–190, 195–198 [In Shankar K (1998). *Exercise Prescription*. Philadelphia, PA: Hanley and Belfus].

Cohen H A, Neuman I, Nahum H (1997). Blocking effect of vitamin C in exercise-induced asthma. *Arch Pediatr Adolesc Med* 151: 367–370 [Cited in Lacroix V J (1999). Exercise-Induced Asthma. http://wwwphyssportsmed.com/issues/1999/11_99/lacroix.htm (accessed 25 August 2005)].

Davis J M, Burgess W A, Slentz C A, *et al.* (1988) Effects of ingesting 6% and 12% glucose/electrolyte beverages during prolonged intermittent cycling in the heat. *Eur J Appl Physiol* 57: 563–569 [In Maughan R J (1998). The sports drink as a functional food: formulations for successful performance. *Proc Nutr Soc* 57: 15–23].

Feinstein R A, LaRussa J, Wang-Dohlman A, *et al.* (1996) Screening adolescent athletes for exercise-induced asthma. *Clin J Sports Med* 6: 119–123 [Cited in Lacroix V J (1999). Exercise-Induced Asthma. http://wwwphyssportsmed.com/issues/1999/11_99/lacroix.htm (accessed 25 August 2005)].

Gatorade. http://www.gssiweb.com/reflib/refs/127/d00000002000001db.cfm

Daries H N, Noakes T D, Dennis S C (2000). Effect of fluid intake volume on 2-h running performances in a 25°C environment. *Med Sci Sports Exerc* 32: 1783–1789.

Hargreaves M, Briggs C A (1988). Effect of carbohydrate ingestion on exercise metabolism. *J Appl Physiol* 65: 1553–1555.

Hollman W (1995). Changes in the capacity for maximal and continuous effort in relation to age. In: Jokl E, Simon E, eds. *International Research in Sport and Physical Education*. Springfield Ill Smith EI. Age: The interaction of nature and nurture.

Horton E S (1991). Exercise in the treatment of NIDDM. *Diabetes* 40(Suppl 2): 175–178.

Hubbard R W, Sandick B J, Matthew W T, *et al.* (1984).Voluntary dehydration and alliesthesia for water. *J Appl Physiol* 57: 868–875.

Kaplan T A (1995). Exercise challenge for exercise-induced bronchospasm. *Phys Sports Med* 23: 47–57.

Kayne S B (2001). Sport and exercise. In: Harman R J, ed. *Handbook of Pharmacy Health Education*, 2nd edn. London: Pharmaceutical Press, 214–215.

Kayne S B, Reeves A (1994). Sports care and the pharmacist – an opportunity not to be missed. *Pharm J* 253: 66–67.

Lamb D R, Brodowicz G R (1986). Optimal use of fluids of varying formulations to mimimise exercise-induced disturbances in homeostasis. *Sports Med* 3: 247–274.

Maughan R J (1991). Fluid and electrolyte loss and replacement in exercise. *J Sports Sci* 9: 117–142.

Milosevic A (1997). Sports drinks hazard to teeth. *Br J Sports Med* 31: 28–30.

Shi X, Summers R W, Schedl H P (1995). Effect of carbohydrate type and concentration and solution osmolarity on water absorption. *J Appl Physiol* 27: 1607–1615.

Smith E I (1995). Age: the interaction of nature and nurture. In: Smith E U, Serfass

R C, eds. *Exercise and Aging. The Scientific Basis.* Englewood Cliffs, NJ: Enslow Publishers, 11–17 [Cited in Lamb D R, Gisolfi C V, Nadel E, eds. (1995). *Perspectives in Exercise Science and Sports Medicine, Vol. 8. Exercise in Older Adults.* Carmel, NY: Cooper Publishing Group, Chapter 2].

Sole C C, Noakes T D (1989). Faster glucose gastric emptying for glucose-polymer and fructose solutions than for glucose in humans. *Eur J Appl Physiol* 58: 605–612 [Cited in Hawley J A, Dennis S C, Noakes T (1992). Oxidation of carbohydrate ingested during prolonged endurance exercise. *Sports Med* 14: 27–42].

Wagenmakers A J M, Brouns F, Saris W H, *et al.* (1993). Oxidation rates of orally ingested carbohydrates during prolonged exercise in men. *J Appl Physiol* 75: 2774–2780.

Further reading

Fentem P H, Turnbull N B, Bassey E J (1990). *Benefits of Exercise: The Evidence.* Manchester: Manchester University Press.

First Aid Manual: The Authorised Joint Manual of St John Ambulance, St Andrew's Ambulance Association and the British Red Cross Society, 8th edn. London: Dorling Kindersley, 2002.

Grisogono V, ed. (1989). *Sports Injuries.* Edinburgh: Churchill Livingstone.

Jamieson R H (1985). Exercises for the Elderly. New York: Emerson Books.

Reents S (2000). *Sport and Exercise Pharmacology.* Champaign, IL: Human Kinetics.

Useful web addresses

Drug information

UK Sport's Drug Information Database (DID), http://www.uksport.gov.uk/did is the most comprehensive and up-to-date sports drug information service available to athletes and support personnel anywhere in the world.

Drugs in sport search, http://www.eirpharm.com/sports/drugs_in_sport_search_result.php is a resource that gives the current status of OTC products.

Specific conditions

Diabetes

Diabetes UK, http://www.diabetes.org.uk/infocentre/p.htm#activity, gives advice on physical activity.

Diabetes and diving, http://www.ukdiving.co.uk/ukdiving/info/medicine/diabetes.htm

International Diabetic Athletes Association, http://www.diabetes-exercise.org/index.asp

Epilepsy

National Society of Epilepsy, http://www.epilepsynse.org.uk/pages/info/leaflets/leisure.cfm

Ostomy patients and sport

http://www.hollister.com/uk/resource_center/ostomy/lifestyle/sports.htm#health

http://www.hollister.com/uk/resource_center/ostomy/lifestyle/sports.htm#contact (contact sports)

http://www.hollister.com/uk/resource_center/ostomy/lifestyle/sports.htm#swimming (swimming)

Studenthealth.co.uk, http://www.studenthealth.co.uk/_sports/archives Index.htm – lists common sports problems with treatments

Education

Centre for Pharmacy Postgraduate Education
http://www.cppe.man.ac.uk

Sportspharmacy
http://www.sportspharmacy.com
Sports pharmacy is a resource for pharmacists in sport highlighting international events, doping control education and drugs in sport.

New Athlete Guide (3rd Edition)
Details of the anti-doping programme and lists of prohibited drugs for the newcomer to sport
http://www.wada-ama.org/rtecontent/document/WADA_Athlete-Guide_ENG.pdf

Useful addresses

Examples of suppliers:

Mobilis Physiotherapy
100 Shaw Rd
Oldham
Lancashire OL1 4AY
Tel: +44 (0)161 678 0233

Porter Nash Medical
Medical Suite
120 Wigmore St
London W1U 3LS
Tel: +44 (0)207 486 1434

John Bell and Croyden
50-54 Wigmore Street
London W1U 2AU
Tel: +44 (0)207 935 5555

Sports organisations with special affinities
British Paralympic Association
9th Floor, 69 Park Lane
Croydon
Surrey CR9 1BG
Tel: +44 (0)20 7662 8882
http://www.paralympics.org.uk/

Central Council for Physical Education (CCPR)
Francis House
Francis Street
London SW1P 1DE
Tel: +44 (0)20 7854 8500
http://www.ccpr.org.uk/
The CCPR is the representative body for National Sports Organisations

Disabled Living Foundation
380–384 Harrow Road
London W9 2HU
Tel: +44 (0)20 7289 6111
http://www.dlf.org.uk/

Exercise training for the elderly and/or disabled Ltd. (EXTEND)
2 Place Farm
Wheathampstead
Hertfordshire AL4 8SB
Tel: +44 (0)1582 832760
http://www.extend.org.uk/
EXTEND provides recreational movement to music for men and women over-sixty and for the less able people of all ages

Keep Fit Association
Astra House Suite 1.05
Arklow Road
London SE14 6EB
Tel: +44 (0)20 8692 9566
http://www.keepfit.org.uk
The Keep Fit Association offers fitness through movement, dance and exercise.

Physical Education Association of the United Kingdom
Ling House Building 25
London Road
Reading RG1 5AQ
Tel: +44 (0)118 931 6240
http://www.pea.uk.com
PEA offers members advice on all matters relating to PE, health and safety and associated professional matters.

Special Olympics UK
The Management Office
Willesborough Industrial Park
Kennington Road
Ashford
Kent TN24 0TD
Tel: +44 (0)233 639910
The aim of Special Olympics is to provide year round training and athletic competition in a variety of well coached Olympic-type sports for individuals with a mental handicap.

St John Ambulance
1 Grosvenor Crescent
London SW1X 7EF
Tel: +44 (0)8700 10 49 50
http://www.sja.org.uk/firstaid/info/

St Andrews Ambulance Association
Strachan House
16 Torphichen Street
Edinburgh EH3 8JB
Tel: +44 (0)131 229 5419
http://www.firstaid.org.uk/

English Sports Association for People with Learning Disability
(ESAPLD)
Unit 9, Milner Way
Ossett
West Yorkshire WF5 9JN
Tel: +44 (0)8451 298992
http://www.esapld.co.uk
The aim of ESAPLD is to campaign for, initiate and provide oppor-
tunities for sport and physical recreation in England for some of the one
million people who have a learning disability.

Index

Page references in *italic* refer to figures and tables.
Page references in **bold** refer to main discussions where there is more than one reference for an entry.